Applied Behavior Analysis-Based Interventions for Autism Spectrum Disorder

Santoshi Halder • Hui-Ting Wang
Karola Dillenburger
Editors

Applied Behavior Analysis-Based Interventions for Autism Spectrum Disorder

Bridging Theory and Practice

Springer

Editors
Santoshi Halder
Department of Education
University of Calcutta
Kolkata, West Bengal, India

Hui-Ting Wang
Department of Special Education
National Taiwan Normal University
Taipei, Taiwan

Karola Dillenburger
Queen's University Belfast, Belfast
Northern Ireland, UK

ISBN 978-981-95-2888-2 ISBN 978-981-95-2889-9 (eBook)
https://doi.org/10.1007/978-981-95-2889-9

This Springer imprint is published by the registered company Springer Nature Singapore Pte Ltd.
The registered company address is: 152 Beach Road, #21-01/04 Gateway East, Singapore 189721, Singapore

Preface

Educational inclusion is an integral part of the right to education and an important condition for social and community participation for all. Worldwide statistics are currently witnessing a sharp peak in the enrolment rate of students with disabilities as never before. However, a huge proportion of students with disabilities are experiencing acute challenges in the sphere of education in terms of dropout, low achievement, performance discrepancy, learning needs, behavioural issues, differences in styles of learning, etc. at almost all levels of education. Autism Spectrum Disorder (ASD), a neurodevelopmental disorder, has increased by 175% over a decade. The global prevalence of autism spectrum disorder (ASD) is estimated at approximately **0.72%** suggesting about **1 in 140 people** worldwide affected by autism. One of the acute challenges of the learners with autism is their behavioural needs as they often exhibit a broad spectrum of challenging behaviours such as self-injury, hyperactivity, aggression, stereotypes, anxiety, or impulsivity three times more frequently than in the general population. Almost half of the learners with autism pose severe challenges for the teacher educators and other stakeholders including parents who interfere with their appropriate education, performance, social interactions with peers, academic achievement, and safety causing hindrances in their way of inclusion and full participation. Exponential changes have taken place in the schools and classrooms in the past few decades in terms of the increase in the range of diversities that needs to be addressed by the teachers in an everyday classroom context.

However, addressing the needs of the learners with autism has been always a challenge for the teachers, practitioners, parents, and other stakeholders due to the associated complexities of the spectrum. Disruptive behaviours pose challenges not only for their own lives but also for the lives of others around them and increase the risk of social isolation and exclusion and is a constant source of stress for teachers in the classroom. Problem behaviours and other behavioural needs of individuals with autism in different contexts, be it at home, school, or other living arrangements significantly impact their overall quality of life and well-being. Lack of definite guidelines, knowledge, awareness, specialized skills, and expertise creates additional barriers for the PwD, their families, and the teachers.

In spite of the differences in ability every child has the potential to learn and progress, if their needs are addressed appropriately with skilled personnel who can take the right decision and implement appropriate strategy at the right time. In an attempt to facilitate positive behavioural outcome various interventions are being practiced all over the world to address the behavioural needs including the various skill deficits such as social, communication, daily living, and play skills through a systematic process whereby teachers create opportunities for children to produce target behaviours through prompts, cues, and reinforcers to shape appropriate behaviour.

Unfortunately, there is an alarming shortage of trained or skilled personnel to specifically understand and implement individualized evidence-based behaviour intervention procedures appropriately. Researchers accentuate the importance of skilled teachers who have the knowledge, ability, and skills to effectively address the needs of all their learners in the classroom successfully. Hence, there is a pertinent need to prepare, train, and orient the teachers and other personnel to cater for the behavioural needs of the diverse learners with autism and thereby create opportunities for participation and inclusion in all walks of life.

Applied Behaviour Analysis (ABA) is an evidence-based science of behaviour analysis has gained ground all over the world for its robust foundation and empirical research findings that show the effectiveness of the various ABA-based strategies in bringing about significant changes in addressing the behavioural needs of the people with diverse needs. The book presents evidence-based practices based on Applied Behaviour Analysis (ABA) by formally trained and skilled Board-Certified Behaviour Analysts (BCBAs) of the world who are researchers, practitioners, educators, teachers in various schools, colleges, universities, centres, and research institutes through this comprehensive book as handbook of evidence-based behaviour analytic interventions for people with autism.

The key areas that the book covers are:

- Conceptual background, and historical trajectory of ABA as an evidence-based science of intervention.
- Practice-based interventions by experts in the specific area.
- Diverse perspectives from across countries touching almost all corners of the globe under one book
- Brings in innovations in the field of ABA from the global north and global south countries
- Captures technology-related work in the field of ABA
- Includes multidisciplinary works intersecting various disciplines, subjects, and fields

The book intends to cover most significant and pertinent topics of behavioural analytic interventions that can be extremely effective for peoples working with learners with autism spectrum disorder including other developmental disabilities to ensure and promote an increase in participation and inclusion of learners with autism. The book is edited by experts from three countries; bringing in expertise and specialists across the globe who are specialized in intervention for autism and formally certified BCBAs from Foreign Board for Behaviour Analysis, USA. The editors of the book have a vast and wide array of experience in the field bringing in divergent thoughts and discourses.

Keywords: Applied behaviour analysis, function-based intervention, people with disabilities, inclusive classroom, challenging behaviour, behavioural needs, inclusion, participation

Kolkata, West Bengal, India — Santoshi Halder
Taipei, Taiwan — Hui-Ting Wang
Northern Ireland, UK — Karola Dillenburger

Acknowledgment

The idea of bringing out this book emerged and shaped eventually and gradually as I met, interacted, and communicated with more and more neurodiverse autistic individuals not only in India but also from various other parts of the world such as the USA, Australia, South Africa, Germany, Hungary, Japan, etc. My concept and understanding have gone through an evolutionary journey since 2011 as a young vibrant Fulbright Nehru Senior Research Fellow (FNSRF) at Indiana University (IU), USA to now as a Fulbright Scholar in Residence (S-I-R) at Bluefield State University (BSU), WV, USA. I am glad that I accepted the invitation from IU for volunteering the autistic children in the home-bound programs that was beyond my Fulbright project goals. I still remember volunteering those children at their homes and my ever-increasing inquisitiveness to know them more; their needs and challenges. Over the years my understanding grew while I came across wonderful strengths that these individuals with autism have. I decided to understand in-depth the unique traits including the atypicalities and find strategic ways to address their needs. I found many myths, gaps, and missing dots regarding autism.

The book is prompted by the needs and challenges I visualized in various countries even the most developed countries like USA where I witnessed the complete lack of specialists, interventionists, and experts to address the needs and challenges of people with autism in school, home, and community. Significant thoughts accumulated over the years prompted the proposal of this book in collaboration with my wonderful colleagues as editors and chapter authors. The concept and understanding of the proposed book got refined and ignited through the discussions and discourses with many specialists worldwide during academic visits, conferences networking, collaborative research projects, etc. It would be extremely difficult and rather impossible to name all of them as there are so many who have directly or indirectly influenced the thought process for further refinement and manifestation in the form of the present book. My special thanks to all the Board-Certified Behaviour Analysts (BCBA) working closely with people with autism and also to Behaviour Analyst Certification Board (BACB), USA.

I am thankful to my home institution *University of Calcutta* for providing me with the scope, and platform, and continuously supporting my research and academic endeavours.

I would like to acknowledge the funding bodies who supported my research and academic endeavours across the globe; *Erasmus EU partnership, United States India Education Foundation (USIEF), International Institute of Education (IIE), Rockefeller Foundation, Shastri Indo-Canadian Institute, Japan Society for Promotion of Science (JSPS), Australian Government, Department of Education and Training, Australian High Commission, Endeavour Australia India Council, Indian Institute of Social Science Research (ICSSR), University Grants Commission (UGC), National Institute for Humanities and Social Sciences (NIHSS), National Research Funding (NRF), South Africa* for their constant trust in me and for providing the funding support for the academic and research endeavours nationally and internationally. These and many more such opportunities provided wonderful scope to get connected to the amazing scholars who stimulated and kindled my thoughts towards addressing some of the pertinent global challenges for facilitating inclusive participation and the agreeableness for accepting, respecting, and embracing all sorts of diversities.

My sincere thanks to my research colleagues *Dr. Hui-Ting Wang, BCBA-D & Prof. Karola Dillenburger, Clin. Psych., BCBA-D the Co-editors* of this book for accepting my invitation to join me for this wonderful partnership and for their time and efforts in assisting me in the book project with their most desired and needful inputs, valuable suggestions, and contribution in all phases and stages of this book. Special thanks also go to several chapter reviewers who together contribute to the quality of this book.

Finally, I would also like to thank my husband Dr. Arindam Talukdar, Principal Scientist, Indian Institute of Chemical Biology (IICB), India, my daughter Mihika, my son Kiaan.

I acknowledge blessings of my (late) parents; my father to provide me an Army environment; a rich, vibrant multi-cultural learning experience, who served the Indian Armed Force (IAF) all his years and my mother for her discipline, hard work, blessings and the foundation that she built in me that constantly energizes and drives me towards some futuristic goal for a better future and to contribute to mankind without all their contributions the book would not have been possible.

The book is the product of the cumulative efforts of so many people who trusted to share their valuable perspectives and agreed to extend their experiences for our readers to facilitate the pathway to creating an inclusive society. Special thanks are due to all those people whom I may have missed out.

Finally, I cannot resist conveying that this is just the beginning of a long amazing journey of making a world that accepts respects and embraces differences.

Santoshi Halder

Contents

About the Editors and Contributors

About the Editors

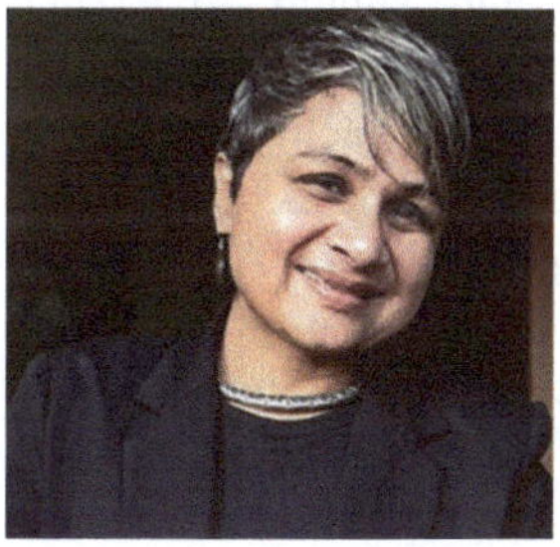

Santoshi Halder Ph.D., is a Professor at the Department of Education, University of Calcutta, India. She is a Board-Certified Behaviour Analyst (BACB, USA) and has a Special Educator license (Rehabilitation Council of India, RCI). She is awarded the prestigious *'Extraordinary Professorship'* by the University of Pretoria, South Africa (2023) and the *Fulbright Scholar-in-Residence (S-I-R), USA (2024).* She has been the recipient of prestigious International awards; *Short-visit, Ludwigsburg University of Education, Germany (2024), Hungarian ICM Erasmus, (2022–2025), Hungarian State bilateral Awardee (2022–2023), Shastri-Indo-Canadian Fellow (2020–2022), Fulbright Academic and Professional Excellence fellow, USA (2020), Rockefeller Fellow*, Italy (2019), *Japan Society for Promotion of Science/ JSPS Fellow, (2019), Endeavour Australia-India Education Research Fellow and Honorary Fellow at Olga Tennison Autism Research Centre (OTARC), La Trobe University, Australia (2015-2016), Endeavour Awards Ambassador* (2018) and *Fulbright Nehru Senior Research Fellow, USA (2011–2012)*. She received the *Governor's Medal (West Bengal, India)* in 2001 for her contribution to the community as a National Cadet (NCC). She has edited and authored international books on Inclusion and Technology *(Springer, Palgrave Macmillan, and Routledge*). She is *Associate Editor* for the *Journal of Disability and Impairment, International Fulbright Chronicle, Indonesian Journal of Disability Studies, and Asian Journal of Inclusive Education. Thirteen Ph.Ds are awarded under her supervision and many currently undergoing. She is in the decision making communities & board members to many Universities and institutions across many countries. She is working as a principal investigator and collaborator to multiple national & internatinal research projects on global agendas. She is passionate to identify the secluded communities from across the world & understanding their needs & challenges to find effective strategic pathways for their inclusion.*

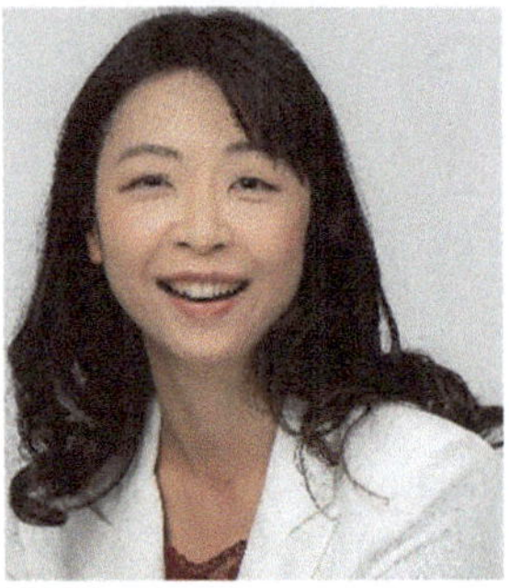

Hui-Ting Tina Wang (王慧婷) is an Associate Professor in the Department of Special Education, National Taiwan Normal University. She is a Licensed Secondary Education Special Educator in Taiwan and a Board-Certified Behaviour Analyst at the Doctoral Level. Hui-Ting serves as the International Member at-large for the Division on Autism and Other Developmental Disabilities of the Council for Exceptional Children, United States.

Hui-Ting's research interests include evidence-based practices (EBPs) and technology-enhanced EBPs for teaching individuals with autism, with a focus on the multi-tiered ecological considerations of teachers, parents, and peers. Her recent innovative national project, leveraging artificial intelligence, reflects her dedication to driving meaningful change by addressing the massive need for decision-making support in emotional and behavioral management and communication skills. This project aligns with the International Classification of Functioning, Disability and Health (ICF) and UNESCO's inclusive education principles.

As a scholar, she strives to maintain a balanced commitment to teaching, research, student advising, and global community service. Her dedication has been recognized through multiple awards, including two Teaching Excellence Awards, the 2030 Young Scholar Research Excellence Award, the Taiwan Education Academic Joint Association Special Education Service Award, and the Outstanding Industrial Cooperation Award.

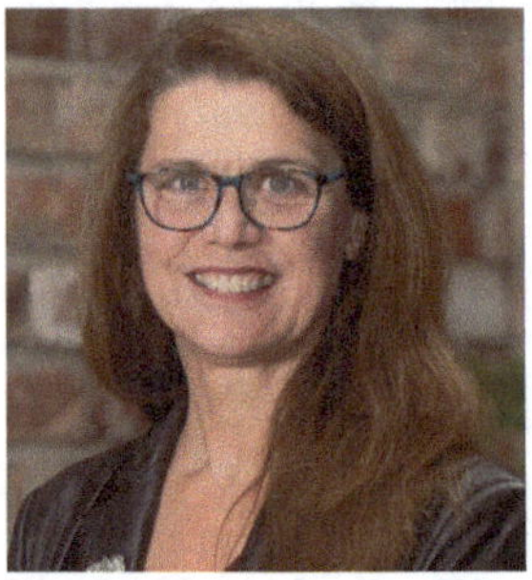

Karola Dillenburger is Professor of Behaviour Analysis and Education and the Founding Director of the Centre for Behaviour Analysis at Queen's University Belfast. She is a Board-Certified Behaviour Analyst-Doctoral (BCBA-D), a certified behaviour analyst with the UK-Society for Behaviour Analysis (UKBAcert. PSA accredited), and a HCPC registered Clinical Psychologist. Professor Dillenburger is a Fellow of the Higher Education Academy (AdvanceHE), and an Associate Fellow of the British Psychological Society and has been adjunct Professor at multiple universities across Europe and Australia. She is International Guest Faculty at the Asia Pacific ABA Network Institute in Japan and international advisor for Behaviour Momentum in India. Her teaching focus is on behaviour analysis, autism, and professionalization. Her research focuses on meeting the needs of the autism community nationally and internationally; developing compassionate behaviour analytic interventions to support vulnerable children and adults, explicating parenting across the lifespan, and elucidating trauma, bereavement, and stress. She has successfully supervised many PhD students and invites applications from those interested in doctoral research in any area of behaviour analysis. She is published widely in high-impact international journals and has delivered invited keynote addresses and lectures in Europe, America, Asia, and Australia. In 2024, she was awarded the Gold Medal from Masarky University, Czech Republic in recognition of her outstanding contribution to science, culture, higher education, and public life, including her commitment to the struggle for human rights and dignity. She is the academic lead for the Memorandum of Understanding (MOU) between Queen's and Masaryk University in the Czech Republic. In 2024, she was elected as the President of the European Association for Behaviour Analysis. In 2025 she was appointed Fellow of the Association for Behavior Analysis International (ABAI).

About the Contributors

Maryam Al Hammadi MEd, is a Family and Community Relations Specialist at the Mohammed bin Rashid Center for Special Education operated by the New England Center for Children in Abu Dhabi, United Arab Emirates.

Miriam C. Boesch is an Associate Professor of Special Education. Her research focuses assessing pre-/in-service special education teacher preparation in augmentative and alternative communication and investigating intervention strategies for autism. She teaches courses in autism, intervention strategies, and behavior management.

Nichola Booth is Senior Lecturer at Queen's University where she is the course director for the MScABA. Her research focuses on improving access to public transport, namely airports, for neurodiverse individuals. Her research interests include using virtual environments to deliver effective training to educators working in all educational settings to increase student engagement.

Kimberly N. Bowers is a Master's Student in the Department of Special Education. Her area of study is in severe disabilities and applied behavior analysis.

Alexandra Candelaria is a Doctoral Student Special Education (Developmental Disabilities and Autism) and a Board-Certified Behavior Analyst. Her research interest focuses on interdisciplinary collaboration between behavior analysts and other autism service professionals.

Traci M. Cihon co-founded and currently co-facilitates the Culturo-Behavior Science Innovation Network, a community of faculty, scholars, and practitioners interested in learning more about Culturo-Behavior Science and advancing the corresponding research and practice through mentorship and collaboration. Dr. Cihon's scholarship focuses on culturo-behavior systems science, building systems to support behavior scientific work on social and cultural issues, developing international and interdisciplinary collaborations, and behavioral education.

Elena Couldrey Dr. Elena R. Couldrey is a dedicated Board-Certified Behavior Analyst and accomplished educator holding a Doctorate in Education. She leverages her extensive experience in diverse settings to support children and adults with learning difficulties. Elena passionately advocates for innovative evidence-based practices, ensuring tailored interventions that foster growth, resilience, and lifelong learning.

M. Alexandra Da Fonte is an Associate Professor of the Practice in the Department of Special Education. Her research evaluates the preparation of special education teachers in augmentative and alternative communication, investigates strategies to support teachers in effective practices, and assesses the reliability of assessment and intervention app tools.

Karola Dillenburger is Professor of Behaviour Analysis and Education and the Founding Director of the Centre for Behaviour Analysis at Queen's University Belfast. She is a Board-Certified Behaviour Analyst-Doctoral (BCBA-D), a certified behaviour analyst with the UK-Society for Behaviour Analysis (UKBAcert. PSA accredited), and a HCPC registered Clinical Psychologist. Professor Dillenburger is a Fellow of the Higher Education Academy (AdvanceHE), and an Associate Fellow of the British Psychological Society and has been adjunct Professor at multiple universities across Europe and Australia. She is International Guest Faculty at the Asia Pacific ABA Network Institute in Japan and international advisor for Behaviour Momentum in India. Her teaching focus is on behaviour analysis, autism, and professionalization. Her research focuses on meeting the needs of the autism community nationally and internationally; developing compassionate behaviour analytic interventions to support vulnerable children and adults, explicating parenting across the lifespan, and elucidating trauma, bereavement, and stress.

Yu-Shan Ding (丁于珊), M.Ed., Doctoral student in the Department of Special Education, National Taiwan Normal University, Taiwan. Her research interests are parent-implemented interventions and autism. Yu-Shan works at Wu-Chang Junior High School in Taiwan.

Karen L. Gischlar Dr. Gischlar has close to 40 years of experience in the field of education. She has taught kindergarten, served as a school psychologist, and currently trains school psychologists at Rider University in New Jersey. Her primary areas of research interest focus on tiered systems of support for academics and behaviors.

Laura Regina Gómez is a third-year PhD student at the University of Florida, researching culturally competent training for providers working with Latinx families of children with autism to promote culturally responsive implementation of evidence-based practices for Latinx children with autism.

Brittney L. Goscicki is a Lecturer in the Department of Special Education, a Board-Certified Behavior Analyst, and former special education teacher. Her current research focuses on the experiences of neurodivergent youth on gender and disability, masking behaviors, disability advocacy, and teacher preparation.

Santoshi Halder Ph.D., is a Professor at the Department of Education, University of Calcutta, India. She is a Board-Certified Behaviour Analyst (BACB, USA) and has a Special Educator license (Rehabilitation Council of India, RCI). She is awarded the prestigious *'Extraordinary Professorship'* by the University of Pretoria, South Africa (2023). She has been the recipient of multiple prestigious international awards. She received the *Governor's Medal (West Bengal, India)* in 2001 for her contribution to the community as a National Cadet (NCC). She has edited and authored international books on Inclusion and Technology *(Springer, Palgrave Macmillan, and Routledge*). She is Associate Editor for the Journal of Disability and Impairment, International Fulbright Chronicle, Indonesian Journal of Disability Studies, and Asian Journal of Inclusive Education. Her research interest is in the inclusion of marginalized communities, disability studies, autism, educational psychology, educational technology, cross-cultural studies, etc. Edited and coauthored multiple books on topics of global importance, she is the Principal Investigator of multiple multi-country projects on inclusion, gender, and well-being of people with disabilities. Her objective is to facilitate inclusion of people who are marginalized through strategic plans and actions globally, nationally and locally.

Sarah C. Hammonds is the T2C Project Coordinator and University Supervisor for the Severe Disabilities Track in the Department of Special Education. She is a former special education teacher and currently engages in teacher preparation, including as a lead coach for special education teachers.

Michelle P. Kelly is an Associate Professor at Emirates College for Advanced Education, a teacher education institute in Abu Dhabi, United Arab Emirates. She is a Board-Certified Behavior Analyst-Doctoral, a Chartered Behavioural Psychologist (Psychological Society of Ireland), and a member of the Research Collaborative for the Special Olympics Global Center for Inclusion in Education.

Sheri Kingsdorf an Assistant Professor at Masaryk University in Czechia and a doctoral-level Board-Certified Behavior Analyst, has worked in the fields of behavior analysis and special education since 2002. Her extensive experience includes implementing the CABAS model, providing bilingual early intervention services, consulting and delivering behavior analytic-based services across four continents, conducting international transdisciplinary research, and focusing on culturally competent telehealth practices, caregiver training, and teacher education to support children's social-emotional and behavioral health.

Tia Martin is a co-founding director of PBS UK and a visiting scholar with Queen's University Belfast. Her PhD centred on behaviour analytic approaches to teach safety skills to autistic and learning-disabled people. Current research interests include wider implementation of Positive Behavioural Support and the impact of language on perceived acceptability of restrictive practices.

Ciara Maye a BCBA and Coordinator of the Positive Behaviour Support Service at the Brothers of Charity Cork, has worked with children and adults with high behaviour support needs since 1999. She is a founding member of the Irish Society for Behaviour Analysis and her primary interests are in the education and support of Social Care students and staff to promote quality of life for people with intellectual disabilities.

Sarah C. Mead Jasperse is an Assistant Professor at Emirates College for Advanced Education, Abu Dhabi, United Arab Emirates. She is a Board-Certified Behavior Analyst-Doctoral with experience applying the science of behavior in a variety of contexts and with a range of populations and behaviors.

Melissa L. Oliver Dr. Melissa L. Oliver is the Director of Education at The Mohammed bin Rashid Center for Special Education operated by the New England Center for Children. A Board-Certified Behavior Analyst and licensed special educator, she applies evidence-based behavioral science to autism education, inclusive practices, and teacher training.

George Pickersgill works for DFN (David Forbes-Nixon) Project SEARCH as a Programme Specialist. He provides consultancy and training for businesses, education providers, and local authorities to implement supported internships in England. His research interests lie in identifying how to transition young people with additional needs into meaningful and competitive employment.

Bertram O. Ploog College of Staten Island & Graduate Center, City U. of New York (CUNY) is a licensed psychologist, licensed behavior analyst, and Board-Certified Behavior Analyst (BCBA-D). My background is in the experimental analysis of behavior and applied behavior analysis. My research has focused on 'stimulus control', which is relevant for the study of stimulus over-selectivity and other atypical attention patterns common in people with autism. Stimulus over-selectivity has implications for the acquisition of social, academic, and communication/language skills. To inform my research with autistic children, I have used various animal models. I also have a private practice and work directly with autistic children providing ABA services.

Laura A. Riffel after years of teaching children and adults, ran a statewide clinic for children with behavioral issues. Her greatest joy was living with an adult friend with autism who taught her how to live a dignified life.

Ronaldo L. Rodas Jara, PhD is an Associate Professor at Universidad Iberoamericana in Asunción, Paraguay. His academic trajectory spans Taiwan, the United Kingdom, and Paraguay, with a focus on inclusive education and neurodevelopmental systems in under-resourced environments. His work emphasizes equitable support for individuals with developmental disabilities. Originally from Yhú, Paraguay, he designs and evaluates evidence-based strategies that translate research into practical applications for educational institutions and community services. He collaborates with educators and policymakers to strengthen sustainable, culturally sensitive models of inclusion.

Liza R. Rodas Jara is an independent researcher in Paraguay whose work centers on psychological distress assessment, evidence-based practices, contextual therapies, and Dialectical Behavior Therapy (DBT). Her medical background underpins her focus on clinically applied, empirically supported mental health research.

Dag Strömberg is a licensed speech-language pathologist, board-certified behavior analyst (BCBA, ACC-A), MS in special education, doctoral student at the Department of Special Education, Stockholm University, Sweden, and president of the Swedish Association for Behavior Analysis. For more than 25 years, he has provided services for individuals diagnosed with autism, intervening directly with children and caregivers, as well as providing supervision and in-service training to staff members in preschools, schools, and habitation centers. Dag is also involved in various international projects, mainly in France, India, and the Nordic countries.

Alan Tennyson is the Positive Behaviour Support Manager with Ability West and a Board-Certified Behaviour Analyst with over 15 years of experience in research, practice, and training in Positive Behaviour Support. He has worked as a behaviour specialist in County Cork and is a co-chair and founding member of the Irish Society for Behaviour Analysis.

Adriana Kaori Terol PhD, Postdoctoral scholar in Psychiatry and Behavioral Sciences, University of California, Davis, United States

Adel A. Wahdain holds a Master of Education in Applied Behavior Analysis from Emirates College for Advanced Education, Abu Dhabi, UAE, and works as an ASD specialist in public schools within the UAE Ministry of Education. He supports students with ASD across 22 schools and is passionate about promoting evidence-based inclusive education.

Hui-Ting Wang Associate Professor, PhD, BCBA-D, Department of Special Education, National Taiwan Normal University, Taiwan. She is a Licensed Secondary Education Special Educator in Taiwan and a Board-Certified Behaviour Analyst at the Doctoral Level. Hui-Ting's research interests include evidence-based practices (EBPs) and technology-enhanced EBPs for teaching individuals with autism, with a focus on the multi-tiered ecological considerations of teachers, parents, and peers.

Part I
Foundations of Applied Behaviour Analysis (ABA)

Chapter 1
Applied Behaviour Analysis: What It Is and What It Isn't

Catriona Gower, Nichola Booth, and Karola Dillenburger

Abstract Contrary to popular myths, ABA *is not* simply a specific therapy for children with autism. Applied behaviour analysis (ABA) is the applied branch of the natural science of behaviour analysis. As with any applied branch of a science, it harnesses the fundamental principles uncovered by the scientific investigation of phenomena, in this case behaviour, with a view to developing effective uses. Applications of behaviour analysis utilise environmental variables shown to reliably impact on behaviour with a view to address socially significant issues. In this chapter, we provide examples of how ABA can help learners achieve a better quality of life. Some of the most common misconceptions of ABA are also discussed.

Keywords Behaviour analysis · Applied behaviour analysis (ABA) · Radical behaviourism · Experimental analysis of behaviour (EAB) · Autism · Misrepresentation

(1) **Applied Behaviour Analysis (ABA)** ***is*** the applied branch of the science of behaviour analysis with the aim of "discovering environmental variables that reliably influence socially significant behaviour and for developing a technology of behaviour change that takes practical advantage of those discoveries" (Cooper et al., 2020, p. 18).
(2) **ABA** ***is not*** a "therapy for autism" (Chiesa, 2006, p. 225).

These two statements may come as a surprise to readers who only ever heard of ABA in connection with autism, and who thought, therefore, that ABA was a specific intervention for autism. It is not. In fact, it is one of the three branches of the science of Behaviour Analysis:

(1) The philosophical and conceptual basis of the science of behaviour analysis.

C. Gower · N. Booth · K. Dillenburger (✉)
Queen's University Belfast, Belfast, Northern Ireland, UK
e-mail: k.dillenburger@qub.ac.uk

S. Halder et al. (eds.), *Applied Behavior Analysis-Based Interventions for Autism Spectrum Disorder*, https://doi.org/10.1007/978-981-95-2889-9_1

(2) The experimental analysis of behaviour (EAB) that focuses on the discovery of the underlying principles of behaviour.
(3) Applied behaviour analysis (ABA), that uses the principles of behaviour to achieve socially important change (Baer et al., 1968; Cooper et al., 2020; Skinner, 1953).

1.1 Conceptual Basis of the Science

Behaviour analysis is a natural science, that, like other natural sciences, aims to understand natural phenomena based on empirical evidence from observation and experimentation. The validity of the findings of a natural science is ensured via repeatability and peer-review. For behaviour analysts, behaviour is the subject matter of their science. Behaviour is defined widely and holistically as the interaction of a person (i.e. a biological organism) with their environment, past and present. Hence, behaviour is defined as anything a person does, that is, anything that can be expressed as a verb (Moore, 2003; Thyer, 1999). This includes all publicly observable actions as well as behaviour that can only be observed by the person themselves, not by others, such as the private activities of thinking and feeling (Keenan, 2015; Keenan & Dillenburger, 2020a; Thyer, 2009). Explanations for private as well as public activities are sought in past as well as the prevailing contingencies (Cooper et al., 2020), in other words, in the past experiences of the person as well as the situation they find themselves in at the time of observation.

When behaviour is defined as anything a person does, circular reasoning and mentalism is avoided (Keenan & Dillenburger, 2020a). Circular reasoning occurs when a verb is turned into a noun (i.e. reification) and this noun then is used to try and explain the behaviour. For example, when someone is feeling angry (verb) the noun "anger" is used in an attempt to explain the behaviour; it is said that he is "feeling angry because of his anger" and anger management might be recommended without any reference to the situation that made him feeling angry in the first place. In effect, this kind of circular reasoning (Questel, 2020) places the cause of the behaviour inside the person (i.e. mentalism; Keenan & Dillenburger, 2020a) and therefore can lead to the illusion that an explanation has been found (i.e. a pseudo-explanation). To stay with the example, in behaviour analysis the noun "anger" would be viewed as a descriptive summary label and the analysis would focus on the environmental contingencies that led to the person feeling angry. Thus conceptually, in behaviour analysis the explanation of behaviour is sought in a person's past and present interactions with their environment (i.e. experiences), not in hypothetical constructs or reifications (Baum, 2004; Cooper et al., 2020; Dillenburger & Keenan, 2009).

1.2 Experimental Analysis of Behaviour

The experimental analysis of behaviour (EAB) originated in the early twentieth century (Watson, 1913; Skinner, 1938b). Experimental behaviour analysts explore basic behavioural processes in the laboratory with relatively naïve organisms, such as rats or pigeons (Catania, 1997) and more composite processes are studied with more complex participants (Skinner, 1953). Experimental behaviour analysts thereby focus on systematically determining the principles and processes that reliably explain behaviour from a natural science perspective without resort to the kinds of mentalistic pseudo-explanations described earlier (Skinner, 1977, 1987). EAB is based on the basic principles of natural sciences: determinism, experimentation, empiricism, reliability, philosophical doubt, and parsimony (Schlinger, 2020).

1. Determinism is the assumption that the universe is a lawful and ordered place, in which "events do not just happen willy-nilly" (Cooper et al., 2020, p.5). In determinism events are viewed as determined by preceding and current environmental contingencies. Consequently, statements, such as "she did this out of the blue" or "he did this for no reason" make no sense. In fact, "if the behavior of organisms were neither completely nor for the most part lawful, scientists would be unable to identify why an individual emits a behavior and thus be unable to modify the behavior" (Fisher et al., 2011, p. 9).
2. The purpose of experimentation is to identify functional relationships between environmental events and behaviour. The purpose is to find out what effect changes in the environment (independent variables) have on behaviour (dependent variable). "A functional relation is said to exist when a change in the independent variable reliably produces a defined change in the dependent behavior" (Fisher et al., 2011, p. 10). In other words, the experimental question is: what happens to the behaviour when something in the environment is changed (either adding or taking away a stimulus).
3. Empiricism means that conclusions drawn as a result of scientific investigation are primarily related to information received by the senses. In other words, the scientist makes decisions based what they observe, rather than on what they hypothesise to be true. This requires objective measurement taken in precise, consistent, and publicly verifiable ways (Cooper et al., 2020).
4. The principle of reliability refers to the gathering of sufficient evidence to warrant trust in drawing conclusions. A single experiment does not offer sufficient evidence to determine the effects of changes in an independent variable on a dependent variable (Johnston & Pennypacker, 2008). A core component of the scientific reliability is the replicability of studies, thus demonstrating that results are robust. If the procedure of a study is described insufficiently, it cannot be replicated accurately, and consequently, results cannot be substantiated. Therefore, a detailed description of the procedures used in laboratory and applied studies lies at the heart of behaviour analysis.
5. Philosophic doubt means that a healthy level of scepticism is retained and that the truthfulness of a fact is continuously questioned (Cooper et al., 2020).

Philosophical doubt requires that data are derived from direct and repeated observations rather than from statistical inferences or verbal reports of events.

6. Parsimony means that where there is more than one possible explanation for a finding, the simpler explanation is to be preferred. For the experimental behaviour analyst, this means that preference is given to the simplest most parsimonious explanation of a behavioural phenomenon, thereby rendering more complicated mentalistic explanations redundant (Johnston & Pennypacker, 2008).

Using these six basic tenets of science, the aim of the experimental analysis of behaviour is to explore and discover natural laws of behaviour. One of the key discoveries found that an "if-then" relationship exists between behaviour and environmental events that happen before and after a behaviour (Skinner, 1938a, 1953). This relationship is called three-term contingency (or ABC contingency), because of the relationship between three variables, **A**ntecedent event/stimulus, **B**ehaviour, and **C**onsequent event/stimulus (Skinner, 1969).

Consequent events/stimuli fall into two main functional categories: if they increase the probability of the behaviour recurring, they are called *reinforcers*; if they reduced the probability of the behaviour, they are called *punishers*. Importantly, reinforcers and punishers are defined by their function (i.e. increasing or decreasing the probability of behaviour), not by their form. This means that the same stimulus (e.g. a child being allowed time on a tablet device) could function as a *reinforcer*, increasing the probability of one behaviour (e.g. doing homework), and as a *punisher*, reduced the probability of another behaviour (e.g. not quarrelling with a sibling) (Heward, 2003).

When stimuli are presented contingent on a behaviour, the process is denoted with a plus sign (+) or the prefix *positive*; when stimuli are removed contingent on a behaviour, the process is denoted with a minus sign (-) or the prefix *negative*. In either case, the function remains the same; positive as well as negative reinforcers increase the probability of the behaviour recurring, while positive as well as negative punishers decrease the probability of the behaviour recurring (Cooper et al., 2020).

1.3 Applied Behaviour Analysis

The application of the science of behaviour analysis to socially important areas is called applied behaviour analysis (ABA) (Cooper et al., 2020; Mayer et al., 2012). Fuller (1949) was one of the first to report applications of behaviour analytic concepts to humans. His research participant was a young man who was so severely physically disabled that he was considered unteachable. Fuller's aim was to show that even this man was able to learn by teaching him a simple new behaviour. Within four teaching sessions, the young man learned to raise his arm to a vertical position. With this simple experiment, Fuller had established that the principles of behaviour discovered in the laboratory could be applied successfully to shape human behaviour (Cooper et al., 2020).

Pioneers like Ayllon and Michael (1959) and Boyle and Greer (1983) showed that ABA-based interventions were effective with individuals who were so profoundly disabled that they required total nursing care. Further research (e.g. Rice et al., 1967) identified the need for a separate applied branch of the science with a dedicated journal. In the inaugural issue of the *Journal of Applied Behavior Analysis (JABA)*, Baer et al. (1968) provided the first official definition of ABA. Since then, Cooper et al.'s (2020) updated defintion is used most widely. They define ABA as the science of

> discovering environmental variables that reliably influence socially significant behaviour and for developing a technology of behaviour change that takes practical advantage of those discoveries. (p. 18)

Baer et al. (1987) stipulated that in order for applied behaviour analytic conduct to be considered good practice, it has to meet seven basic principles; it has to be applied, behavioural, analytic, technological, conceptually systematic, effective, and generalisable.

1. *Applied*: To be applied means that the target behaviour must be socially and/or clinically valid, import, and significant, such that it results in an improved quality of life for the learner, their families, and/or society. If the intervention shows merely that it is possible to teach or modify a behaviour that is of no social importance, the procedure is not considered ABA. It is the responsibility of the behaviour analyst in close collaboration with the learner (and their social support circle) to monitor the relevance of the behaviour being targeted, to ensure that together they prioritise what behaviour should be the primary focus of any ABA-based intervention.
2. *Behavioural*: Outcomes of ABA-based interventions have to be behaviourally quantifiable. This means that primary data are collected via direct observation of clearly defined target behaviour along a specific dimension, such as frequency, duration, latency, product, or rate. Indirect, incidental, or proxy measures, such as clinical records, interviews, or self-reports, may be used but are not considered sources of primary data (Hrisos et al., 2009). In fact, there has to be explicit evidence that the behaviour change occurred for the learner and that this change is due to the intervention (Cooper et al., 2020).
3. *Analytic*: As an inductive science, ABA utilises intra-subject comparison to evidence functional relationships between independent environmental variables and dependent behaviour change. For the most part, data are displayed using single system research designs (SSRD), including reversal, multi-element, and multiple baseline designs (Johnston & Pennypacker, 2008). In SSRD, individual baseline data are collected prior to the interventions and compared against data collected during and after the intervention. This methodology stands in contrast to the kinds of deductive group comparison methodologies that commonly are used in medical and social sciences, where group designs and statistical analysis generalisations overshadow individual data (Keenan & Dillenburger, 2011).

4. *Technological*: Being technological means that procedures have to be transparent and in concord with the science. To be replicable, the intervention has to be based on a clear and operational definition of the target behaviour, the use of instruments/research tools has to be clearly described, and an accurate account of the procedures that were used and to be incorporated, and evidence of procedural integrity/fidelity, lack of bias, and/or conflict of interest has to be included. To be technical means that scientific terms have to be defined very clearly to ensure that scientists can communicate very precisely. To the lay person, not trained in a science, this need for precision can lead to the perception that scientific language is jargon.
5. *Conceptually systematic*: Given the conceptual basis of behaviour analysis described earlier, it is important that interventions are conceptually systematic. This means that behaviour is defined broadly, including public and private behaviour, and that explanations for behaviour are sought in an analysis of the context (i.e. environmental contingencies) of which they are a function and not in mental or cognitive constructs or hypothetical pseudo-explanations (Baum, 2004; Chiesa, 1984; Keenan, 2015; Keenan & Dillenburger, 2020a).
6. *Effective*: ABA-based interventions have to be based on evidence of effectiveness (Dillenburger, 2011, 2015). Rather than using statistical analysis or algorithms, the effectiveness of ABA-based interventions is determined by inter-observer agreement and visual data displays, such as graphs. Effectiveness, generally, is determined according to intra-subject, individual data (i.e. baseline data compared to intervention data), rather than averages across a population (Keenan & Dillenburger, 2011).
7. *Generality*: Behaviour analytic interventions have to ensure behaviour change generalises to other settings, other caregivers, and/or other behaviour. Additionally, the behaviour change must be maintained after the intervention. Procedures to ensure generalisation and maintenance of behaviour change should be included into the intervention programme (Cooper et al., 2020).

The main difference between ABA and the experimental analysis of behaviour (EAB) is that while the EBA is focussed on the discovery and exploration of behavioural principles, ABA is concerned with utilising these principles to bring about socially important/clinically significant improvements. In ABA, social validity has to be evidenced on three levels (Wolf, 1978, p207):

- *The social significance of the goals*: Are the specific behavioural goals really what individual wants and needs?
- *The social appropriateness of the procedures*: Do the ends justify the means? That is, do learners, caregivers, and other consumers consider the treatment procedures acceptable?
- *The social importance of the effects*: Are consumers satisfied with the results? Are all the results, including any unpredicted ones, important?

ABA-based programmes are tailored individually to the needs of the specific learner at a particular point in time; they must be closely monitored and adjusted as necessary (e.g. Martin & Dillenburger, 2019). The question of which socially important behaviour to target with the intervention has to be decided in close collaboration with the learner and/or their caregivers, if the learner is a very young child. Vulnerable young people, or very severely disabled adults, may need skilled support to enable them to voice their choices, but this does not mean that they should not be included in decision making about target behaviours (Dillenburger et al., 2019; Hanley, 2020).

To avoid confusion, the target behaviour needs to be identified, defined precisely, and assessed properly before ABA-based supports are put in place. It is important that the intervention focuses on skills development. ABA-based supports and interventions do not aim to "change the person", "cure their autism", or "make anyone more normal", as some people have asserted (Milton, 2012; The Skeptical Advisor, 2014). The aim of ABA-based supports is to enhance skills that lead to empowerment, active participation, and the greatest possible level of independence.

Behaviour can be measured on different dimensions, such as frequency, duration, latency, or product. When the behaviour has a distinct beginning and end point, it can be measured in terms of *frequency*, such as simple counts of incidents of behaviour during a specified time period. When a behaviour lasts for a while, it should be measured in terms of *duration* (i.e. the time spent being engaged in a behaviour). When the behaviour has a particular start point, a measurement of *latency* might be appropriate (e.g. the time between an instruction and the compliant behaviour). If the behaviour produces a distinct outcome, it would be measured along the dimension of *product of behaviour* (e.g. the number of bottles that were recycled during a week; Jacob Keller, 2010). The dimensions used to measure the target behaviour depend on the definition and assessment of the behaviour and the purpose of the intervention (Cooper et al., 2020; Johnston & Pennypacker, 2008; Keenan & Dillenburger, 2020a).

1.4 Assessment Procedures

There are three main assessment procedures that are common in most ABA-based programme. Foremost, functional assessments and/or functional analyses are conducted to assess which behaviour requires consideration and what kind of intervention may be advised (Hanley et al., 2003; Iwata et al., 1994). In addition, repeated preference and/or reinforcer assessments are carried out throughout the programme to ensure that the stimuli used as reinforcers are effective (Cló & Dounavi, 2020; Elliott & Dillenburger, 2014). Once the target behaviour is identified, the collection of stable baseline data is an important aspect of the programme because it allows for a thorough assessment of the behaviour prior to the intervention and thus allows for a comparison between data collected before the intervention and data collected during/after intervention data (Johnston & Pennypacker, 2008).

Functional Assessment Determining the function of a behaviour refers to the process of identifying the reason why a behaviour occurs and why it is maintained in certain circumstances or settings (Dillenburger & Keenan, 1997; Skinner, 1938a). Functional assessments (FA) are used to identify the variables that maintain the target behaviour prior to ABA-based supports being put in place. FAs are used most frequently in programmes that target particularly challenging behaviour, such as extreme task avoidance, violence against staff or family, or self-injurious behaviour, however they also are useful more generally (Hanley et al., 2003; Iwata et al., 1994).

Functional assessments include direct observation, standardised assessment tools, such as tests or schedules, interviews, and experimental functional analysis (Keenan & Dillenburger, 2020a; Schlinger & Normand, 2013). Data collected in FAs ensure that supports focus on the specific function of the target behaviour, thus increasing the prospect of successful outcomes. It is important that those who conduct an FA and design interventions based on an FA are well trained and experienced behaviour analysts (BACB, 2020; Dillenburger, 2016; Dillenburger et al., 2016; Hughes & Shook, 2007).

Preference and/or Reinforcer Assessment A preference and/or reinforcer assessment is a test to see if the learner has preferences for specific stimuli that could function as effective reinforcers. This can include indirect assessments by simply asking a caregiver or learner for suggestions of what stimulus might work or direct assessment through systematic exposure to a variety of stimuli while recording the learners' responses. Direct reinforcer assessment can be approach-based to find out which stimulus is preferred when two or more are available or engagement-based to assess which potential reinforcer the learner engages with for longer (Cló & Dounavi, 2020; Hagopian et al., 2004).

It is important to carry out preference and/or reinforcer assessment frequently, because even well-established reinforcers can lose effectiveness (satiation); for example, food may not function as a reinforcer directly after a big meal. On the other hand, new reinforcing stimuli may become established or gain in effectiveness (deprivation), for example, if an attractive toy is only used during the intervention and is not available during free play, time to play with that toy can become an effective reinforcer for more demanding behaviour (Cooper et al., 2020).

Baseline Assessment Taking a baseline is a necessary part of the assessment process prior to any ABA-based intervention. It is important that enough behavioural data are taken for the baseline to be considered "stable" (Cooper et al., 2020). This means that baseline data are not ascending (rising) or descending (dropping) across time. The basic premise is that baseline data that are stable before the intervention would continue to be the same or similar if nothing were done to change them. Therefore, it would be safe to conclude that if the data change once the intervention is introduced, the change can be attributed to the intervention and not to other external factors or maturation.

Of course, experimentally, it would be necessary to return to baseline after the intervention to ensure that it was the intervention and nothing else that caused the change; however, usually this is not possible or desirable in applied setting. Therefore, a number of other data collection designs are used commonly in ABA-based interventions, including multiple baseline designs (Johnston & Pennypacker, 2008). The choice of monitoring or data collection system depends on the target behaviour as well as the intervention procedures.

1.5 Basic ABA-Based Support Procedures

Given that ABA-based programmes are grounded in the science of behaviour analysis, this allows for the development of individually tailored procedures (Luce et al., 1996). Consequently, there is no specific or definitive number of ABA-based support procedures or interventions. However, some tried and tested methods are included frequently in behaviour analytic programmes. These include the use of discrete learn units, shaping and chaining, token economies, and modelling (further procedures are described in other chapters of this book).

Discrete Learn Units Discrete learn units include all three aspects of the three-term contingency (Greer & McDonough, 1999). An antecedent stimulus is presented, the behaviour is emitted (prompted, if necessary), and a consequent stimulus is provided as a potential reinforcer. This three-step process is used often early in a programme when very basic skills are taught. The formalised procedure is known as Discrete Trial Training (DTT; Booth & Keenan, 2018; Keenan & Dillenburger, 2020a). DTT usually is conducted on a table, with the teacher on one side and the learner on the other side of the table or on a mat on the floor. The teacher sets out the task, such as learning colours and shapes, or imitation skills, the child responds, and the teacher delivers the reinforcing stimulus. However, learn units also can be provided in more natural settings by creating or utilising naturally occurring learning opportunities in Natural Environment Training (NET) (Luce et al., 1996).

Shaping and Chaining As tasks become more difficult and behaviour more refined, new behaviour may have to be taught in small steps. The process is called shaping. Shaping consists of systematically reinforcing successive approximations towards the target behaviour (Cooper et al., 2020; Keenan & Dillenburger, 2020a). "Operant conditioning shapes behavior as a sculptor shapes a lump of clay... The final product seems to have a special unity or integrity of design, but we cannot find a point at which this suddenly appears... it is the result of a continuous shaping process" (Skinner, 1953, p. 91).

In order to develop a successful shaping programme, it is important to choose and define the target behaviour as well as determining the learner's skills level (Booth et al., 2018). It is necessary early in the programme to identify all of the steps that are essential for the behaviour or skill to be learned successfully. Teaching starts when the learner engages in an approximation of the behaviour and this is reinforced immediately. Then, the next step is reinforced, and so on. Shaping is a useful technology that can be easily combined with other procedures, such as chaining, to develop more complex behaviour.

A behaviour chain is defined as "a sequence of responses that are functionally linked to the same terminal reinforcer" (Kuhn et al., 2006, p. 263). The individual elements of the chain are determined by a task analysis (Booth & Keenan, 2018; Keenan & Dillenburger, 2020a), that clearly identifies the discrete steps that are required to perform the complex target behaviour. Chaining begins either with learning the first step (forward chaining) or last step in the chain (backward chaining) (Cooper et al., 2020). In some circumstances it may be appropriate to train the whole task at once (concurrent chaining or total-task presentation). Chaining can be used to teach many tasks, from self-care, cooking, and gardening, to job skills (Dillenburger et al., 2019; Shrestha et al., 2013; Williams & Burkholder, 2008).

Token economy In a token economy, tokens are used as conditioned reinforcers immediately after the behaviour (Cló & Dounavi, 2020). Usually, a pre-determined number of tokens has to be earned before the larger reinforcer is delivered. As such, tokens are used to serve as backup reinforcers and bridge the time between the behaviour and the delivery of the final reinforcer. Tokens can be anything, like stickers, marbles, or simply a star drawn on a piece of paper or a blackboard. In a token economy

1. The target behaviour must be defined very clearly.
2. A sufficient number of tokens must be available.
3. The schedule must be clear, e.g. one token for three correct matching tasks.
4. The number of tokens required for the final reinforcer must be clearly specified.
5. It has to be clear, when and where tokens can be exchanged for the final reinforcer.
6. The preferred back-up reinforcers must be identified and available once the required number of tokens has been earned.
7. A decision has to be made as to whether or not a response-cost element (loosing tokens for undesired behaviour) is incorporated into the token economy.

Token economies are highly structured procedures resulting in consistency in the delivery of positive reinforcers and as such they can be employed usefully where many teachers or therapists are involved with the same learner. Token economies also can be used to develop a learner's self-management skills (Petscher & Bailey, 2006).

Modelling or Imitation Modelling, imitation, or observational/vicarious learning are terms used when, after the learner has observed the behaviour of a visual (physical) model in vivo or on video, they are able to engage in the behaviour (Nikopoulos & Keenan, 2006). In fact, learning via imitation is an important developmental skill (Lindsay et al., 2013). Most children learn this skill very early, often within weeks or months of birth, however, not all children do and generalised imitation skills may have to be taught (SimpleSteps, 2020).

Four factors that need to be considered for behaviour to be imitative:

1. Any physical movement may function as a model for imitation.
2. An imitative behaviour must immediately follow the presentation of the model.
3. Both the model and the imitative behaviour must have 'formal similarity'. 'Formal similarity' refers the model and learner resembling one another as much as possible.
4. The imitation must occur because of the model; in other words, the model must be the controlling variable for the imitative behaviour (Cooper et al., 2020).

Once someone has learned to imitate, they can learn new and adaptive behaviour very quickly (Greer et al., 2006). In fact, there is evidence that "modelling is more effective in producing changes in parenting behaviour than either direct instruction or group discussion" (Johnson & Brown, 1969).

1.6 Correcting Misrepresentations

When people are not trained in the science of behaviour analysis, confusion about ABA can occur (Dillenburger & Keenan, 2023). This has led to misunderstandings that are quite widespread across Europe (Keenan et al., 2014; Kelly et al., 2018). In fact, some people still consider behaviour analysis as being of historical interest only, despite incredible advances of the science in the 21st century (Baron-Cohen, 2014; The Skeptical Advisor, 2014).

Despite repeated publications to correct erroneous reporting (Heward, 2003; Keenan & Dillenburger, 2020b; Morris, 2009), misunderstandings persist. This is due mainly because behaviour analysts are not included in guideline development and review or policy making bodies (Dillenburger et al., 2014; Keenan & Dillenburger, 2018, 2023) and because those not trained in the science teach the next generation of students (Howlin, 2013; Jordan, 2001). These students then go on to think that ABA is just a therapy for autism (Dillenburger et al., 2016; Fennell & Dillenburger, 2018). It is important to correct misrepresentations in the media (social media, radio, newspapers, or television) or elsewhere to ensure that only accurate information about ABA is disseminated.

1.7 Conclusion

ABA-based programmes and procedures have a long-standing, well-founded research base and are considered established and evidence-based for a variety of applications in business, sport, general education, medicine, and special education (APBA, 2020; Dillenburger & Coyle, 2019; Gormley et al., 2017; Levy et al., 2016; McGrath et al., 2018; Quinn et al., 2015). The focus of all ABA-based supports and interventions, as has been pointed out repeatedly, is the enhancement of socially significant behaviour and skills (Baer et al., 1968; Cooper et al., 2020).

In this chapter, the three branches of the natural science of behaviour analysis were outlined and examples given of a range of applications. Despite some persistent misconceptions, more and more students and practitioners are beginning to realise the potential of this science to enhance socially important behaviour. While much of this work is conducted with individuals on the autism spectrum, this does not mean that ABA is effective only with this population. There is a significant body of research showing the successful application of behavioural strategies and principles for teaching new skills, reducing challenging behaviour, and improving quality of life for a multitude of learners (Dillenburger, 2015). Therefore, behaviour analysts need to be part of any multidisciplinary professional team (Dillenburger et al., 2014; NICE, 2015).

In sum, ABA is not a therapy for autism. Instead, ABA is the applied branch of the science of behaviour analysis. ABA is underpinned conceptually by the philosophy of science and utilises behaviour change mechanisms that were discovered in the experimental analysis of behaviour. This means that ABA avoids pseudo-explanations and ensures that behavioural goals are socially significant, that procedures are socially appropriate, and that the effects of ABA-based supports are socially valid and important.

Acknowledgements This chapter was previously published by the Czech Republic's Department of Education in the Czech language. Gower, C. & Booth, N., & Dillenburger, K. (2022). *Aplikovaná behaviorální analýza: co to je a co to není*. In A. Markova & A. CIibulková (ed.). Užití prvků aplikované behaviorální analýzy ve školním prostředí. Praha: Národní pedagogický institut České republiky, (*Applied Behaviour Analysis in education settings*. Czech Department of Education), ISBN: 978-80-7578-080-5. Permission was granted to publish the English original.

This chapter is based in part on the 1st author's PhD thesis, supervised by the 3rd author.

We acknowledge helpful review comments by Prof. Mickey Keenan.

References

APBA. (2020). Identifying applied behavior analysis interventions. Association of Professional Behavior Analysts White paper. Retrieved April 21, 2020, from http://www.apbahome.net/

Ayllon, T., & Michael, J. (1959). The psychiatric nurse as a behavioral engineer. *Journal of the Experimental Analysis of Behavior, 2*(4), 323–334. https://doi.org/10.1901/jeab.1959.2-323

BACB. (2020). Behavior Analyst Certification Board. Retrieved April 2, 2021, from www.bacb.com

Baer, D. M., Wolf, M. M., & Risley, T. R. (1968). Some current dimensions of applied behavior analysis. *Journal of Applied Behavior Analysis, 1*(1), 91–97.

Baer, D. M., Wolf, M. M., & Risley, T. R. (1987). Some still-current dimensions of applied behavior analysis. *Journal of Applied Behavior Analysis, 20*(4), 313–327. https://doi.org/10.1901/jaba.1987.20-313

Baron-Cohen, S. (2014). What scientific idea is ready for retirement? Radical behaviourism. Retrieved April 2, 2018, from https://www.edge.org/response-detail/25473

Baum, W. (2004). *Understanding behaviorism: Behavior, culture, and evolution*. Blackwell Publishing Ltd.

Booth, N., & Keenan, M. (2018). Discrete Trial Teaching: A study on the comparison of three training strategies. *Interdisciplinary Education and Psychology, 2*(2), 3.

Booth, N., Keenan, M., & Gallagher, S. (2018). Autism, interventions and parent training. *Psichologija, 57*, 74–94. https://doi.org/10.15388/Psichol.2018.0.11904

Boyle, M. E., & Greer, R. D. (1983). Operant procedures and the comatose patient. *Journal of Applied Behavior Analysis, 16*(1), 3–12. https://doi.org/10.1901/jaba.1983.16-3

Catania, C. A. (1997). *Learning*. Pearson Publishing.

Chiesa, M. (1984). Radical behaviorism: The philosophy and the science. Retrieved December 5, 2015, from http://www.amazon.com/Radical-Behaviorism-The-Philosophy-Science/dp/0962331147

Chiesa, M. (2006). ABA is not 'A Therapy for Autism. In M. Mickey Keenan, K. D. Henderson, & K. P. Kerr (Eds.), *Applied behaviour analysis and autism building a future together* (pp. 225–240). Jessica Kingsley Publishers.

Cló, E., & Dounavi, K. (2020). A systematic review of behaviour analytic processes and procedures for conditioning reinforcers among individuals with autism, developmental or intellectual disability. *Behaviour Interventions*. https://doi.org/10.1080/15021149.2020.1847953

Cooper, J., Heron, T., & Heward, W. (2020). *Applied behaviour analysis* (3rd ed.). Pearson Prentice Hall.

Dillenburger, K. (2011). The Emperor's new clothes: Eclecticism in autism treatment. *Research in Autism Spectrum Disorders, 5*(3), 1119–1128. https://doi.org/10.1016/j.rasd.2010.12.008

Dillenburger, K. (2015). Evidence-based management and intervention for autism spectrum disorders. In M. Fitzgerald (Ed.), *Autism* (1st ed., p. 10.5772/58983). Intech. Retrieved April 2, 2021, from https://www.intechopen.com/books/autism-spectrum-disorder-recent-advances/evidence-based-management-and-intervention-for-autism-spectrum-disorders

Dillenburger, K. (2016). Staff training. In J. Matson (Ed.), *Handbook of autism treatments* (pp. 95–109). Springer US.

Dillenburger, K., & Coyle, C. (2019). Education for all: The Good Inclusion Game (GIG). https://doi.org/10.1002/bin.1671

Dillenburger, K., & Keenan, M. (1997). Human development: A question of structure and function. In K. Dillenburger, M. O'Reilly, & M. Keenan (Eds.), *Advances in behaviour analysis* (pp. 3–22). University College Dublin Press.

Dillenburger, K., & Keenan, M. (2009). None of the as in ABA stand for autism: Dispelling the myths. *Journal of Intellectual & Developmental Disability, 34*(2), 193–195. https://doi.org/10.1080/13668250902845244

Dillenburger, K. & Keenan, M. (2023). Autism and behavior analysis: From dissonance to dialogue. *International Electronic Journal of Elementary Education. Special Issue editors* J. Cihon, E. Kazemi, J. Leaf., *15*(3), 199–208.

Dillenburger, K., Matuska, E., de Bruijn, M., & Röttgers, H.-R. (2019). *Job coaches for adults with disabilities: A practical guide*. Jessica Kingsley Publishers.

Dillenburger, K., McKerr, L., & Jordan, J.-A. (2014). Lost in translation: Public policies, evidence-based practice, and Autism Spectrum Disorder. *International Journal of Disability, Development and Education, 61*(2), 134–151. https://doi.org/10.1080/1034912X.2014.905059

Dillenburger, K., McKerr, L., Jordan, J.-A., & Keenan, M. (2016). Staff training in autism: The one-eyed wo/man.... *International Journal of Environmental Research and Public Health, 13*(7), 716. https://doi.org/10.3390/ijerph13070716

Dillenburger, K., Röttgers, H.-R., Dounavi, K., Sparkman, C., Keenan, M., Thyer, B., & Nikopoulos, C. (2014). Multidisciplinary teamwork in autism: Can one size fit all? *Australian Educational and Developmental Psychologist, 31*(2), 1–16. https://doi.org/10.1017/edp.2014.13

Elliott, C., & Dillenburger, K. (2014). The effect of choice on motivation for young children on the autism spectrum during discrete trial teaching. *Journal of Research in Special Educational Needs, 16*(3), 187–198. https://doi.org/10.1111/1471-3802.12073

Fennell, B., & Dillenburger, K. (2018). Applied behaviour analysis: What do teachers of students with autism spectrum disorder know. *International Journal of Educational Research, 87*, 110–118. Retrieved April 2, 2021, from http://www.sciencedirect.com/science/article/pii/S088303551630057X

Fisher, W. W., Piazza, C. C., & Roane, H. S. (2011). *Handbook of applied behavior analysis*. GIlford Press.

Fuller, P. R. (1949). Operant conditioning of a vegetative human organism. *American Journal of Psychology, 62*, 587–590.

Gormley, G., Dillenburger, K., Lydon, S., Byrne, D., Walsh, I., Brennan, C., et al. (2017). Precision teaching: Opening new doors in health profession education? In *INMED - Irish network of medical educators, collective competence for healthcare practitioners: Preparing for real world practice* (pp. 27.02–01.03).

Greer, R. D., Dudek-Singer, J., & Gautreaux, G. (2006). Observational learning. *International Journal of Psychology*. https://doi.org/10.1080/00207590500492435

Greer, R. D., & McDonough, S. H. (1999). Is the learn unit a fundamental measure of pedagogy? *The Behavior Analyst, 22*(1), 5–16.

Hagopian, L. P., Long, E. S., & Rush, K. S. (2004). Preference assessment procedures for individuals with developmental disabilities. *Behavior Modification, 28*(5), 668–677. https://doi.org/10.1177/0145445503259836

Hanley, G. (2020). A perspective on today's ABA. Retrieved June 7, 2020, from https://practicalfunctionalassessment.com/2020/06/04/a-perspective-on-todays-aba-by-dr-greg-hanley/?fbclid=IwAR2WAfpDxCfSUokPi4_DREeAMvLHLOtvvTU3D-UfCbsSKpQFYTOMY-UklQQ

Hanley, G. P., Iwata, B. A., & McCord, B. E. (2003). Functional analysis of problem behavior: A review. *Journal of Applied Behavior Analysis, 36*(2), 147–185. https://doi.org/10.1901/jaba.2003.36-147

Heward, W. L. (2003). Ten faulty notions about teaching and learning that hinder the effectiveness of special education. *The Journal of Special Education, 36*(4), 186–205. https://doi.org/10.1177/002246690303600401

Howlin, P. (2013). 70 Years of autism research: How far have we come? *Autism Europe Newsletter, Dec.* https://doi.org/10.1197/jamia.M1749

Hrisos, S., Eccles, M. P., Francis, J. J., Dickinson, H. O., Kaner, E. F., Beyer, F., & Johnston, M. (2009). Are there valid proxy measures of clinical behaviour? A systematic review. *Implementation Science, 4*(1), 39. https://doi.org/10.1186/1748-5908-4-37

Hughes, C. J., & Shook, G. L. (2007). Training and certification of behaviour analysts in Europe: Past, present, and future challenges. *European Journal of Behavior Analysis, 8*(2), 239–249.

Iwata, B. A., Dorsey, M. F., Slifer, K. J., Bauman, K. E., & Richman, G. S. (1994). Toward a functional analysis of self-injury. *Journal of Applied Behavior Analysis, 27*(2), 197–209. https://doi.org/10.1901/jaba.1994.27-197

Jacob Keller, J. (2010). The recycling solution: How I increased recycling on dilworth road. *Behavior Analyst, 33*(2), 171–173. https://doi.org/10.1007/bf03392212

Johnson, S. M., & Brown, R. A. (1969). Producing behaviour change in parents of disturbed children. *Journal of Child Psychology and Psychiatry, 10*(2), 107–121. https://doi.org/10.1111/j.1469-7610.1969.tb02073.x

Johnston, J., & Pennypacker, H. (2008). *Strategies and Tactics of Behavioral Research*, 3rd edn. Retrieved July 18, 2014, from http://www.amazon.com/Strategies-Tactics-Behavioral-Research-Edition/dp/0805858822

Jordan, R. (2001). Parents' Education as Autism Therapists: Applied Behaviour Analysis in Context. By M. Keenan, K. Kerr & K. Dillenburger. Jessica Kingsley Publishers, London. pp. 175. £13.95 (pb). *Journal of Child Psychology and Psychiatry*, *42*(3), 421–423. https://doi.org/10.1017/S0021963001216795

Keenan, M. (2015). Private Events (Part 1, Part 2 and Part 3). Retrieved April 2, 2021, from https://www.youtube.com/watch?v=LFVykFNOGdw&t=292s

Keenan, M., & Dillenburger, K. (2011). When all you have is a hammer …: RCTs and hegemony in science. *Research in Autism Spectrum Disorders, 5*(1), 1–13. https://doi.org/10.1016/j.rasd.2010.02.003

Keenan, M., & Dillenburger, K. (2018). How "fake news" affect autism policies. *Societies, 2018030238*. https://doi.org/10.20944/preprints201803.0238.v1

Keenan, M. & Dillenburger, K. (2020a). *Behaviour analysis: A primer*. Retrieved January 30, 2021, from www.behaviouranalysis.eu.com

Keenan, M. & Dillenburger, K. (2020b). *Drama in the courtroom: Defending the rights of children diagnosed with autism*. Retrieved December 2, 2020, from https://www.barristermagazine.com/drama-in-the-courtroom-defending-the-rights-of-children-diagnosed-with-autism/

Keenan, M. & Dillenburger, K. (2023). Advocacy and open science in the UK: Case studies in the Autism wars. *Behavior Analysis in Practice*. https://link.springer.com/article/10.1007/s40617-023-00881-2

Keenan, M., Dillenburger, K., Röttgers, H.-R., Dounavi, K., Jónsdóttir, S. L., Moderato, P., et al. (2014). Autism and ABA: The gulf between North America and Europe. *Review Journal of Autism and Developmental Disorders, 2*(2), 167–183. https://doi.org/10.1007/s40489-014-0045-2

Kelly, M., Martin, N., Dillenburger, K., Kelly, A., & Miller, M. M. (2018). Spreading the news: History, successes, challenges and the ethics of effective dissemination. *Behavior Analysis in Practice*. https://doi.org/10.1007/s40617-018-0238-8

Kuhn, S. A. C., Lerman, D. C., Vorndran, C. M., & Addison, L. (2006). Analysis of factors that affect responding in a two-response chain in children with developmental disabilities. *Journal of Applied Behavior Analysis, 39*(3), 263–280. https://doi.org/10.1901/jaba.2006.118-05

Levy, I. M., Pryor, K. W., & McKeon, T. R. (2016). Is teaching simple surgical skills using an operant learning program more effective than teaching by demonstration? *Clinical Orthopaedics and Related Research®, 474*(4), 945–955. https://doi.org/10.1007/s11999-015-4555-8

Lindsay, C. J., Moore, D. W., Anderson, A., & Dillenburger, K. (2013). The role of imitation in video-based interventions for children with autism. *Developmental Neurorehabilitation, 16*, 283–289. https://doi.org/10.3109/17518423.2012.758185

Luce, S. C., Green, G., & Maurice, C. (1996). Behavioral intervention for young children with autism: Retrieved February 4, 2015, from http://www.amazon.co.uk/Behavioral-Intervention-Young-Children-Autism/dp/0890796831

Martin, C., & Dillenburger, K. (2019). Behavioural water safety and autism: A Systematic review of interventions. *Review Journal of Autism and Developmental Disorders, 6*, 356–366. https://doi.org/10.1007/s40489-019-00166-x

Mayer, G. R., Sulzer-Azaroff, B., & Wallace, M. (2012). *Behavior analysis for lasting change*. Sloan Publications.

McGrath, C., McCourt, C., Corry, A., Dounavi, K., Dillenburger, K., & Gormley, G. (2018). The use of "Precision Teaching" in enhancing medical students' dermatological diagnostic skills. *MedEdPublish, 7*(2). https://doi.org/10.15694/mep.2018.0000091.1

Milton, D. (2012, September 10). The normalisation agenda and the psycho-emotional disablement of autistic people. *Autonomy, the Critical Journal of Interdisciplinary Autism Studies*. Retrieved April 2, 2021, from http://www.larry-arnold.net/Autonomy/index.php/autonomy/article/view/AR3/21

Moore, J. (2003). Behavior analysis, mentalism, and the path to social justice. *The Behavior Analyst / MABA, 26*(2), 181–193. Retrieved April 2, 2021, from http://www.pubmedcentral.nih.gov/articlerender.fcgi?artid=2731454&tool=pmcentrez&rendertype=abstract

Morris, E. K. (2009). A case study in the misrepresentation of applied behavior analysis in autism: The Gernsbacher lectures. *The Behavior Analyst, 32*(1), 205–240. https://doi.org/10.1007/BF03392184

NICE. (2015). *Challenging behaviour and learning disabilities: Prevention and interventions for people with learning disabilities whose behaviour challenges: Methods, evidence and recommendations (NICE Guideline 11)*. Retrieved August 3, 2015, from http://www.nice.org.uk/guidance/ng11/evidence/full-guideline-60708493

Nikopoulos, C., & Keenan, M. (2006). *Video modelling and behaviour analysis: A guide for teaching social skills to children with autism*. Jessica Kingsley Publishers.

Petscher, E. S., & Bailey, J. S. (2006). Effects of training, prompting, and self-monitoring on staff behavior in a classroom for students with disabilities. *Journal of Applied Behavior Analysis, 39*(2), 215–226. https://doi.org/10.1901/jaba.2006.02-05

Questel, M. (2020). *Avoiding the pitfalls of circular reasoning*. Retrieved April 2, 2021, from https://asatonline.org/for-parents/becoming-a-savvy-consumer/pitfalls-of-circular-reasoning/?utm_source=Newsletter+Subscribers&utm_campaign=538b97be62-EMAIL_CAMPAIGN_2020_11_28_03_59&utm_medium=email&utm_term=0_a219af0e1e-538b97be62-2251025

Quinn, M. J., Miltenberger, R. G., & Fogel, V. A. (2015). Using tagteach to improve the proficiency of dance movements. *Journal of Applied Behavior Analysis, 48*(1), 11–24. https://doi.org/10.1002/jaba.191

Rice, H. K., McDaniel, M. W., Stallings, V. D., & Gatz, M. J. (1967). Operant behavior in vegetative patients II. *The Psychological Record, 17*, 449–460.

Schlinger, H. D. (2020). *A behavior-analytic theory of child development*. Retrieved April 2, 2021, from https://doi.org/10.1002/9781119171492.wecad050

Schlinger, H. D., & Normand, M. P. (2013). On the origin and functions of the term functional analysis. *Journal of Applied Behavior Analysis, 46*(1), 285–288. https://doi.org/10.1002/jaba.6

Shrestha, A., Anderson, A., & Moore, D. W. (2013). Using point-of-view video modeling and forward chaining to teach a functional self-help skill to a child with autism. *Journal of Behavioral Education, 22*(2), 157–167. https://doi.org/10.1007/s10864-012-9165-x

SimpleSteps. (2020). *Simple Steps Autism: The online teaching platform for the treatment of Autism*. Retrieved October 29, 2014, from www.simplestepsautism.com

Skinner, B. F. (1938a). *Behavior of organisms*. D. Appleton-Century Company, Inc.

Skinner, B. F. (1938b). *The behavior of organisms: An experimental analysis*. Appleton-Century.

Skinner, B. F. (1953). *Science and human behavior*. Simon and Schuster. Retrieved April 2, 2021, from https://books.google.com/books?hl=en&lr=&id=Pjjknd1HREIC&pgis=1

Skinner, B. F. (1969). *Contingencies of reinforcement: A theoretical analysis. Behavior Therapy*. Appleton-Century-Crofts. https://doi.org/10.1016/S0005-7894(70)80039-9

Skinner, B. F. (1977). Why I am not a cognitive psychologist. *Behaviorism, 5*, 1–10. Retrieved April 2, 2021, from http://www.jstor.org/stable/27758892?seq=1#page_scan_tab_contents

Skinner, B. F. (1987). Whatever happened to psychology as the science of behavior? *American Psychologist, 42*(8), 780–786. https://doi.org/10.1037/0003-066X.42.8.780

The Skeptical Advisor. (2014). *Simon Baron-Cohen's fantastically false article on Radical Behavior: An example of valid, but false premises*. Retrieved November 11, 2014, from http://theskepticaladvisor.wordpress.com/2014/01/21/simon-baron-cohens-fantastically-false-article-on-radical-behavior-an-example-of-valid-but-false-premises/

Thyer, B. (1999). *The philosphical legacy of behaviorism*. Springer Science & Business Media.

Thyer, B. (2009). Epistemology: A behavior analytic perspective. *Humana Nente, 3*(11), 45–63.

Watson, J. B. (1913). Psychology as the behaviourist views it. *Psychological Review, 20*(2), 158–177. https://doi.org/10.1037/h0074428

Williams, W. L. & Burkholder, E. (2008). Response chaining. In *Cognitive behavior therapy: Applying empirically supported techniques in your practice* (2nd Ed.).

Wolf, M. M. (1978). Social validity: The case for subjective measurement or how applied behavior analysis is finding its heart. *Journal of Applied Behavior Analysis, 11*(2), 203–214. https://doi.org/10.1901/JABA.1978.11-203

Chapter 2
Contemporary Applied Behavior Analysis: A Shift to an Ecologically Valid Natural Learning Paradigm

Bertram O. Ploog

Abstract Ever since its inception in the 1950s, Applied Behavior Analysis (ABA) has been the occasional target for criticism by the developmental disability community, psychiatrists, psychologists, and others that view ABA as a mechanistic and unnatural intervention. Sometimes, the general public has outrightly rejected ABA as an unethical and traumatizing intervention. These critiques stem from several misconceptions but also, to be fair, from an accurate portrayal of some early implementations of ABA that in fact, by today's standards, would be considered at best unacceptable. In addition, what is often offered as "ABA" is not what properly trained behavior analysts would consider high-quality, bona fide ABA. In this chapter, first, the origins of ABA will be reviewed, with experimental behavior analysis as its foundation, followed by a discussion of early challenges that may have led to approaches in ABA that today are rightfully considered unacceptable. Next, the discrete-trial training (DTT) approach (a common target for criticism and often seen, incorrectly, as representing the entire field of ABA) will be contrasted with the Natural-Learning Paradigm (NLP), even though the DTT approach may still be the intervention of choice for some individuals. Finally, a person's Right to Effective Treatment along with ethical considerations will be discussed, as well as NLP in relation to neurodiversity and ABA's appreciation of unequivocal respect for individual dignity and self-determination.

Keywords Autism · Contemporary applied behavior analysis · Experimental behavior analysis · Radical behaviorism · Natural learning paradigm · Discrete-trial training · Neurodiversity · Critique of ABA · A person's right to effective treatment

B. O. Ploog (✉)
Department of Psychology, 4S-105, College of Staten Island and Graduate Center, City University of New York, Staten Island, NY, USA
e-mail: bertram.ploog22@login.cuny.edu

S. Halder et al. (eds.), *Applied Behavior Analysis-Based Interventions for Autism Spectrum Disorder*, https://doi.org/10.1007/978-981-95-2889-9_2

2.1 Introduction

When the general public (i.e., not professional behavior analysts), including laypersons, educators, and politicians, make a reference to “ABA,” portrayals of contemporary Applied Behavior Analysis (ABA) range from patently incorrect and ideological characterizations to blameless misconceptions and, at best, to a vague appreciation of what ABA may have to offer to persons with autism spectrum disorders (e.g., Devita-Raeburn, 2016; Winter, 2024; Rozsa, 2025). This book chapter represents an attempt to clarify the role of contemporary ABA from the perspective of behavior analysis based on radical behaviorism. Points of discussion will be the origins (going back at least 70 years) and scope of ABA (it is not just for autism), its philosophical underpinnings (radical behaviorism with its *explicit inclusion* of cognition, emotion, language, and complex social behavior), a critique of ABA where appropriate, the contemporary practice of true ABA (much beyond the application of discrete-trial procedures, far from just being simplistic “training”), and its unequivocal support of neurodiversity and respect for the individual including any individual’s right to effective treatment, dignity, and self-determination.

2.2 Origins of ABA

2.2.1 Behavior Analysis, Radical Behaviorism, and Natural Science

In the most general terms, behavior analysis is the science of studying and identifying the contingencies that result in the ontogeny of a living being (e.g., Skinner, 1966), under consideration of biological constraints. Unfortunately, biological constraints were largely ignored until Garcia and Koelling (1966). Early behavior analysis comprised mostly studies that employed the experimental analysis of behavior (EAB; Skinner, 1938) with radical behaviorism as its philosophical foundation (Watson, 1930/1970; Zilio, 2016). Thus, EAB followed the principles of a natural science like other natural sciences (e.g., biology, chemistry, physics), which embrace a Newtonian view of science (Popper, 2005).

Radical behaviorism *explicitly includes* complex human behavior such as language and thought (Skinner, 1957) and emotion (Watson, 1930/1970). *Radical* behaviorism stands in contrast to *methodological* behaviorism which limits its scope of investigation to only the directly observable (see Moore, 2001[1]). When subscribing to strict methodological behaviorism, it is fair to say that much of human behavior is seen through a skewed, narrow scope and that ABA practitioners

[1]The criticism of “behaviorism” of assuming a “Black Box” while ignoring its content may be justified with regards to methodological but not with regards to radical behaviorism. Radical behaviorism does not subscribe to any notion of a “Black Box.”

may not do justice to individuals with all their human complexities. It is also true that much of ABA is, in practice, based on methodological behaviorism as the practitioner's immediate interest is in finding interventions "that work," that is, have immediate applicability to improve the individual's quality of life.

In the natural-science approach to scientific discovery (thus, also true for behavior analysis based on radical behaviorism), the first step is an observation of a phenomenon of interest, which then leads to the formulation of a question to be experimentally addressed: Why did [*phenomenon*] occur? The why-question is then further formalized as a scientific hypothesis putting cause and effect in relation. In experimental terminology, the "cause" is the independent variable to be manipulated freely by the experimenter, whereas the "effect" is the dependent variable as it is hypothesized that the dependent variable changes systematically depending on the value of the independent variable. Once the hypothesis is formalized, experiments are conducted with at least two values of the independent variable. If the dependent variable changes systematically with the independent variable (i.e., internal validity is high), then support of the hypothesis is gained and is used to expand the knowledge base that is specific to the phenomenon that was studied.[2] If, in contrast, there is no clear, systematic relationship between the independent and dependent variables (i.e., internal validity is low), then the original hypothesis is not supported, which then must lead to revising the hypothesis and to continuing the hypothesis testing reiteratively until a cause-and-effect relationship can be identified.

An example will illustrate this approach: A teacher observes that a child is aggressive. Based on the why-question "Why is Anthony aggressive towards his classmates?", one hypothesis could be "Anthony hits his classmate because it gets him out of having to do his math work"—hitting being the effect (dependent variable) and being presented with math work and a chance to avoid math work being at least one of the possible causes (independent variable) for Anthony's aggression. Many other hypotheses or combinations of different independent variables or causes could be explored: Does aggression occur only with a particular classmate, only at a particular time of the day, only with math but not with history, only with a particular teacher, or only when Anthony's para-educator is not paying attention to him? Aggression is then assessed under at least two conditions that relate to the hypothesis: 15 min before presentation of the math work and then for 15 min after the introduction of the math work. If hitting reliably increases as soon as math work is introduced, the hypothesis is supported. If hitting occurs regardless of whether math work is presented or not, the hypothesis is not supported, and other hypotheses need to be considered.

---

[2] In this light, behavior analysis is a cumulative science, just like the other natural sciences. A cumulative science expands a body of knowledge through continued scientific study by generating new data and revealing discoveries that become commonly accepted facts. For example, the discovery of the law of gravity became a part of the general body of knowledge with regards to physics as much as the law of effect (reinforcement principle) has become a part of the general body of knowledge with regards to the natural science of behavior.

Three points about such hypothesis-testing are important: (1) The variables need to be precisely defined (e.g., "aggression" is too vague as it might refer to verbal threats, throwing objects at a person, making threat gestures, or physical assault which itself can take many forms such as hitting, kicking, or spitting. Even "hitting" may be too vague. It could be tapping, lightly touching, pushing, or a full-blown punch). Precise definitions are critical so that high interobserver agreement can be achieved (cf. Essig et al., 2023). (2) A hypothesis needs to be falsifiable, which means that the data to be collected will allow us to either reject or accept the hypothesis. An example of a non-falsifiable hypothesis might be "If Anthony is presented with math work, he will either control himself or be aggressive." No matter what Anthony's behavior will be (either he shows or does not show aggression), the data will not allow one to reject the hypothesis because the absence of aggression is taken as evidence of self-control and supports the hypothesis anyway, even if there is no outward sign of aggression. Also, in general, poorly defined variables lead to non-falsifiable hypotheses because the data cannot be interpreted clearly as either being or not being in support of the hypothesis. (3) As there are likely many causes for any given behavior (Matson et al., 2003) and most of them might remain unknown, the preferred term in ABA for an independent variable is "functional variable" (Madden et al., 2021). A functional variable can be identified by performing a functional analysis or assessment (Davison, 2019). It is understood that the functional analysis may only identify one of many possible causes in the form of the functional variable. However, it is still true that the functional variable reliably affects the target behavior. In other words, a functional variable can be seen as an "on/off switch" for the target behavior and thus informs an effective intervention.[3]

2.2.2 Experimental Analysis of Behavior (EAB)

There are two main branches of behavior analysis, EAB and ABA, with ABA having grown out of EAB. Thus, EAB is considered the foundation of ABA. Both have been represented for decades by the *Society for the Experimental Analysis of Behavior* in two flagship journals: The *Journal of the Experimental Analysis of Behavior*, first published in 1958, and the *Journal of Applied Behavior Analysis* first published in 1968. The *Association for Behavior Analysis International* was founded in 1974 and publishes six other journals with focus on behavior analysis (*Behavior Analysis in Practice, Behavior and Social Issues, Education and Treatment of Children, Perspectives on Behavior Science, The Analysis of Verbal Behavior*, and *The Psychological Record*). Initially, EAB's almost exclusive focus was on work with animals such as pigeons and rats, not humans. This preference was predicated in part by the tight experimental control that could only be obtained with

[3] In applied settings, scientific rigor may be loosened (i.e., not all causes need to be identified) in favor of practical considerations (i.e., one variable was identified that "works" for an effective intervention).

nonhumans (e.g., being able to account for an animal's nearly complete learning history across its entire lifespan; low intersubject variability; fewer ethical concerns). An obvious drawback was, and still is, that animal studies may be low in external validity (i.e., limited in that findings may not generalize to humans, especially when complex, such as social or verbal, behaviors are studied[4]). But it was also understood from early on that behavior analysis was invaluable because of its implications for understanding human behavior in all its complexity, and that basic research findings from EAB could offer powerful insights in how to translate those findings into applications with the goal of improving the quality of life for human individuals and society at large. Specifically, possibilities for developing interventions and clinical applications for people in need were recognized early on.

There have been early EAB studies that involve humans (e.g., Razran, 1934; Fuller, 1949) and also throughout the following decades (e.g., Baron et al., 1969; Galizio, 1979; Case et al., 1990; cf. Baron et al., 1991; Fantino & Savastano, 1996; Ribeiro & de Souza, 2024) but they were not studies with an explicit goal to modify human behavior for the direct benefit of the individual or society as would be the case for true ABA studies.

2.2.3 Applied Behavior Analysis (ABA)

The idea that behavior analysis can be employed to modify human behavior for the improvement of individuals and societies sparked the beginnings of ABA (Skinner, 1938, 1953, 1954, 1958; Lindsley & Skinner, 1954; Isaacs et al., 1960). Skinner, in particular, related behavior analysis to the field of education (Skinner, 1954, 1958, 1961) and society at large. His book, *Walden Two*, is a fictional novel about a society that is built on the principles of behavior analysis (Skinner, 1948). Based on *Walden Two*, a community by the name "*Los Horcones*" was founded with the goal of implementing the principles of behavior analysis to build a modern, just, and egalitarian society. Members refer to their community as a "cultural laboratory" which reflects the community's roots in, and commitment to, behavior analysis and science.

John B. Watson also recognized and proposed the principles of behavior analysis to improve human society (Watson, 1930/1970). His best-known experiment involving "Little Albert" (Watson & Rayner, 1920) was inspired by his desire to develop an effective treatment of phobias based on empirical science. To do so, Watson and Rayner felt that a scientist needed to know the person's learning history that resulted in a phobia, which in most cases remains unknown or speculative at best. So, they first established a phobia to then eliminate it, which was their primary goal to begin

[4] In this light, "mouse models of autism" (e.g., Zerbi et al., 2021) may be limited to genetic marker studies that attempt to link autism to some clear biological factors but do not address uniquely human behaviors such as deficits in language, abstract cognition, and complex social skills (all known to be among the diagnostic criteria for autism).

with. Nine-month-old Albert's phobia was induced by pairing the presentation of a rat or another small, furry animal with a loud noise, produced by hitting a steel bar with a hammer. The loud noise elicited unconditionally (i.e., innate, not learned) crying and other emotional fear reactions in Albert. The rat, even though it initially did not elicit any observable fear reactions, did eventually do so after a few presentations of the rat followed by the loud noise. By current standards, Little Albert's treatment is considered entirely unethical, and no behavior analyst would advocate for an experiment of this sort. Regardless, Watson's work did in fact have a great clinical impact on the development of behavioral treatments of phobias. Mary Cover Jones, for example, had attended one of Watson's lectures and was inspired to develop interventions to treat phobias (Jones, 1924), which in turn lead to the formal development of systematic desensitization to treat phobias (Wolpe, 1961). Systematic desensitization in its various forms can be understood within the framework of behavior analysis—involving high-order classical conditioning, extinction, learning by observation, and negative reinforcement—and is still considered one of the most effective behavioral therapies today for the treatment of phobias.

Baer et al. (1968) formalized the "dimensions" of ABA as (1) applied (i.e., relevant for issues concerning an individual or society), (2) behavioral (i.e., can be measured scientifically), (3) analytic (i.e., an analysis breaks down a compound product—like functional relationships or behaviors—into its critical components), (4) technological (i.e., the procedure/intervention has to be described and defined in such a way that it is replicable), (5) conceptually systematic (i.e., based on principles that are founded on a body of knowledge, reaffirming ABA as a cumulative science), (6) effective (i.e., bring about real, beneficial, and empirical changes), and (7) general (i.e., the effected change holds up over time and place).

A current characterization of ABA was offered by Madden et al. (2021), framed as a behavior analyst's two main goals: The first goal is to accurately predict behavior (i.e., having identified a functional variable; the "on/off" switch). The second goal is to positively influence behavior (e.g., by changing the antecedents or consequences to a behavior). The public may understand the formulation of these two goals more easily than the formulation by Baer et al. (1968), and as such this formulation may be more powerful when ABA is to be presented and explained to the public. But this characterization is also open to interpretation that can lead to misunderstandings and controversies. Specifically, "positively influence behavior" may come across as "manipulation/bribery," and it begs the question for whom it is "positive." Critics of ABA have argued that ABA is used to "normalize" persons, and that it is contrary to the goals of the neurodiversity movement. After all, the "positive influence" may only refer to what society deems convenient and conforming, thus deny an individual's wishes and autonomy.

For a history of applied behavior analysis regarding autism specifically, see Munno et al. (2022). Here, very briefly, only a few studies that precede the publication of the first issue of the *Journal of Applied Behavior Analysis* in 1968 will be presented, just to give a flavor of the early ABA studies that were still very much in the tradition of EAB but also embraced the goals of the budding branch of ABA.

For example, Mowrer and Mowrer (1938), like Watson and Rayner (1920), employed a classical conditioning paradigm to study and treat nocturnal enuresis referring to age-inappropriate nightly bed-wetting. In contrast to common psychodynamic interpretations at the time, which interpreted enuresis as a neurotic behavior triggered by childhood trauma, Mowrer and Mowrer (1938) approached enuresis from the perspective of behavior analysis after exclusion of a medical diagnosis. The sensation of the full bladder preceded the sounding of an alarm (triggered by the urine closing an electric circuit) that would wake up the child. After several pairings of these two stimuli (first, sensation of the full bladder, then sound of the alarm), the sensation of the full bladder alone would wake up the child before urination and before the alarm occurred. This intervention became known as the "wet-pad method," and the device to implement this intervention became widely popular and commercially available. This intervention represented the spirit of ABA in that its goal was to improve the child's quality of life (no teasing by peers, prevention of social ostracization) and of the parents (uninterrupted sleep, no soiled bedsheets, less irritation and other negative emotional behavior that might undermine the parent-child relationship) by applying the principles of behavior analysis to a socially relevant problem.

In another example, using operant conditioning techniques, Ayllon and Michael (1959) trained psychiatric nurses to deliver reinforcers such as cigarettes or candy (obviously not acceptable nowadays) to patients who displayed desirable behaviors and to ignore (extinguish) undesirable ones according to a specific schedule of reinforcement. The goal to make life on the ward safer and more productive for both, nurses and patients, was again in the spirit of ABA.

Ayllon and Azrin (1965) provide an early implementation of a token economy (also operant conditioning), which means that tokens (conditioned reinforcers) could be earned and then exchanged later for socially acceptable, healthy backup reinforcers. Again, psychiatric patients participated with a goal of improving their quality of life. Patients could choose to perform different types of jobs (e.g., helping with laundry, cleaning, serving meals, clerical work such as typing or answering phones) and earn tokens for performing the tasks. A specified number of tokens could be exchanged for backup reinforcers such as choice of bedroom, eating group, personal locker, personal chair, or room divider. These type of jobs and backup reinforcers may seem puny or even demeaning in today's world. However, this early study needs to be evaluated in context of a typical day on a psychiatric ward in the 1960s where patients would aimlessly spend their time without anything to do and with no freedom of making meaningful choices. At that time, most psychiatric patients (including children with autism who were sometimes labeled "psychotic" or "schizophrenic") were solely treated with psychopharmacological medication, with little or no access to psychotherapy, educational or vocational options, or meaningful leisure activities (cf. Geraldo Rivera's video exposé, *Willowbrook: The Last Great Disgrace*). Thus, the study by Ayllon and Azrin (1965) should also be seen in the true spirit of ABA with a goal of improving a person's quality of life by offering freedom of making choices and being accountable for making them. Alternative treatments based on psychodynamic theory, for example, offered no hope (e.g., Bettelheim, 1967; Cohmer, 2013) and put the blame solely on faulty parenting.

Ferster (1961) also used operant conditioning techniques (reinforcement and extinction) to overcome behavioral deficits that are common in autistic children such as deficits in language (either mute or echolalic) and social behavior (e.g., solitary activities instead of social, interactive play), and behavioral excesses such as self-stimulatory behaviors, self-injurious behaviors, and tantrums. What made his study unique was that he not only addressed the children's behaviors but also anticipated that parents can become effective caregivers for their own children. He wrote "we must look for conditions influencing the parents' behavior, which will alter the parental performances, in turn providing reinforcement of the child's performances" (p. 444). Since then, parent training, especially in the autism community, has grown, and continues to grow, into one of the most important developments in contemporary ABA (for review see Schreibman & Koegel, 2005).[5] The importance of parent training lies in the fact that (1) parents can provide support to their own children on a continuous basis, not limited to intermittent, professional therapy sessions, (2) effective parenting can be taught by using ABA, (3) families have direct control over ABA interventions with regard to their own family members, and (4) parent-provided ABA is relatively cost-effective, thus accessible even for families with limited income. In this sense, parent training based on behavior analysis has contributed to some degree to the democratization of public health.

Risley and Wolf (1967) conducted a study that demonstrated the effectiveness of establishing functional speech in echolalic children. Echolalia refers to vocal behavior with prosody and vocabulary partially intact but with its repetitive speech not being functional in the sense of not allowing speakers to communicate with others in a reciprocal manner; therefore, echolalia represents severe limits in social behavior. This study is an excellent example of ABA in that Risley and Wolf (1967) used several of the well-established techniques of behavior analysis: differential reinforcement, extinction, shaping, stimulus fading, and time-out procedures. This study is also noteworthy as it shows ABA's success in overcoming a deficit in a complex, uniquely human, and socially relevant behavior, such as language, in autistic children.

Lovaas (1987) serves as a last example to show the effectiveness of ABA. In this study, two groups were approximately matched by diagnosis (autism), age, and IQ. One group received 40 hours of ABA per week; the other group received 10 hours or less per week. One of the most striking results was that 47% of the children in the 40-hour group achieved "normal intellectual and educational functioning" whereas only 2% of the other group achieved this level. Because of its striking

[5] Numerous versions of parent training, many with an explicit ABA framework, are available nowadays. (A review is beyond the scope of this chapter; cf. Dawson-Squibb et al., 2020). The common feature is that with relatively few training sessions, the parents or other caregivers (including all family members) can acquire the basics of the program, including ABA principles, and then implement them in the daily caregiving of their children with developmental disabilities. This point will be discussed again in context of the Natural Learning Paradigm.

success, ever since its publication, there have been criticisms of this study, either because of some suspected methodological flaws, because of overstated results, or because ABA was generally rejected as a legitimate approach. Lovaas and Wright (2006) provided a response to these criticisms. They state: "... with over 500 scientific articles on autism and ABA between 1985 and 2006, why do authors continue to pick apart single articles without placing them in the context of the whole?" It remains unchallenged that ABA offers a very effective approach to support children with autism and their families.

2.3 Two Approaches to Implement ABA

2.3.1 Discrete-Trial Training (DTT)

The Lovaas (1987) study is also significant as it provides a good representation of the discrete-trial training (DTT) paradigm, which was almost exclusively employed in that study. To about the mid 1980s, DTT had been the predominant ABA approach. The following example from early film footage illustrates DTT: One boy was taught to say his name. The therapist gives a prompt (the start of a trial): "What is your name?" The child answers (the target behavior): "Buh" [Billy]. The therapist reinforces the response by praise and other reinforcers. This concludes one trial that would then be repeated many times, perhaps with increasingly stringent criteria for reinforcement. (This method is called "shaping by successive approximations" in which first the response "Buh" may get reinforced but on successive trials only "Buh-ee" results in reinforcement because it represents a better approximation of "Billy.") One trial is based on one instance of the "three-term contingency" (Skinner, 1938; cf. Moxley, 1996, for an in-depth analysis of this concept). The three-term contingency is captured by the relationship between a so-called discriminative stimulus (S^D), which sets the occasion for the response (R) to occur, and when it occurs, to be reinforced (S^R). In less formal ways, the three-term contingency has been referred to as the "ABC pattern" (Antecedent, Behavior, Consequence). For a comprehensive review of DTT see Lerman et al. (2016). The characteristics of the DTT approach are: It is highly structured; each trial has a clear beginning and end; trials are repeated many times successively; trials are relatively immutable; trials are typically presented in a specific learning environment (e.g., learner and ABA provider sit across from each other at a desk); stimulus materials are preplanned and vary little; a reinforcer is anything that is motivating to the child (e.g., edibles, praise, opportunity to play a computer game, tokens that can be exchanged for backup reinforcers after the training session). It is easy to see why this approach may be ideal for some learners (e.g., learners that initially need to acquire very basic skills, like eye contact, imitation, sitting in a chair while paying attention, suppressing self-stimulatory behavior while learning academic skills). It is also easy to see why this approach may *not* be ideal for other learners (e.g., parents and children experience DTT as exhausting, as mechanistic, as aversive and repetitive "drill" sessions that result in lack of motivation for both, parent and child; reinforcers are seen as contrived, unnatural, and/or unhealthy; the rigid structure of trials does not foster generalization). The negative experience of DTT is still one common critique of ABA. Furthermore, commonly but incorrectly, DTT is seen as the only "technique" that contemporary ABA supposedly employs. It should be noted here that for more than the past three decades, alternatives to DTT have been developed, and it is not correct anymore to equate ABA with DTT, even though DTT is still commonly used for many learners to supplement other approaches (see Steege et al., 2007). For example, Lerman et al. (2016) point out that since Lovaas (1987), DDT is often integrated in other approaches such as "natural environment teaching" (p. 47). These authors also emphasize that DTT in its rigidity may characterize Lovaas's "UCLA Programming Model" but not contemporary ABA approaches. To address these drawbacks of DTT, natural learning paradigms (NLP) have been developed and employed.

2.3.2 Natural-Learning Paradigm (NLP)

Fahmie et al. (2023) reviewed and discussed the various usages of the term "ecological validity." These authors defined ecological validity as the degree to "how closely an experiment aligns with real-world phenomena" (p. 302). Frequently, also the term "natural environment" has been used in the literature. In this writing, the term "natural" and "naturalistic" will be used interchangeably with the term of ecological validity.

Koegel et al. (1987) appear to offer one of the first formal and published implementation of natural learning in context of ABA and language. As their primary goal was to teach functional language, their approach was called "natural language (teaching) paradigm." They employed a multiple-baseline design across participants in which two autistic children were first exposed to traditional DTT sessions (baseline sessions). Then, in accordance with the multiple-baseline design, the natural language teaching paradigm was introduced for one child after 2 months and for the other after 19 months. This version of NLP differed critically from DTT in the following ways: (1) Instead of the practitioner selecting the stimulus items to be used in the session, the child could choose with which materials to engage. (2) Instead of presenting the same stimulus successively and repetitively, to hold the child's interest, the children were presented with an array of stimuli that the children could choose from. (3) Instead of presenting invariable, repetitive prompts (e.g., "Say 'giraffe'"), the practitioner and child were engaged in a play-like situation in which the practitioner would model a response (e.g., "Giraffe! Look, a giraffe!"). (4) If the child made no attempt at vocalizing, the practitioner would model a verbal response again. (5) Any of the child's attempts to vocalize, were reinforced (i.e., reinforcement was not based on the child producing a criterion response, as would be typically required in DTT). (6) Finally, in addition to praise, a reinforcer consisted of access and opportunity to play with the toy chosen for the current interaction. Compared to baseline measures, Koegel et al. (1987) reported under the NLP condition increased rates in each child's imitative utterances, spontaneous speech, and utterances outside the clinical setting. Note that correct utterances were scored using the same criteria as under the baseline (DTT).

This approach can still be conceptualized as one that uses effective three-term contingencies (e.g., S^D = "Giraffe! Look, a giraffe!"; R = Any attempt to vocalize; S^R = Being allowed to pick up the toy giraffe and play with it) but with a less rigid structure, and most importantly, giving the child some control over the situation to maintain motivation, and a meaningful, "natural" context in which the learning occurs. Also, this approach integrates generalization strategies that were formally outlined by Stokes and Baer (1977). Koegel et al. (1987) reported successful generalization as evident in increased rates of "outside the clinical setting" utterances. Lack of generalization has been known to be a drawback of strict DTT unless specific measures were taken to promote generalization of treatment effects (Stokes & Baer, 1977).

Laski et al. (1988) followed Koegel et al.'s (1987) prescriptions for implementing NLP and extended their study by including four nonspeaking children and four echolalic children diagnosed with autism, again employing a multiple-baseline design. Most importantly, the children's parents received training to implement NLP themselves, thus the utility of parent training in ABA could be studied. In fact, this study could be presented as a promising, new parent-training program. Laski et al. (1988) found clear increases in child *and* parent vocalizations/verbalizations when assessed in three generalization settings: a large-play room in the clinic but not associated with therapy or training, a free-play setting at the child's home, and in the break room in the clinic. Furthermore, the findings showed that parents generalized their skills even to the siblings of the autistic children. Finally, a decrease in echolalic speech was also observed in the free-play setting.

It is easy to see how the NLP approach can be embedded in a family's daily life especially if the parents are trained in this approach. For example, when the family sits around the dinner table, natural conversations can continue as always but special attention is given to the child with autism. Instead of just serving the food on the child's plate, a parent or sibling can ask: "Would you like some chicken [S^D]?" The child might respond with "Ch-ch [R]." The sibling then responds by saying "Great! You want more chicken. Here it is!" and serves the chicken [S^R] on the child's plate.

Koegel et al. (1996) discussed the benefits of a "naturalistic paradigm" in context of parent training and teaching so-called pivotal responses. Parent training is invaluable as it allows the parents continued opportunity to teach their child in their own home (natural) environment for many more hours than would be affordable if professionals were to be hired to provide the entire ABA intervention. Pivotal responses are responses that, when mastered, allow access to an array of other skills to be acquired. Language, for example, is a pivotal response because mastery of functional language represents an array of possibilities regarding social and communication skills. NLP, however, is not restricted to language learning. For example, teaching a child self-help skills like being able to use money appropriately is considered a pivotal response. Once the child learned how to manage money, the child can then start to learn how to use public transportation, go to stores, visit a friend, go to the ice cream parlor, or buy groceries. Using public transportation safely is another pivotal skill itself that offers opportunities to build a social network (e.g., go on a date; go to the mall to hang out with friends; commute to a specific school or workplace; go to the bank). Teaching how to use public transportation can, in fact should, be taught in a naturalistic context. The natural reinforcer at the end of using public transportation might be a visit to the ice cream parlor. In the spirit of NLP, when training a given skill, any attempt should be reinforced (e.g., the reinforcer being real money that then allows the child to pay for the ice cream). Furthermore, in the spirit of NLP, the child should be able to choose between different possibilities (e.g., ice cream parlor, meet with a friend, go to school like a "big kid" without parents around) with reinforcers that are meaningful in this context (e.g., get ice cream, have a great play date, pride to be independent).

Schreibman et al. (2015) summarize the idea of NLP, not limited to language, and refer to this approach as "naturalistic developmental behavioral interventions." Their approach is entirely consistent with the NLP principles as originally outlined for language by Koegel et al. (1987): implementation occurs in a natural setting, involves shared control between child and practitioner in context of learning new skills, uses natural contingencies (e.g., "If you count out the money correctly, then you can buy your own ice cream"), and avoids the repetitiveness of DTT that often diminishes motivation in both the child and parent who may perceive DTT sessions as an aversive chore. Similarly, many studies have embraced the NLP approach in one variation or other (e.g., Weiss, 2001; LeBlanc et al., 2006; Peterson, 2007; de Matos et al., 2020).

2.4 Criticisms of ABA

Previously, a few points of criticism were already addressed in context (for criticism by the public, see again Devita-Raeburn, 2016; Winter, 2024; Rozsa, 2025): Methodological behaviorism, which is common in ABA, sometimes takes an agnostic stance with respect to some human qualities that are not directly observable (e.g., private thoughts and feelings such as anxiety or low self-esteem, identity, and mental processes in general are not acknowledged). Also, one goal of ABA, that is, to "positively influence" behavior, can be construed as an unjust manipulation and as an attempt to normalize people with autism to fit the expectation of the dominant culture for convenience's sake. In other cases, the unimaginative use of only edibles as reinforcers (in early studies even cigarettes) is certainly a concern. Furthermore, as also mentioned above, DTT is seen as a tool to mechanistically train people to perform behaviors that conflict with their identity.[6] Contemporary ABA, performed by board-certified and licensed behavior analysts, however, attempts to address these legitimate points by use of natural learning paradigms, by acknowledging mental and emotional processes (e.g., Cognitive Behavior Therapy and Dialectical Behavior Therapy are derived from ABA), and by highly individualizing any intervention while being vigilant of the precept "*not* one glove fits all." In fact, during the functional analysis, which should precede the development of any ABA program anyway, behavioral strengths as well as behavioral weaknesses are considered in order to carefully customize any intervention for a given individual. The overall goal is to provide an individual with as many skills as possible to live a life worth living, in the context of society at large.

A major controversy is ABA's use of "punishment." In the general public's view, "punishment" is categorically rejected as an unacceptable form of coercion that should never be a part of any intervention, therapy, or education because "punishment" conjures images of corporal punishment and other severe physical abuse. In ABA, "punishment" refers to very specific procedures that can take two forms: *Positive punishment* refers to the contingent *presentation* of an aversive (undesirable) stimulus and *negative punishment* ("penalty") refers to the contingent *removal* of an appetitive (desirable) stimulus following a behavior. Both forms result in a reduction or elimination of a specific target behavior compared to the "before-punishment" frequency (baseline) of the behavior. By this definition, contingent electric shock is in fact *positive* punishment but so is a sharp "No!" or adding an extra math problem to homework, if it can be shown that these consequences result in a future reduction of the target behavior. Another form of positive punishment is called "overcorrection" which incorporates the concept of reasonable restitution (i.e., a natural consequence instead of an arbitrary punishment, thus consistent with the natural learning paradigm). For example, a child that threw food on the wall may be required to not only wipe and clean the wall but also must clean his and his classmates' lunch tables. The time-out procedure is an example of *negative* punishment. For example, a child might be removed for a short time-period from a reinforcing situation (e.g., an enjoyable, fun classroom) whenever the undesirable target behavior (e.g., hitting a classmate) occurred.[7] In other words, the target behavior results in

[6] Sometimes ABA, as an approach, has been compared to "conversion therapy" (Rozsa, 2025 #2400). The use of electric shock has been equated with torture.

[7] For time-out "to work," it is imperative that the learning situation from which the child is removed is truly enjoyable (i.e., reinforcing) to the child. The implication of this is that it is the teacher's or therapist's responsibility to make the learning situation as enjoyable as possible (one aspect of NLP). If the child experiences the learning situation as aversive to begin with, then removing the child from it results in strengthening instead of decreasing the undesirable target behavior due to negative reinforcement (i.e., the child's behavior results in escape from an aversive situation and is thus strengthened).

the removal of reinforcement. Another version of negative punishment is referred to as "response cost" (e.g., Jenna loses a previously earned gold star for pulling out her hair or scratching herself bloody). These methods (excluding electric shock or corporal punishment) are uses of punishment that are generally accepted in our society: Drivers may have to pay a fine for speeding, an athlete may have to sit in the penalty box for a foul, not filing taxes may result in a having to pay a fine, and a vandal gets sentenced to provide community service to clean up a community. Note, however, that behavior analysts have advocated for decades that society should refrain from coercion and aversive control,[8] if it can be avoided at all, because of the ethical implications and also because of questions of its effectiveness (e.g., Sidman, 1989).

The experiment by Watson (1930/1970) introduced in Sect. 2.2 is probably one of the earliest reasons for criticism of behaviorism and, by association, of ABA. Indisputably, the Little Albert experiment is by today's standards unacceptable and unethical. Watson's and behavior analysis's reputation was further marred by persistent rumors that Little Albert was traumatized and psychologically damaged for the rest of his life. This is not true as it has been documented that Albert and his mother moved for a better job opportunity, thus couldn't complete the participation in the experiment that would have removed the fear (Beck et al., 2009). By this account, Little Albert continued to be a typical child but most likely died at an early age of meningitis that was not linked to Watson's experiment. Furthermore, it seems unlikely that exposure to a rat and loud noises would lead to lifelong trauma. Many one-year-old children experience popping balloons, slamming doors, fireworks, or loud noises from falling objects, yet they are not traumatized for the rest of their lives even though they may never like balloons again, which is not so uncommon among young children.

The most damaging criticism of ABA might stem from his book *Behaviorism* (Watson, 1930/1970), which is persistently misrepresented. For one, the philosophy of behaviorism supposedly excludes enormously important human attributes such as emotions. Watson's radical behaviorism does not. Note that Watson wrote: "Apparently it never occurred to [William] James, or to any of his followers for that matter, to speculate, much less experiment, upon the genesis of the emotional forms of response. […] By this […] James robbed psychology of perhaps its most beautiful and most interesting field of research" (p. 142). In fact, Watson's *Behaviorism* dedicates *two* entire chapters to emotions. Secondly, Watson's polemic quote "Give me a dozen healthy infants […] my own specified world [and] I'll guarantee to take any one at random and train him to become any type of specialist […] doctor, lawyer, artist, merchant-chief and, yes, even beggar-man and thief […]" (p. 104–105) is frequently presented without context as if it unequivocally meant that biology and

[8] Aversive control refers to procedures that involve the use of positive or negative punishment but also includes negative reinforcement (see Footnote 7), which is the removal of an aversive stimulus contingent upon the occurrence of a target behavior. For example, a parent's nagging until the child agrees to complete their homework is a form of aversive control because the aversive nagging only stops once the child agrees to do their homework.

heredity do not play any role in the development or behaviors of a person. Note that Watson (1913/1996) wrote: "The psychology which I should attempt to build up would take as a *starting point* [italics added], first, the observable fact that organisms, man and animal alike, do adjust themselves to their *environment by means of hereditary* [italics added] and habit equipments" (p. 250). Even in his later writing, as a direct follow-up to his (in)famous "Give me a dozen healthy infants ..." quote, Watson acknowledges heredity as an important factor albeit deplorably in context of supposed racial superiorities and inferiorities (Watson, 1930/1970, pp. 104–105).

The controversy further escalated with Lovaas et al. (1965) and other studies using aversive stimuli in ABA interventions. In this study, which is frequently cited to condemn ABA for its abuses, electric shock was used to teach social behavior such as approaching adults to avoid shock (negative reinforcement) and to suppress (positive punishment) undesirable behaviors such self-stimulatory behavior, self-injurious behavior, and tantrums. This treatment was deemed effective because it could be shown that social behavior increased and undesirable behaviors decreased but, clearly, this study does not represent contemporary ABA. Skinner (1953) pointed out as early as 1953 that punishment procedures need to be evaluated with caution because of the negative side-effects of them (also see Bettelheim, 1967). For a comprehensive review of ABA's use of electric shock up to 1976, see Lichstein and Schreibman (1976). These authors acknowledge that up to 1976 not much systematic, reputable research had been done to fully evaluate the positive and negative side-effects of the use of electric shock. They summarize their review by stating that electric shock was effective in decreasing behaviors such as dangerous self-injury, disabling, uncontrollable, and stigmatizing self-stimulation, and aggression towards others. However, they also concluded that there were clear negative side-effects (e.g., negative emotions such as fear and a possible increase of other maladaptive behaviors), even though not serious and long-term if electric shock was appropriately used.

2.5 Ethics, Neurodiversity, and a Person's Right to Effective Treatment, Identity, Autonomy, and Dignity

Skinner (1976) explicitly outlined that it was ABA's responsibility to help people. Already in 1972, B. F. Skinner was named the Humanist of the Year by the *American Humanist Association* for advocating for people who often lacked protection from abuse or did not possess the skills necessary for effective counter-control (e.g., the elderly, children, prisoners, people with disabilities). These facts need to be emphasized as Skinner himself had been the target of criticism because of common misunderstandings and misconceptions particularly for his notion of determinism and his rejection of bona fide "free will" (cf. Grünbaum, 1952, 1972, for a defense of determinism). Skinner wrote the aforementioned *Walden Two* (Skinner, 1948) as a portrayal of a fictional egalitarian and just society that attempted to maximize positive reinforcement and minimize aversive control. This novel consists in large parts of dialogues between Frazier, the founder of the community "Walden Two" that is based on Skinner's behavior analysis, and Frazier's foil, Professor Castle, a philosophy professor who challenges Frazier throughout the novel, giving the author Skinner a platform of addressing popular criticism and promoting behavior analysis. Considering Skinner's advocacy, it seems fair to argue that ABA has been a long-term advocate of social justice. In addition, *The Association for Behavior Analysis International* (ABAI) presents yearly an Award for Distinguished Contributions to Diversity, Equity, and Inclusion (DEI) at ABAI's annual convention to a person who has emphasized "effective models of action in DEI." But it is also fair to acknowledge that at times ABA in practice and in research has fallen short of these aspirations, and that it continues to be ABA's responsibility to correct any shortcomings and to strives to improve its practice with particular emphasis on compassion and humbleness, and to pursue justice, dignity, and equity for the persons that choose ABA.

Allen et al. (2024) published a remarkably comprehensive, nuanced, and honest review of the historical and contemporary practice of ABA (and what it should be). Their message was a call for "neurodiversity-affirming" ABA. To do justice to all the critical points that were addressed in their paper is beyond this chapter. Therefore, in this last section, only a limited selection of points will be presented: Briefly, ABA is not only for autism nor is it a cure. Some behavior analysts are not properly trained as graduate schools often do not address the issues surrounding neurodiversity and its movement. Ableism and implicit bias are still prevalent in the practice of ABA. Furthermore, because much of ABA is now regulated through health insurance, ABA is seen in the framework of a medical model (e.g., autism as a pathology) and not following a social model. According to Allen et al. (2024), the social model of disability "focuses on the need for society or the *environment* to adapt and accommodate rather than the individual needing to change."

This last point warrants some elaboration because the social model must be seen as pursuing a balance of pros and cons between an individual's and society's liberties, cultural norms, and safety. Allen et al. (2024) consider elimination of innocuous self-stimulatory behavior through ABA as unnecessary and possibly discriminatory, and as not honoring an individual's dignity, identity, and autonomy. On the other hand, one must consider that even innocuous self-stimulatory behavior can have serious consequences for the individual who engages in self-stimulatory behavior. For example, absorption in self-stimulatory behavior may exclude the individual from learning critical skills such as participating in communal activities; or when an individual publicly engaging in self-stimulatory behavior is seen as odd, even threatening, the consequences can range from social shunning (e.g., not being offered a job, not getting a date, or not being invited to social gatherings) to drawing attention of the police with subsequent, possibly fatal, altercations. Thus, a stance of feeling at liberty to present one's true, not masked, identity without regard of the context—perhaps not having learned to regard the context—may not be safe and healthy. Good ABA would focus on helping the individual by teaching them to exhibit or suppress a given behavior depending on the context. This notion applies to anyone, and people with disability are not singled out. In some sense, holding autistic people to different standards than allistic people may in fact reflect a discriminatory attitude that is to be avoided. Thus, consistent with the social model, ABA attempts to help any individual, who seeks help, by teaching as many skills as possible from which the individual can freely choose whether, when, and how to use them in any given situation. This attitude is opposite to the notion of "normalizing" an autistic person. Instead, it is the attitude of explicitly respecting the autonomy and dignity of the person to live in a social context where they can choose how to present themselves rather than being limited without choice because of lack of skills. Through a functional analysis, the individual's strengths and weaknesses are assessed as well as the learning style of the individual (recognizing the diversity among learners), and then a highly individualized intervention is designed to provide those skills that would maximize the person's quality of life within the societal context.

Honoring diversity is also a focus point within the disability community itself, thus also within the autism community. The prefix "dis" originally meant to indicate "not" or "opposite." Thus, the term "disability" implies somehow a quantification of more or fewer skills. Furthermore, the assumption is made that autism has at least in part a brain organic origin and is not a free choice of identity or way of life. It follows that persons with this diagnosis should be afforded with proper accommodations. In this spirit, the social model, as mentioned above, advocates a society that is open to change for people with disabilities. For example, it is not controversial to having accessibility laws to accommodate persons using a wheelchair. However, a person who uses a wheelchair may request physical therapy to possibly improve mobility. Analogously, whether one sees autism as a disability or not, ABA can offer interventions or skills training that lift an individual with special needs up without taking away dignity or identity, broadening a person's repertoire, rather than abandoning a person in a situation where they behave in a certain way because they cannot help it.

The use of acceptable language is an important topic in our society with regards to using language to include all groups with a given identity, including individuals having an identity as an autistic person. Allen et al. (2024) point out that even within the autism community, there is diversity with regards to use of appropriate language. If one subscribes to the person-first language, one refers to an individual as "a person with autism." With identity-first language, the same person is referred to as "an autistic person" (possibly with capital "A"). Clearly, there is no "correct" language, Instead, one should be tolerant to different perspectives if it is with the intent of respecting the identity and dignity of a person. Another controversy with regards to language is the use of the labels "low-" vs. "high-functioning" autism. Allen et al. (2024) point out the absurdity of these labels by asking why these labels should be used for autistic but not for allistic individuals acknowledging that everybody has strengths and weaknesses. ABA's approach can avoid such labels as each person is seen as an individual of whom a portfolio or profile of strengths and weaknesses can be assessed, and there is no notion that there is such a thing as a "typical" or "average" autistic person. The same view is also reflected in ABA's commonly used research designs. Instead of group or between-subject designs, which are based on a comparison of arithmetic means, ABA research generally prefers "small-n" designs (with within-subject comparisons) that respect individuals by making them their own reference point for changes in behavior.

In the significant second portion of their paper, Allen et al. (2024) formalize "Calls to Action." Here's a summary: ABA must honor disability, identity, and intersectionality (i.e., many people with autism are also diverse in their gender identity and sexuality); ABA must honor an open-minded discussion about the terminology and language that is being used; ABA must honor dignity, choice, and self-determination; ABA needs to be compassionate and humble; ABA needs to improve on the concepts of informed consent and assent (which are commonly used by Institutional Review Boards for formal research but not in the general practice of providing ABA services); ABA needs to incorporate participatory approaches (as opposed to seeing autistic people as passive research "subjects"); the selected target behaviors for a possible intervention have to agree with the learner's or the legal guardian's concerns; and ABA should incorporate social validation to a larger degree. They conclude that to be neurodiversity-affirming, ABA needs to be culturally humble and compassionate, encourage participatory approaches, and continue an introspective path with origins in the 1990s. It seems that few would disagree with these points. They are certainly consistent with contemporary ABA.

The "Right to Effective Treatment" is the last point to be addressed in this chapter. As early as 1988, van Houten et al. (1988) proposed that recipients of ABA have a right to a "therapeutic environment"; ABA should focus on personal welfare; the service provider has to be competent and properly trained; goals should be those that represent functional skills; the effectiveness of interventions should be empirically documented; and the most effective treatment should be available if chosen freely and without coercion. These guidelines are similar to those in the medical field. For example, a patient with cancer has the right to choose an aggressive chemotherapy or a risky surgery, even if major negative side-effects are anticipated, if and only if the patient chooses the treatment after having received extensive debriefing and being able to balance the chances of a positive outcome with possibly severe side-effects. Generally, the public does not reject the entire field of medicine based on the drawbacks of medical procedures that are commonly used. This should be no different with regards to ABA. It is possible that a given ABA procedure does not only promise desirable outcomes but that there is a chance of undesirable side-effects. The client (learner, consumer, patient) should be able to choose a given procedure after being fully informed of the possible pros and cons. If the client is an adult, the free choice, without coercion, is documented in an informed consent. If the client is not of legal age, informed assent must be secured. In most cases using ABA, the known negative side-effects are minimal, given that the intervention is provided by a competent and caring professional. However, there are cases that create very difficult conflicts that perhaps cannot ever be resolved, and that ultimately must be resolved with an entirely personal judgment call. For example, the *Judge Rotenberg Educational Center* has come under fire for their use of electric shock until a legal battle that started in 2020 banned it. It is not the intention here to resolve the issue, neither legally nor ethically, but this last discussion is intended to shed light on two opposing views: On one hand, the use of electric shock can be categorically rejected as torture with no good to come out of it. On the other hand, some parents have argued that everything was tried to protect their child from dangerous, sometimes severely damaging or even fatal self-harm. The argument in support of using drastic methods like electric shock is that this may be the only method left that has been unexplored, that all other methods have failed. So, given the choice for a life in physical restraints under continuous sedation versus the use of shock which may represent one last option for "effective treatment," parents may demand the right to choose. However, this is only acceptable under very special conditions: No other known treatment is available; federal, state, and local agencies (in particular ethics review boards) need to be consulted; the procedure needs to be implemented by trained professionals; the treatment cannot be considered a "maintenance treatment" (i.e., go on for an unlimited time period); success has to be empirically demonstrated, and if no improvement is seen, then the procedure has to be stopped immediately; and finally, negative side-effects need to be monitored, and if they occur, immediately treated.

2.6 Conclusion

This chapter was an attempt to present contemporary ABA as an ethical and effective treatment choice that offers support and improved quality of life to persons who, without coercion, wish to receive it. Contemporary ABA focuses on natural learning paradigms within the framework of scientific behavior analysis. Finally, as Allen et al. (2024) phrased it succinctly, ABA should be neurodiversity affirming.

References

Allen, L. L., Mellon, L. S., Syed, N., Johnson, J. F., & Bernal, A. J. (2024). Neurodiversity-affirming applied behavior Anaysis. *Behavior Analysis in Practice*. https://doi.org/10.1007/s40617-024-00918-0

Ayllon, T., & Azrin, N. H. (1965). The measurement and reinforcement of behavior of psychotics. *Journal of the Experimental Analysis of Behavior, 8*, 357–383.

Ayllon, T., & Michael, J. (1959). The psychiatric nurse as a behavioral engineer. *Journal of the Experimental Analysis of Behavior, 2*, 323–341.

Baer, D. M., Wolf, M. M., & Risley, T. R. (1968). Some current dimensions of applied behavior analysis. *Journal of the Applied Behavior Analysis, 1*, 91–97.

Baron, A., Kaufman, A., & Stauber, K. A. (1969). Effects of instructions and reinforcement-feedback on human operant behavior maintained by fixed-interval reinforcement. *Journal of the Experimental Analysis of Behavior, 12*, 701–712.

Baron, A., Perone, M., & Galizio, M. (1991). The experimental analysis of human behavior: Indispensable, ancillary, or irrelevant? *The Behavior Analyst, 14*, 145–155.

Beck, H. P., Levinson, S., & Irons, G. (2009). Finding Little Albert. *American Psychologist, 64*, 605–614.
Bettelheim, B. (1967). *The empty fortress*. Free Press.
Case, D. A., Ploog, B. O., & Fantino, E. (1990). Observing behavior in a computer game. *Journal of the Experimental Analysis of Behavior, 54*, 185–199.
Cohmer, S. (2013). *Early infantile autism and the refrigerator mother theory (1943-1970)* [Report]. In: Embryo Project Encyclopedia. Arizona State University, School of Life Sciences, Center for Biology and Society.
Davison, G. C. (2019). A return to functional analysis, the search for mechanisms of change, and the nomothetic-idiographic issue in psychosocial interventions. *Clinical Psychological Science, 7*, 51–53.
Dawson-Squibb, J., Davids, E. L., Harrison, A. J., Molony, M. A., & de Vries, P. J. (2020). Parent education and training for autism spectrum disorders: Scoping the evidence. *Autism, 24*, 7–25.
de Matos, D. C., Araújo, P. M. S., Silva, F. D. M. A. M., Firmo, W. D. C. A., & de Matos, P. G. S. (2020). Effects of access to a naturally reinforcing activity on the acquisition of repertoires in autistic learner. *Research on Humanities and Social Sciences, 10*, 46–52.
Devita-Raeburn, E. (August 11, 2016). Is the most common therapy for autism cruel? *The Atlantic*.
Essig, L., Rotta, K., & Poling, A. (2023). Interobserver agreement and procedural asymmetry. *Journal of Applied Behavior Analysis, 56*, 78–85.
Fahmie, T. A., Rodriguez, N. M., Luczynski, K. C., Rahaman, J. A., Charles, B. M., & Zangrillo, A. N. (2023). Toward an explicit technology of ecological validity. *Journal of the Applied Behavior Analysis, 56*, 302–322.
Fantino, E., & Savastano, H. I. (1996). Humans' responses to novel stimulus compounds and the effects of training. *Psychonomic Bulletin & Review, 3*, 204–207.
Ferster, C. B. (1961). Positive reinforcement and behavioral deficits of autistic children. *Child Development, 32*, 437–456.
Fuller, P. R. (1949). Operant conditioning of a vegetative human organism. *American Journal of Psychology, 62*, 587–590.
Galizio, M. (1979). Contingency-shaped and rule-governed behavior: Instructional control of human loss avoidance. *Journal of the Experimental Analysis of Behavior, 31*, 53–70.
Garcia, J., & Koelling, R. A. (1966). Relation of cue to consequence in avoidance learning. *Psychonomic Science, 4*, 123–124.
Grünbaum, A. (1952). Causality and the science of human behavior. *American Scientist, 40*, 665–676.
Grünbaum, A. (1972). Free will and laws of human behavior. In H. Feigl, W. Sellars, & K. Lehrer (Eds.), *New readings in philosophical analysis* (pp. 605–627). Appleton-Century-Crofts.
Isaacs, W., Thomas, J., & Goldiamond, I. (1960). Application of operant conditioning to reinstate verbal behavior in psychotics. *Journal of Speech and Hearing Research, 25*, 8–12.
Jones, M. C. (1924). A laboratory study of fear: The case of Peter. *Pedagogical Seminary, 31*, 308–315.
Koegel, R. L., Bimbela, A., & Schreibman, L. (1996). Collateral effects of parent training on family interactions. *Journal of Autism and Developmental Disorders, 26*, 347–359.
Koegel, R. L., O'Dell, M. C., & Koegel, L. K. (1987). A natural language teaching paradigm for non-verbal autistic children. *Journal of Autism and Developmental Disorders, 17*, 187–200.
Laski, K. E., Charlop, M. H., & Schreibman, L. (1988). Training parents to use the natural language paradigm to increase their autistic children's speech. *Journal of Applied Behavior Analysis, 21*, 391–400.
LeBlanc, L. A., Esch, J., Sidener, T. M., & Firth, A. M. (2006). Behavioral language interventions for children with autism: Comparing applied verbal behavior and naturalistic teaching approaches. *The Analysis of Verbal Behavior, 22*, 49–60.
Lerman, D. C., Valentino, A. L., & LeBlanc, L. A. (2016). Discrete trial training. In R. Lang, T. Hancock, & N. Singh (Eds.), *early intervention for young children with autism Spectrum disorder. Evidence-based practices in behavioral health* (pp. 47–83).

Lichstein, K. L., & Schreibman, L. (1976). Employing electric shock with autistic children. A review of the side effects. *Journal of Autism and Childhood Schizophrenia, 6*, 163–173.
Lindsley, O. R., & Skinner, B. F. (1954). A method for the experimental analysis of the behavior of psychotic patients [Abstract]. *American Psychologist, 9*, 419–420.
Lovaas, O. I. (1987). Behavioral treatment and normal educational and intellectual functioning in young autistic children. *Journal of Consulting and Clinical Psychology, 55*, 3–9.
Lovaas, O. I., Schaeffer, B., & Simmons, J. Q. (1965). Building social behavior in autistic children by use of electric shock. *Journal of Experimental Research in Personality, 1*, 99–109.
Lovaas, O. I., & Wright, S. (2006). A reply to recent public critiques…. *Journal of Early and Intensive Behavior Intervention, 3*, 234–236.
Madden, G. J., Reed, D. D., & DiGennaro Reed, F. D. (2021). *Introduction to behavior analysis*. John Wiley & Sons, Inc..
Matson, J. L., Kuhn, D. E., Dixon, D. R., Mayville, S. B., Laud, R. B., Cooper, C. L., Malone, C. J., Minshawi, N. F., Singh, A. N., Luke, M. A., Lott, J. D., & Matson, M. L. (2003). The development and factor structure of the functional assessment for multiple causality (FACT). *Research in Developmental Disabilities, 24*, 485–495.
Moore, J. (2001). On distinguishing methodological from radical behaviorism. *European Journal of Behavior Analysis, 2*, 221–244.
Mowrer, R. R., & Mowrer, W. M. (1938). Enuresis: a method for its study and treatment. *American Journal of Orthopsychiatry, 8*, 436–459.
Moxley, R. A. (1996). The import of Skinner's three-term contingency. *Behavior and Philosophy, 24*, 145–167.
Munno, R., Thomson, K., & Pear, J. (2022). A brief history of contributions of applied behaviour analysis to autism treatment. In J. L. Matson & P. Sturmey (Eds.), *Handbook of autism and pervasive developmental disorder: Assessment, diagnosis, and treatment* (pp. 761–778). Springer International Publishing.
Peterson, P. (2007). Promoting generalization and maintenance of skills learned via natural language teaching. *The Journal of Speech and Language Pathology – Applied Behavior Analysis, 2*, 97–138.
Popper, K. (2005). *The logic of scientific discovery* [Original in German, 1935; First English Edition, 1959]. Routledge/Taylor-Francis e-Library.
Razran, G. H. S. (1934). Conditioned withdrawal responses with shock as the conditioning stimulus in adult human subjects. *Psychological Bulletin, 31*, 111–143.
Ribeiro, G. W., & de Souza, D. G. (2024). Evidence of precurrent responses expanding equivalence classes in a delayed matching-to-sample task. *Journal of the Experimental Analysis of Behavior, 121*, 151–162.
Risley, T., & Wolf, M. (1967). Establishing functional speech in echolalic children. *Behavior Research and Therapy, 5*, 73–88.
Rozsa, M. (2025, February 5). *A controversial autism therapy is gaining prominence, but some say it hurts neurodiverse people*. Salon.
Schreibman, L., Dawson, G., Stahmer, A. C., Landa, R., Rogers, S. J., McGee, G. G., Kasari, C., Ingersoll, B., Kaiser, A. P., Bruinsma, Y., McNerney, E., Wetherby, A., & Halladay, A. (2015). Naturalistic developmental behavioral interventions: Empirically validated treatments for autism spectrum disorder. *Journal of Autism and Developmental Disorders, 45*, 2411–2428.
Schreibman, L., & Koegel, R. L. (2005). Training for parents of children with autism: Pivotal responses, generalization, and individualization of interventions. In E. D. Hibbs & P. S. Jensen (Eds.), *Psychosocial treatments for child and adolescent disorders: Empirically based strategies for clinical practice* (2nd ed., pp. 605–631). American Psychological Association.
Sidman, M. (1989). *Coercion and its fallout*. Authors Cooperative, Inc. Publishers.
Skinner, B. F. (1938). *The behavior of organisms*. Appleton-Century-Crofts.
Skinner, B. F. (1948). *Walden Two*. Hackett Publishing Company.
Skinner, B. F. (1953). *Science and human behavior*. Macmillan.

Skinner, B. F. (1954). The science of learning and the act of teaching. *The Harvard Educational Review, 24*, 86–97.
Skinner, B. F. (1957). *Verbal behavior*. Appleton-Century-Crofts, Inc.
Skinner, B. F. (1958). Teaching machines. *Science, 128*, 969–977.
Skinner, B. F. (1961). Why we need teaching machines. *Harvard Educational Review, 31*, 377–398.
Skinner, B. F. (1966). The phylogeny and ontogeny of behavior. Contingencies of reinforcement throw light on contingencies of survival in the evolution of behavior. *Science, 153*, 1205–1213.
Skinner, B. F. (1976). The ethics of helping people. *The Humanist, 36*, 7–11.
Steege, M. S., Mace, F. C., Perry, L., & Longenecker, H. (2007). Applied behavior anaysis: Beyond discrete trial teaching. *Psychology in the Schools, 44*, 91–99.
Stokes, T. F., & Baer, D. M. (1977). An implicit technology of generalization. *Journal of Applied Behavior Analysis, 10*, 349–367.
van Houten, R., Axelrod, S., Bailey, J. S., Favell, J. E., Foxx, R. M., Iwata, B. A., & Lovaas, O. I. (1988). The right to effective behavioral treatment. *Journal of Applied Behavior Analysis, 21*, 381–384.
Watson, J. B. (1970). *Behaviorism* [Reprint of Watson, 1930]. W. W. Norton & Company, Inc.
Watson, J. B. (1996). Psychology as the behaviorist views it [Reprint of Watson, 1913]. *Psychological Review, 101*, 248–253.
Watson, J. B., & Rayner, R. (1920). Conditioned emotional reactions. *Journal of Experimental Psychology, 3*, 1–14.
Weiss, M. J. (2001). Expanding ABA intervention in intensive programs for children with autism: The inclusion of natural environment training and fluency based instructions. *The Behavior Analyst Today, 2*, 182–186.
Winter, J. (2024, February 12). The argument over a long-standing autism intervention. *The New Yorker*.
Wolpe, J. (1961). The systematic desensitization treatment of neuroses. *The Journal of Nervous and Mental Disease, 132*, 189–203.
Zerbi, V., Pagani, M., Markicevic, M., Matteoli, M., Pozzi, D., Fagiolini, M., Bozzi, Y., Galbusera, A., Scatonni, M. L., Provenzano, G., Banerjee, A., Helmchen, F., Basson, M. A., Ellegood, J., Lerch, J. P., Rudin, M., Gozzi, A., & Wenderroth, N. (2021). Brain mapping across 16 autism mouse models reveals a spectrum of functional connectivity subtypes. *Molecular Psychiatry, 26*, 7610–7620.
Zilio, D. (2016). On the autonomy of psychology from neuroscience: A case study of Skinner's radical behaviorism and behavior analysis. *Review of General Psychology, 20*, 155–170.

Chapter 3
No-One Left behind: Adulthood, Autism, and Applied Behaviour Analysis

Nichola Booth, George Pickersgill, and Karola Dillenburger

Abstract Since autism was first recognised as a distinct diagnostic category, prevalence rates have increased considerably. This chapter is aimed specifically for professionals who work with adults with autism who have high support needs. The chapter outlines some of the key issues that may cause obstacle for these adults, such as social relationships and self-advocacy, education, training, and employment, as well as housing and living conditions. Given that most of the available research evidence endorses interventions that are based on the science of Applied Behaviour Analysis (ABA), this chapter describes some concrete examples of these practices for people who require support to achieve their full potential. The chapter closes with specific recommendations for policy and practice.

Keywords Adults · Autism · Applied behaviour analysis · Transition · Employment · Social skills

Autism Spectrum Disorder (ASD) originally was thought of as a relatively rare childhood disorder (Wing & Gould, 1979; Murphy et al., 2016). However, prevalence rates for children have risen to an estimated 2.8% in the USA (CDC, 2023) and 3.5–4.2% in the UK (Dillenburger et al., 2015; DoH, 2020). Statistics for adults with autism[1] are more difficult to find, but it has been suggested that at least 1.1% of all adults are on the autism spectrum (Brugha et al., 2012). While officially autism is a medical diagnosis based on the *Diagnostic Statistical Manual of Mental Disorders*, fifth edition (DSM-5; APA, 2013) or the *International Classification of Mental and Behavioural Disorders-11* (ICD; WHO, 2020), there are no known

[1] The terms that are used in relation to autism differ (Kenny et al., 2015). While some adult self-advocates prefer identity-first terms, such as "Autistics" or "autistic person", most professionals use person-first language, e.g. "a person with a diagnosis of autism".

N. Booth · G. Pickersgill · K. Dillenburger (✉)
Queen's University Belfast, Belfast, Northern Ireland, UK
e-mail: k.dillenburger@qub.ac.uk

S. Halder et al. (eds.), *Applied Behavior Analysis-Based Interventions for Autism Spectrum Disorder*, https://doi.org/10.1007/978-981-95-2889-9_3

biological or medical markers. In fact, the diagnosis is based entirely on behaviour observations and reports of behavioural experiences and/or observations with regards to issues related to the ability to initiate and to sustain reciprocal social interaction and social communication, and a number of restricted, repetitive, and inflexible patterns of behaviour, interests or activities.

For a diagnosis to be confirmed, these behaviours have to be identified as "sufficiently severe to cause impairment in personal, family, social, educational, occupational or other important areas of functioning and are usually a pervasive feature of the individual's functioning observable in all settings, although they may vary according to social, educational, or other context" (WHO, 2020). The DSM-5 (APA, 2013) categorises support needs on three levels (dimensions):

Level 1: Requiring support. Someone who is considered to be at Level 1 experiences challenges with social interactions and probably requires some support to make friends or engage with colleagues, transitioning to new environments, or maintaining conversations.

Level 2: Requiring substantial support. Someone who is considered to be at Level 2 has more significant support needs than someone at Level 1, and even with substantial support, is likely to have problems with communication and change of routines.

Level 3: Requiring very substantial support. Someone who is considered to be at Level 3 has severe difficulties in understanding and using verbal and non-verbal communication and may avoid or limit interaction with others altogether. They may also experience high levels of distress when faced with changes to routine or exposure to crowds or loud noises and there may be evidence of repetitive behaviours that interfere with functioning.

Usually, support needs are greatest if a person has one or more co-occurring conditions (Simonoff et al., 2008). The most common co-occurring conditions are intellectual disabilities (approx. 86%; DoH, 2020), epilepsy (20%; Besag, 2018), sleep problems (approx. 80%; Papadopoulos 2017), gastrointestinal (GI) problems (approx. 70%; Chaidez et al., 2014), challenging behaviour (approx. 64%; Hutchins & Prelock, 2014), or mental health concerns, such as depression, anxiety, or obsessional compulsive disorder (approx. 79%; Lever & Geurts, 2016). The high co-occurrence of these conditions means that most people with autism are involved with a considerable number of professionals and interventions (NICE, 2012, 2014).

Early intensive Applied Behaviour Analysis (ABA)-based interventions (Dillenburger, 2015; Luce et al., 1996) play a major role with regards to developmental trajectories (Orinstein et al., 2014). Effective ABA-based interventions have been developed also for adults with autism who require support. Commonly, these interventions focus on general social and life skills training, such as personal and home hygiene, cooking, paying bills, health and safety skills, and health awareness (Partington & Mueller, 2012); building successful social relationships and self-advocacy; transitioning from school to employment and learning to live independently (Rosenwasser & Axelrod, 2001); and essential skills, like reading and comprehension (Nicolosi & Dillenburger, 2024).

3.1 Autism and Adulthood

Growing up involves changes in social relationships, independence and self-advocacy, adult partnerships and intimacy, education, training and employment, and housing and living conditions. Of course, these changes affect everybody, but for young people on the autism spectrum transitioning to adulthood can be particularly challenging. Many skills, even those that were well-established in childhood, require adjustments to facilitate new social contexts and new skills related to self-sufficiency and independence have to be learned. Therefore, successful transitions into adulthood may require structured planning, bespoke interventions (Shattuck et al., 2012), and the development of substantial networks of social support (Ditchman et al., 2018).

Social Relationships Eventually, most young adults leave the relative safety of the family environment to engage with peers in the community. While at first, this may be voluntary, later it becomes unavoidable when aging parent caregivers become unable to provide necessary supports (Dillenburger & McKerr, 2014).

Due to pervasive communication issues (see DSM-5), young persons with autism tend to experience challenges with making and maintaining reciprocal peer relationships. Even if a person had been taught good communication skills as a child, these strategies may not be effective for the adult. A lack of functional communication skills can lead to frustration and non-adaptive or challenging behaviours, including self-injurious behaviour (Howlin et al., 2014). Therefore, effective future planning should include functional communication skills training where this is needed (Luiselli et al., 2008).

Additional complications might arise especially for those who engage in unusual, restricted, repetitive, and inflexible patterns of behaviour (APA, 2013). Peers may consider these behaviours strange or excessive and misinterpret the behaviour of the young person with autism, which increases the complexities of navigating around changing social relationships and situations (Dillenburger & McKerr, 2009). Consequently, those who have significant support needs, usually require bespoke interventions to enable them with the necessary skills to engage in constructive and beneficial social relationships.

Independence and Self-Advocacy Self-advocacy is an important skill to learn for a young person on the autism spectrum. It includes "the ability to assertively state wants, needs and rights, determine and pursue needed supports and conduct your own affairs" (Izzo & Lamb, 2002, p. 6). Clearly, good advocacy skills should be taught early. They are linked to independence, better adult relationships, and increased success in education and employment (Kinney & Eakman, 2017), while a lack of these skills leads to poorer outcomes generally (Fleischer, 2012). Self-advocacy skills include knowledge of rights (Stein & Dillenburger, 2017; UNCRC, 2001; UNCRPD, 2006), responsibilities, and leadership (Test et al., 2005).

Challenging the traditional medical view of autism, the neurodiversity movement provides a powerful example of the use of self-advocacy skills (Dillenburger & Keenan, 2023). The term "neurodiversity" was coined by the Australian autism self-advocate and sociologist Judy Singer (1998). She rejected the notion of autism as a disorder and thought instead that autism should be celebrated as an inseparable aspect of a person's identity. She viewed autism as a neurological difference rather than a disability and advocated that it should be recognised as a definite category, alongside gender, class, and ethnicity.

> The neurodiversity claim contains at least two different aspects. The first aspect is that autism, among other neurological conditions, is first and foremost a natural variation. The other aspect is about conferring rights and in particular value to the neurodiversity condition, demanding recognition and acceptance (Jaarsma & Welin, 2012, p. 20).

Although the neurodiversity movement has led to significant advance in public awareness of autism, it is not without its critics. For example, adults with autism and parents whose children are affected severely worry that the strong lobbying influence that the movement has had on government policies could lead to a situation where services are withheld from those who need them urgently (Russell, 2020). Jaarsma & Welin (2012) recognised that the neurodiversity movement does not represent everyone on the autism spectrum and argued that "[o]nly a narrow conception of neurodiversity, referring exclusively to high-functioning autists, is reasonable" (p. 20). The American autism self-advocate Jonathan Mitchell (2019) agreed when he wrote, "[i]t concerns me greatly that the neuro-diversity movement now wields such influence. I worry that it will prevent the scientific research that might help me and others more severely afflicted" (p. 1). His concern reflects the fact that all too often, autism research presents a picture askew in favour of participants with few support needs (OAR, 2015) and that this has led to a situation where there is some debate about whether or not interventions are necessary at all (Mitchell, 2019). This controversy has gained momentum, so much so, that Stedman et al. (2019) worried that "[i]nadequate representation of the full autism spectrum in the literature could lead to an unbalanced picture of ASD and leave behind those with arguably the greatest need" (p. 1378).

Adult Partnerships and Intimacy By and large, adults with autism are as interested in having intimate peer relationships as anyone else (Stein & Dillenburger, 2017) and empowered with behavioural skills and competences, they can navigate the adult world, including establishing adult relationships and becoming parents (Bush, 2020). However, more often than not they remain single as a prospective partner may perceive romantic advances as blunt, inappropriate, too intense, or ill-timed (Warrier et al., 2020).

Appropriate sexuality and relationship education can help (Stein et al., 2017), but of course, as in teaching generally, it is important that sexuality education is tailored to the needs of the student, that it considers cognitive and adaptive functioning, is communicated sensitively, and is delivered in collaboration with the autistic person, their support staff, educators, and parents or caregivers. Topics taught should include anatomy and body awareness, reproduction and birth control, sexual health, hygiene across the lifespan, male/female sexual behaviour, dating, marriage, parenting, relationships, boundaries, and abuse (Schaafsma et al., 2017; Travers & Whitby, 2014).

There is very little research about adults on the spectrum becoming parents or the experiences of their children (Bush, 2020). More is known about parents of children on the spectrum (Dillenburger et al., 2012; Munteanu & Dillenburger, 2009). At times these parents seek a diagnosis for themselves after their children are diagnosed, especially when their child's behaviour reminds them of difficulties they may have experienced during their own childhood. Prior to their autism diagnosis, many of these parents had been diagnosed with other clinical conditions, such as anxiety, depressions, obsessive-compulsive disorder, or personality disorders (Lai & Baron-Cohen, 2015). In fact, Pohl et al. (2020) found that the life experiences of nearly a quarter of parents of children on the autism spectrum fit the criteria of a "broader autism phenotype" (p. 2). Therefore, there may be many parents with undiagnosed autism who are parenting children with or without autism. Clearly, more research is needed to better understand the true nature of being a parent with autism or having an autistic parent.

Education, Training, and Employment Gainful employment is an aspiration of almost everyone with a diagnosis of autism and with sufficient training and reasonable structural adjustments this could be achieved for most (Van Bourgondien & Woods, 1992). Job skills training and employment planning are key behaviours to be targeted as is staff autism training for potential bosses and colleagues (Dillenburger et al., 2019). A number of firms are recognising the potential of autistic employees and seek them for specific jobs (Felicetti, 2021).

Yet, it is estimated that only about 15–20% of adults on the autism spectrum are in gainful employment (Lallukka et al., 2020; Hedley et al., 2017; Rosenblatt, 2008). Up to 45% of these adults never experience full-time work (Eaves & Ho, 2008), despite the fact that most of them have had some kind of post-secondary training (Dillenburger et al., 2016; Shattuck et al., 2012). Undoubtedly, behavioural challenges can cause barriers to training and employment. They can cause stress (Berkman & Meyer, 1988) and this can have many negative outcomes, including isolation, disciplinary action, and termination of employment.

The "Supported Employment Model" (EUSE, 2009) is used widely across Europe to guide the process of finding and maintaining employment for people with disabilities more broadly. The Supported Employment Model includes five stages:

Stage 1: Assessment and relationship building and creating the client's vocational profile.

Stage 2: Open labour market research, job finding, and job position analysis.

Stage 3: Client–employer matching, which means direct contact with the employer, induction, and where necessary, work environment adaptation.

Stage 4: Workplace introduction and on-site training.

Stage 5: Ongoing support, formally and, where necessary, off-site support (EUSE, 2009).

The Supported Employment Model was developed in the late 1970s by researchers who were determined to demonstrate that adults with disabilities who require sustained support can achieve competitive employment (Keel et al., 1997; Marshall et al., 2014). Through the model it is recognised that when someone is placed in a work setting, support may need to be provided for certain activities, including supervision, training, and transport. It is the role of the job coach to support and facilitate preparation for work and secure employment for adults with autism and other conditions (Dillenburger et al., 2019).

Housing and Living Conditions Just like everyone else, adults with autism require appropriate residential arrangements that meet their needs, preferences, and choices. While some adults on the autism spectrum live fully independent lives, with or without an adult partner and their own children (4%), about one third live semi-independently (30%), in group homes or sheltered housing. The vast majority (60+%), however, continue to live with their aging parents (Dillenburger & McKerr, 2009). When speaking to young adults with disabilities, Dillenburger and McKerr (2014) found that, "[l]iving at home was seen as a positive experience for most, and they expressed that they had acquired a sense of independence and confidence about their skills" (p. 5).

Ageing parents enjoy the company of their adult sons and daughter with disabilities, although they worry much about their future care and accommodation arrangements (Dillenburger & McKerr, 2009). Sooner or later, when parents are no longer able to care or are deceased, these young adults have to move to new accommodation and this transition can add to the trauma of bereavement (Dillenburger & Keenan, 2005). Therefore, it is vitally important that future planning starts as early as possible (Dillenburger & McKerr, 2011). Future planning does not only involve accommodation and legal arrangements at the time of transition, it starts much earlier; it starts with the supports and interventions necessary for learning functional, social, and life skills.

3.2 Evidence-Based Interventions for Adults with Autism

There is ample evidence that early intensive ABA-based interventions can help young children with autism achieve significant developmental goals (Eldevik et al., 2010, Hampton & Kaiser, 2016; Virués-Ortega, 2010). In fact, generally speaking, ABA-based programmes outperform other intervention methods in terms of positive long-term outcomes and therefore have been recommended widely (Myers & Johnson, 2007; Surgeon General, 1999; Warren et al., 2011; York State Department of Health, 2011). ABA-based interventions also can benefit adults with autism who require supports (Rausa et al., 2016). In fact, ABA-based interventions can be designed to enhance anyone's socially important skills repertoire (Baer et al., 1968, 1987), thereby improving choice, independence, and confidence (Chiesa, 2006; Dillenburger & Keenan, 2009).

Before describing specific procedures and to prevent misunderstandings, it is important to point out some basic facts about ABA (Gower et al., 2021; Keenan & Dillenburger, 2018, 2020a). ABA is the applied branch of the science of behaviour analysis and therefore ABA-based interventions are not limited to a specific diagnostic labels (Baer et al., 1968, 1987; Cooper et al., 2020). ABA is not a therapy for autism (Chiesa, 2006); ABA does not aim to cure autism; ABA does not aim to change the personality of the person with autism (Keenan & Dillenburger, 2020b, 2023). The aim of ABA is to ensure that a person is empowered with new skills and, ultimately, achieves their full potential, whatever that may be. Consequently, the behaviours that are targeted with ABA-based procedures differ significantly from person to person.

3.3 Target Behaviour[2]

ABA-based interventions are tailored to the behavioural goals that are socially significant and important for each learner (Baer et al., 1968). It is not up to behaviour analysts or other professionals to decide what skills a person may or may not want or need to learn. The target behaviour for any intervention should be identified in close collaboration with the autistic learner and, where necessary, their caregivers (Stein et al., 2017). Given that in this chapter the focus is on adults with significant support needs, the behavioural goals should be identified together by finding out, for example, what the autistic adult would like to be able to do socially and behaviourally (Gerhardt, 2020).

To help determine the aims of the intervention a number of useful assessments tools are available, such as "The Assessment of Functional Living Skills" (AFLS) (Partington & Mueller, 2012). The AFLS is a criterion-referenced skills assessment tool that is used to identify skills gaps in terms of independent living skills, which, if addressed, would enhance independence and quality of life for learners. AFLS lists target behaviours in a range of different skill domains and proposes specific teaching strategies and interventions to help the learner master these skills.

Initially, the targets for most interventions are likely to be basic tool skills, that is, skills that need to be in one's behavioural toolkit before more complex skills can be acquired. For example, in order to learn to hand-write one's own name, one needs to be able to hold a pen and draw single letters. Many other behaviours, such as communication, social skills, and self-regulation are essential basic skills for long-term goals, such as successful adult relationships, employment, and independence.

[2] "Target behaviour" is the term used in ABA for the behaviour that is the focus of the intervention.

Ultimately, before choosing a new skill to learn, it is important that the aims, procedures, and outcomes are appropriate, significant, and generally socially valid. In other words, target behaviours should be focused on skills that empower the learner and aid their independence and social inclusion (Wolf, 1978).

Most people with a diagnosis of autism who have high support needs respond well to behavioural skills training, errorless learning, and differential reinforcement procedures that are linked to activity reinforcers, such as extra time on a games console, going for a coffee, or playing a game of chess (Gerhardt & Lainer, 2010).

Whilst we are describing some of these methods here, this should not be read as a "how to do it" guide. It is simply meant as a brief, initial introduction to the thinking behind the design of interventions so as to encourage special education professionals and other staff to learn more about the scope of ABA-based interventions (Keenan & Dillenburger, 2020a, 2023).

3.4 Behavioural Skills Training (BST)

Behavioural skills training (BST) is a multicomponent training package that is used to teach social and life skills (Miltenberger, 2012). In a BST programme, competence is achieved when a predetermined criterion is reached; for example, when the learner is able to use the new skill with 90% accuracy across three consecutive days or tasks. BST ensures that the learner practises the skill until they can use it successfully when and where they need it. In technical terms, behaviour analysts say that fluency has been achieved when the learner can engage in the new skill accurately and at the required speed (Binder, 1987; Kubina & Yurick, 2021).

A BST programme consists of instruction, modelling, behavioural rehearsal, and feedback. After jointly identifying the target skill and discussing the rationale for learning this skill with the learner and their caregivers, a detailed description of the new skill is necessary to share information on when and where (and when not) to use the skill (Engelmann & Carnine, 1991). This instruction phase may be conducted by vocal tuition, via pictures, or written scripts, whichever is the most effective way to communicate with the learner.

For the next phase, the teacher models exactly how to perform the skill. Modelling can be achieved in-vivo where the learner observes the teacher directly or via video modelling (Nikopoulos & Keenan, 2006). Video modelling is used widely, for example, on social media channels to teach people how to cook a new recipe, how to carry out car maintenance, or how to enhance gaming or dancing skills. In the context of BST, video models are more likely to be tailor-made for a specific learner and a specific skill using actors or peers by either showing the whole skill (i.e. total task presentation) or by breaking the skill down into smaller steps (i.e. shaping and chaining; Lindsay et al., 2013). Importantly, suitable models must be available who can role-play or model the behaviour (Nuernberger et al., 2013). It is best if the model is as similar to the learner as possible, in terms of age, gender, ability, and ethnicity. It is also possible to edit a video of the learner themselves engaged in the target behaviour as best they can early in the learning process. By cutting out footage where they may hesitate or make a mistake, this creates a video clip of themselves engaged in the target behaviour fluently. This video then can be used as a bespoke teaching aide (Lindsay et al., 2013).

The behaviour rehearsal phase ensures that the new skill is rehearsed to ensure that the learner practises it until they are able to perform it fluently (with accuracy and at the required speed; Binder, 1987; Kubina & Yurick, 2021; McGrath et al., 2018). Where possible, practice and rehearsal should be carried out in-situ, that is, in the environment in which the skill is needed. Finally, corrective feedback and positive reinforcers are provided frequently during the whole process of BST.

BST has been used successfully with all kinds of learners acquiring all sorts of skills. Learners who have few pre-requisite skills can learn to follow simple instructions, imitation skills, and basic communication skills. For these learners, the skill usually is taught via shaping or chaining, in which behaviours are taught in small steps. BST is particularly useful when someone needs to learn new functional and adaptive social and life skills (Miltenberger et al., 2017). Key skills that are important to achieve good quality of life (Ayers et al., 2011) include communication, choice-making, safety, self-care, leisure and recreation, and vocational skills. Key skills needed to live as independently as possible include road safety skills (PEAT, 2020) and other travel skills (Ruddy et al., 2015), eating out in a restaurant and using community schedules, like reading timetables for public transport (Taylor et al., 2004), and job interview skills (Roberts et al., 2020). BST also has been used to teach behaviour safety skills, such as how to respond in the presence of dangerous stimuli (Rossi et al., 2017), firearms safety (Jostad et al., 2008), stranger abduction prevention (Summers et al., 2011), community safety skills, such as seeking assistance when lost (Rizzi & Dibari, 2019), and water safety (Martin & Dillenburger, 2019).

In sum, BST is a well-established ABA-based intervention programme that enables learners to acquire new skills, irrespective of their age or level of ability. However, there are many other programmes and procedures that utilise behaviour analytic principles to teach new skill, specially to learners with more support needs. Errorless learning is such a teaching procedure that can be used to develop a range of important basic skills in a way that reduces frustration and increases confidence in the learner.

3.5 Errorless Learning

Errorless learning is an effective way to teach new skills, from basic life skills to skills needed to secure and maintain employment and navigate the social and physical environment (Kern et al., 2003; Lloyd et al., 2009). The idea behind errorless learning is that if errors occur during the learning process, they are more likely to occur also in real-life situations, when the skill is needed (Sidman, 1989). For this reason, in errorless learning errors are prevented in the first place by ensuring that the learner always responds correctly. Technically, errorless learning procedures function as "one or more motivating operations, maintaining the frequency of responses on the part of learners which have resulted in access to currently available reinforcers and reducing the frequency of responses which have resulted in access to escape or avoidance as reinforcers" (McGreevy, 2016, p. 1).

Errorless learning is highly effective with a range of different learners, including those with acquired brain injury, memory impairment, developmental disabilities, and psychoses (Haslam et al., 2012). It is particularly useful for learning basic life skills, including personal hygiene, shopping and cooking, home-making, such as cleaning and tiding the home, and employment and leisure skills. It is also used to enhance leisure and other functional skills that open access to enjoyable activities and peer interaction. Reducing the likelihood of errors during the learning process reduces frustration-induced challenging behaviour, such as aggression, avoidance, or self-injury, and increases enjoyment and confidence for the learner.

The errorless learning process starts with the identification and very clear definition of the new skill to be learnt to ensure that two or more observers would agree whether or not the skill has occurred, thereby assuring good interobserver agreement (IOA) (Babel et al., 2008). The teacher or therapist then presents the antecedent stimulus, such as the instruction or cue for the skill and immediately, with a zero-time delay, provides a prompt that results in accurate responding. The prompt can be physical as in hand-over-hand prompting, vocal, pictorial, or gestural (Reinecke et al., 2016). Prompts must be appropriate to the skill as well as to the individual preference; an individual who is hyper-sensitive to touch may respond to vocal prompts better than to tactile prompts.

As in all ABA-based interventions, the exact procedure must be based on the preferences of the learner. Therefore, the prompts used are based on an individually tailored prompt hierarchy and, initially, the least intrusive prompt is used with more precise prompts applied only if necessary. Ultimately, the most appropriate prompt is the one that ensures that the errorless target response occurs. Importantly, to avoid prompt dependency (Lang et al., 2014), prompts need to be faded throughout the learning process. The intervention is completed when the learner has acquired the new skill without errors and without any prompts (Love et al., 2009).

Given that there are no opportunities for making mistakes, reinforcers can be made available frequently. Early on in the programme, reinforcers need to be delivered instantly when the learner engages in the target response. Later on, access increases to natural reinforcers that are available only to anyone who engages in the target skill fluently.

Errorless learning can be used in combination with other ABA-based procedures to teach the target skills. Jerome, Frantino, and Sturmey used errorless learning and backward chaining to teach Internet skills to adults with autism and Cannella-Malone et al. (2016) utilised video modelling to teach physical activities to adolescents with significant disabilities. As always, it is important to identify effective bespoke reinforcers, because if the activity is not enjoyable or interesting for the learner, by definition, it is not a leisure activity and unlikely to occur spontaneously for pleasure outside of the teaching session.

While errorless learning is very useful in situations where difficult new skills are the target, when changes in existing behaviour patterns are required there are other ABA-based methods that can be effective, such as those based on differential reinforcement.

3.6 Differential Reinforcement

This section covers differential reinforcement procedures which are particularly effective to achieve changes of behaviour patterns and address challenging behaviour. Similar to previous sections of this chapter, the following descriptions are to be viewed as a brief introduction, not a full training manual.

Basically, differential reinforcement involves the differential provision of reinforcers for one behaviour (i.e. the socially important target behaviour) and not for another behaviour (i.e. the challenging or non-preferred behaviour; Cooper et al., 2020). There are four main types of differential reinforcement: differential reinforcement of incompatible behaviours (DRI), differential reinforcement of alternative behaviours (DRA), differential reinforcement of other behaviour (DRO), and differential reinforcement of low rates of behaviour (DRL).

Differential Reinforcement of Incompatible Behaviours DRI means that a behaviour is reinforced that is incompatible with the challenging behaviour. For example, if the challenging behaviour to be reduced is "biting", singing or speaking or simply keeping the mouth closed could be selected as the incompatible behaviour to be reinforced, because people cannot bite while they are singing, speaking, or keeping their mouth closed. This means that incompatible behaviour is reinforced and biting is not reinforced. If a DRI procedure is applied successfully, incompatible behaviour increases and biting decreases, although behaviour analysts would expect that early in the process there may be an extinction burst of biting (Pace et al., 1993).

Differential Reinforcement of Alternative Behaviours DRA means that reinforcers are provided for any alternative, socially important behaviour while reinforcers are not provided for the challenging behaviour. Alternative behaviours are not necessarily incompatible with the challenging behaviour which means that DRA is a little more flexible than DRI in the selection of the behaviour that is to be differentially reinforced. In both procedures (DRI and DRA), the substitute behaviour should be in the learner's repertoire already, require less response effort than the challenging behaviour, and allow access to natural reinforcers.

Differential Reinforcement of Other Behaviour In DRO, any other behaviour is reinforced, irrespective of its topography, under the condition that the challenging behaviour does not occur within a particular time period or at a specific time. For example, if DRO is used to reduce spitting behaviour, reinforcers become available after a specified time period under the condition that there was no spitting. Any other behaviour (i.e. other than spitting) that occurs during this time period is reinforced.

Differential Reinforcement of Low Rates of Behaviour DRL is used when the target behaviour is socially relevant but happens too often; DRL involves reducing the rate of this behaviour (Wright & Vollmer, 2002). For example, DRL could be used if someone asks the same question over and over again, for example the question, "What time is it?". The question itself is not the problem, however, if this question is asked 10 times during a 10-minute interval, the frequency may be considered too high and probably thought of as inappropriate. In this case, DRL can be used to reinforce a lower rate of the questioning behaviour, for example, it may be deemed appropriate to ask the question again after 30 min (obviously, the exact details of the time scale depend on the learner). Therefore, the time interval would be set at 30 min. If the target behaviour occurs (e.g. the question is asked), before the time is up, the clock is reset and the response is ignored (i.e. the question is not answered). However, if the target behaviour occurs after the time is up (i.e. after 30 min.) it is reinforced (i.e. an answer to the question is provided). The DRL procedure is not applicable for behaviour where the goal is complete elimination of a behaviour rather than a reduction in the occurrence of a behaviour. As such, it would not be appropriate to use DRL for self-injurious behaviour or aggression towards others.

In sum, differential reinforcement procedures can be used effectively in a number of settings to reduce undesired behaviours or behaviour that challenges. These procedures are essentially positive and dynamic behavioural supports that facilitate quality of life, self-sufficiency, and independence.

3.7 Generalisation and Maintenance

As with all interventions, behaviour changes achieved through ABA-based interventions for adults with autism are only as good as their generalisation and maintenance. Generalisation has occurred when a skill that was learned in one condition, with one particular teacher or therapist, or in one specific environment is fluent also under different conditions, with different people, or in new environments (Baer et al., 1968). While generalisation might occur naturally without additional training, this cannot be assumed. For example, if a person is taught to respond to the question "What is your name?" with "My name is Mark", they also need to be able to answer the question correctly when it is changed slightly, and they are asked "What are you called?", or when someone else asks the same question, or when they are asked the question in an unfamiliar situation. Generalisation has occurred only if they are able to answer this question correctly in all these settings, otherwise, more work is warranted.

A well-planned intervention programme includes procedures to ensure generalisation takes place, regardless of the skills targeted. This can be done by incorporating variability of the antecedent stimuli in the early stages of the programme, by training loosely through using a variety of words, tones, presenting stimuli at different angles, working in different settings, varying reinforcers, changing the time of the teaching session, changing the setting, or using a different behaviour analyst (Baer, 1981, 1999).

Once changes are generalised to different settings, people, and behaviour, it is important that they are maintained. Maintenance considerations need to be programmed into an intervention early by incorporating stimuli and features of the natural environment into the teaching setting. This means that initial teaching is carried out in a safe, controlled environment to allow for repeated practice until mastery is achieved and then transferring the new skills to the natural environment. This would be the case when teaching shopping skills, selecting goods, counting money, and paying for the groceries. These are practised in the clinic setting using real money and real goods and once the skills are learned, the skills would be transferred to a real-life setting by going to a real shop. In sum, generalisation and maintenance are important considerations when designing an ABA-based intervention programme for anyone, including someone with a diagnosis of autism.

Applied behaviour analytic interventions that are used to support adults with autism look very different from those that are used with children, although, of course, the basic behavioural principles remain the same (Nicolosi & Dillenburger, 2024). While formal preference assessments are recommended to identify effective reinforcers, the element of self-determination and choice is increasingly important for adults (Elliott & Dillenburger, 2014). For example, high pitch verbal praise may be used successfully for young children, but adults generally prefer a more natural and mature tone of voice. Physical contact reinforcers, such as high fives, should be used only if the adult has expressed a clear preference for these kinds of stimuli. Formalised token economies may be useful for some adults, however, they should be used sparingly and reviewed frequently and regularly. Contingency contracts can be very useful tools when working with adults, especially if the necessary skills are in their repertoire already but are not used at the necessary time or with the appropriate frequency (McCoy et al., 1977).

Ultimately, interventions for adults on the autism spectrum who have high support needs require flexibility and creativity from the staff or caregivers who support these adults. It is important to remember that like in any ABA-based programme, interventions must be individualised to the needs of the person, target an expansive range of behaviours that are of social importance, and remain based on the fundamental principles of behaviour analysis. Incorporating an element of self-management into teaching is a useful strategy, as the adult moves towards independence in relation to living arrangements, employment, and self-advocacy. This may involve the use of activity schedules or checklists, self-recording, video modelling, and self-reinforcement (Lattimore et al., 2008). This process avoids the traditional "train and hope" approach (Stokes & Baer, 1977), where the teacher just tells the student what to do and then simply hopes that the new skill will be learned (McCarton et al., 2009).

3.8 Conclusion

This chapter provided a brief glimpse into how a science of behaviour can be harnessed in such a way as to be of benefit in the life of adults with autism. In this context, it is important to remember that the diagnostic label of autism is based purely on the categorisation of specific behaviours that are assessed via observation and verbal reports (APA, 2013). ABA-based interventions have been used extensively and successfully for a very long time for teaching important life skills related to independence, social relationships, and employment (Chiesa, 2020). As with any intervention or support, professionals should adopt an ethically sound, culturally aware human rights-based approach to ensure that the needs of the individual learner are front and centre. Policymakers, practitioners, and caregivers should ensure that adults with autism have access to any evidence-based behaviour analytic services they may need, if and when needed (Keenan & Dillenburger, 2023), thereby ensuring that no-one is left behind.

Acknowledgements This chapter was previously published by the Czech Republic's Department of Education in the Czech language. Booth, N., Pickersgill, G, & Dillenburger, K. (2022). *Na nikoho nezapomenout: Dospělí, autismus a aplikovaná behaviorální analýza.* In A. Markova & A. Clibulková (ed.). Užití prvků aplikované behaviorální analýzy ve školním prostředí. Praha: Národní pedagogický institut České republiky, (*Applied Behaviour Analysis in education settings.* Czech Department of Education), ISBN: 978-80-7578-080-5. Permission was granted to publish the English original.

This chapter is based in part on the 2nd author's Masters thesis, supervised by the 1st author. We acknowledge helpful review comments by Prof. Mickey Keenan.

References

American Psychological Association (APA). (2013). *Diagnostic Statistical Manual of Mental Disorders (DSM-5).* https://doi.org/10.1176/appi.books.9780890425596.744053.

Ayers, K. M., Lowery, K. A., Douglas, K. H., & Sievers, C. (2011). I can identify Saturn but I can't brush my teeth: What happens when the curricular focus for students with severe disabilities shifts. *Education and Training in Autism and Developmental Disabilities, 46*(1), 11–21.

Babel, D. A., Martin, G. L., Fazzio, D., Arnal, L., & Thomson, K. (2008). Assessment of the reliability and validity of the discrete-trials teaching evaluation form. *Developmental Disabilities Bulletin, 36*(1–2), 67–80.

Baer, D. M. (1981). *How to plan for generalization.* Pro-Ed.

Baer, D. M. (1999). *How to plan for generalization.* Pro-Ed.

Baer, D. M., Wolf, M. M., & Risley, T. R. (1968). Some current dimensions of applied behavior analysis. *Journal of Applied Behavior Analysis, 1*(1), 91–97. Retrieved from http://www.pubmedcentral.nih.gov/articlerender.fcgi?artid=1310980&tool=pmcentrez&rendertype=abstract

Baer, M., Wolf, M. M., & Risley, T. R. (1987). Some still-current dimensions of applied behavior analysis. *Journal of Applied Behavior Analysis, 20*(4), 313–327. https://doi.org/10.1901/jaba.1987.20-313

Berkman, K. A., & Meyer, L. H. (1988). Alternative strategies and multiple outcomes in the remediation of severe self-injury: Going 'all out' nonaversively. *Journal of the Association for Persons with Severe Handicaps, 13*(2), 76–86. https://doi.org/10.1177/154079698801300204

Besag, F. M. C. (2018). Epilepsy in patients with autism: Links, risks and treatment challenges. *Neuropsychiatric Disease and Treatment, 14*, 1–10. https://doi.org/10.2147/NDT.S120509

Binder, C. (1987). *Fluency building*. Retrieved August 7, 2017, from http://binde1.verio.com/wb_fluency.org/Unpublished/Binder1987.pdf

Brugha, T., Cooper, S. A., McManus, S., Purdon, S., Smith, J., Scott, F., & Tyrer, F. (2012). *Estimating the prevalence of Autism Spectrum Conditions in adults: Extending the 2007 Adult Psychiatric Morbidity Survey*. Retrieved December 3, 2016, from http://content.digital.nhs.uk/catalogue/pub05061/esti-prev-auti-ext-07-psyc-morb-surv-rep.pdf

Bush, H. H. (2020). *AsperDad: Growing up with a parent on the autism spectrum (maybe)*. Retrieved November 13, 2020, from https://www.mghclaycenter.org/parenting-concerns/families/asperdad-growing-up-with-a-parent-on-the-autism-spectrum-maybe/

Cannella-Malone, H. I., Miller, O., Schaefer, J. M., Jimenez, E. D., Page, E. J., & Sabielny, L. M. (2016). Using video prompting to teach leisure skills to students with significant disabilities. *Exceptional Children, 82*, 463–478. https://doi.org/10.1177/0014402915598778

CDC. (2023). *Data & Statistics on Autism Spectrum Disorder*. Retrieved January 5, 2025 from https://www.cdc.gov/ncbddd/autism/data.html

Chaidez, V., Hansen, R. L., & Hertz-Picciotto, I. (2014). Gastrointestinal problems in children with autism, developmental delays or typical development. *Journal of Autism and Developmental Disorders, 44*(5), 1117–1127. https://doi.org/10.1007/s10803-013-1973-x

Chiesa, M. (2006). ABA is not 'a therapy for autism.'. In M. Keenan, K. Henderson, Dillenburger, & K. P. Kerr (Eds.), *Applied behaviour analysis and autism building a future together* (pp. 225–240). Jessica Kingsley Publishers.

Chiesa, M. (2020). *Behaviour analysis, autism and learning disability: Fact and fiction*. Retrieved November 20, 2020, from https://uk-sba.org/wp-content/uploads/2021/04/Behaviour-Analysis-Fact-or-Fiction.pdf

Cooper, J., Heron, T., & Heward, W. (2020). *Applied behaviour analysis* (3rd ed.). Pearson Prentice Hall.

Dillenburger, K. (2015). Evidence-based management and intervention for autism spectrum disorders. In M. Fitzgerald (Ed.), *Autism* (1st ed.). Intech. https://doi.org/10.5772/58983. Retrieved from https://www.intechopen.com/books/autism-spectrum-disorder-recent-advances/evidence-based-management-and-intervention-for-autism-spectrum-disorders

Dillenburger, K., Jordan, J.-A., & Mc Kerr, L. (2016). School's out forever: Postsecondary educational trajectories of students with autism. *Australian Psychologist, 4*, 304–315. https://doi.org/10.1111/ap.12228

Dillenburger, K., Jordan, J.-A., McKerr, L., & Keenan, M. (2015). The millennium child with autism: Early childhood trajectories for health, education and economic wellbeing. *Developmental Neurorehabilitation, 18*, 37–46. https://doi.org/10.3109/17518423.2014.964378

Dillenburger, K., & Keenan, M. (2005). Bereavement: a D.I.S.C. analysis. *Behaviour and Social Issues, 14*, 92–112.

Dillenburger, K., & Keenan, M. (2009). None of the as in ABA stand for autism: dispelling the myths. *Journal of Intellectual & Developmental Disability, 34*(2), 193–195. https://doi.org/10.1080/13668250902845244

Dillenburger, K. & Keenan, M. (2023). Autism and behavior analysis: From dissonance to dialogue. *International Electronic Journal of Elementary Education. Special Issue editors* J. Cihon, E. Kazemi, J. Leaf.*, 15*(3), 199–208.

Dillenburger, K., Keenan, M., Doherty, A., Byrne, T., & Gallagher, S. (2012). ABA-based programs for children diagnosed with autism Spectrum disorder: Parental and professional experiences at school and at home. *Child and Family Behavior Therapy, 34*(2). https://doi.org/10.1080/07317107.2012.684645

Dillenburger, K., Matuska, E., de Bruijn, M., & Röttgers, H.-R. (2019). *Job coaches for adults with disabilities: A practical guide*. Jessica Kingsley Publishers.
Dillenburger, K., & McKerr, L. (2009). "40 Years is an awful long time": Parents caring for adult sons and daughters with disabilities. *Behavior and Social Issues, 18*, 1–21. Retrieved from http://ojs-prod-lib.cc.uic.edu/ojs/index.php/bsi/article/view/2449
Dillenburger, K., & McKerr, L. (2011). "How long are we able to go on?" Issues faced by older family caregivers of adults with disabilities. *British Journal of Learning Disabilities, 39*(1), 29–38.
Dillenburger, K., & McKerr, L. (2014). Echoes of the future: Adults with disabilities living at home with their parents. *The Journal of Neuropsychiatry and Clinical Neurosciences, 1*(2), 1–10.
Ditchman, N. M., Miller, J. L., & Easton, A. B. (2018). Vocational rehabilitation service patterns: An application of social network analysis to examine employment outcomes of transition-age individuals with autism. *Rehabilitation Counseling Bulletin, 61*(3), 143–153. https://doi.org/10.1177/0034355217709455
DoH (formerly DHSSPS). (2020). Prevalence of Autism (including Asperger Syndrome) in School Age Children in Northern Ireland. Retrieved May 22, 2020, from https://www.health-ni.gov.uk/sites/default/files/publications/health/asd-children-ni-2020.pdf
Eaves, L. C., & Ho, H. H. (2008). Young adult outcome of autism spectrum disorders. *Journal of Autism and Developmental Disorders, 38*(4), 739–747. https://doi.org/10.1007/s10803-007-0441-x
Eldevik, S., Hastings, R. P., Hughes, J. C., Jahr, E., Eikeseth, S., & Cross, S. (2010). Using participant data to extend the evidence base for intensive behavioral intervention for children with autism. *American Journal on Intellectual and Developmental Disabilities, 115*(5), 381–405. https://doi.org/10.1352/1944-7558-115.5.381
Elliott, C., & Dillenburger, K. (2014). The effect of choice on motivation for young children on the autism spectrum during discrete trial teaching. *Journal of Research in Special Educational Needs, 16*(3), 187–198. https://doi.org/10.1111/1471-3802.12073
Engelmann, S., & Carnine, D. (1991). *Theory of instruction: Principles and applications*. National Institute for Direct Instruction NIFDI Press.
EUSE. (2009). *European Union of Supported Employment position paper: On and off job support*. Retrieved February 1, 2018, from http://www.euse.org/content/position_papers/On-and-Off-Job-Support.pdf
Felicetti, K. (2021). *These major tech companies are making autism hiring a priority*. Retrieved from https://www.monster.com/career-advice/article/autism-hiring-initiatives-tech
Fleischer, A. S. (2012). Support to students with Asperger syndrome in higher education - The perspectives of three relatives and three coordinators. *International Journal of Rehabilitation Research, 35*(1), 54–61. https://doi.org/10.1097/MRR.0b013e32834f4d3b
Gerhardt, P. (2020, November). *Individuals with ASD, sexuality and sexuality education and what you need to know*. UK-SBA conference.
Gerhardt, P. F., & Lainer, I. (2010). Addressing the needs of adolescents and adults with autism: A crisis on the horizon. *Journal of Contemporary Psychotherapy, 41*(1), 37–45. https://doi.org/10.1007/s10879-010-9160-2
Gower, C., Booth, N., & Dillenburger, K. (2021). Applied behaviour analysis: What it is and what it isn't. In A. Markova (Ed.), *Applied behaviour analysis*. National Pedagogical Institue of the Czech Republic.
Hampton, L. H., & Kaiser, A. P. (2016). Intervention effects on spoken-language outcomes for children with autism: A systematic review and meta-analysis. *Journal of Intellectual Disability Research: JIDR, 60*(5), 444–463. https://doi.org/10.1111/jir.12283
Haslam, C., Bazen-Peters, C., & Wright, I. (2012). Errorless learning improves memory performance in children with acquired brain injury: A controlled comparison of standard and self-generation techniques. *Neuropsychological Rehabilitation, 22*(5), 697–715. https://doi.org/10.1080/09602011.2012.686820
Hedley, D., Cai, R., Uljarevic, M., Wilmot, M., Spoor, J. R., Richdale, A., & Dissanayake, C. (2017). Transition to work: Perspectives from the autism spectrum. *Autism, 22*(5), 528–541. https://doi.org/10.1177/1362361316687697

Howlin, P., Savage, S., Moss, P., Tempier, A., & Rutter, M. (2014). Cognitive and language skills in adults with autism: A 40-year follow-up. *Journal of Child Psychology and Psychiatry, and Allied Disciplines, 55*(1), 49–58. https://doi.org/10.1111/jcpp.12115

Hutchins, T. L., & Prelock, P. A. (2014). Using communication to reduce challenging behaviors in individuals with autism Spectrum disorders and intellectual disability. *Child and Adolescent Psychiatric Clinics of North America, 23*(1), 41–55. https://doi.org/10.1016/j.chc.2013.07.003

International Statistical Classification of Diseases and Related Health Problems (11th ed,; ICD-11; World Health Organization, 2020).

Izzo, M., & Lamb, M. (2002). *Self-determination and career development: Skills for successful transitions to postsecondary education and employment.*

Jaarsma, P., & Welin, S. (2012). Autism as a natural human variation: Reflections on the claims of the neurodiversity movement. *Journal of Health Philosophy and Policy. Health Care Analysis (HCA), 20*(1), 20–30. https://doi.org/10.1007/s10728-011-0169-9

Jostad, C. M., Miltenberger, R. G., Kelso, P., & Knudson, P. (2008). Peer tutoring to prevent firearm play acquisition, generalization, and long-term maintenance of safety skills. *Journal of Applied Behavior Analysis, 41*(1), 117–123. https://doi.org/10.1901/jaba.2008.41-117

Keel, P. K., Fulkerson, J. A., & Leon, G. R. (1997). Disordered eating precursors in pre- and early adolescent girls and boys. *Journal of Youth and Adolescence, 26*(2), 203–216. https://doi.org/10.1023/a:1024504615742

Keenan, M., & Dillenburger, K. (2018). How "fake news" affect autism policies. *Societies*, 2018030238. https://doi.org/10.20944/preprints201803.0238.v1

Keenan, M., & Dillenburger, K. (2020a). *Behaviour analysis: A primer.* Retrieved January 30, 2021, from www.behaviouranalysis.eu.com

Keenan, M., & Dillenburger, K. (2020b). *Drama in the courtroom: Defending the rights of children diagnosed with autism.* Retrieved December 2, 2020, from https://www.barristermagazine.com/drama-in-the-courtroom-defending-the-rights-of-children-diagnosed-with-autism/

Keenan, M., & Dillenburger, K. (2023). Advocacy and open science in the UK: Case studies in the autism wars. *Behavior Analysis in Practice* https://link.springer.com/article/10.1007/s40617-023-00881-2

Kenny, L., Hattersley, C., Molins, B., Buckley, C., Povey, C., & Pellicano, E. (2015). Which terms should be used to describe autism? Perspectives from the UK autism community. *Autism*, 1–21. https://doi.org/10.1177/1362361315588200

Kern, R. S., Green, M. F., Mintz, J., & Liberman, R. P. (2003). Does 'errorless learning' compensate for neurocognitive impairments in the work rehabilitation of persons with schizophrenia? *Psychological Medicine, 33*(3), 433–442. https://doi.org/10.1017/s0033291702007298

Kinney, A. R., & Eakman, A. R. (2017). Measuring self-advocacy skills among student veterans with disabilities: Implications for success in postsecondary education. *Journal of Postsecondary Education and Disability, 30*(4), 343–358.

Kubina, R. M., & Yurick, K. K. L. (2021). *The precision teaching book.* Greatness Achieved Publishing.

Lai, M. C., & Baron-Cohen, S. (2015). Identifying the lost generation of adults with autism spectrum conditions. *The Lancet. Psychiatry, 2*(11), 1013–1027. https://doi.org/10.1016/S2215-0366(15)00277-1

Lallukka, T., Pietiläinen, O., Jäppinen, S., Laaksonen, M., Lahti, J., & Rahkonen, O. (2020). Factors associated with health survey response among young employees: A register-based study using online, mailed and telephone interview data collection methods. *BMC Public Health, 20*(1), 184. https://doi.org/10.1186/s12889-020-8241-8

Lang, R., Harbison Tostanoski, A., Travers, J., & Todd, J. (2014). The only study investigating the rapid prompting method has serious methodological flaws but data suggest the most likely outcome is prompt dependency. *Evidence-Based Communication Assessment and Intervention, 8*(1), 40–48. https://doi.org/10.1080/17489539.2014.955260

Lattimore, L. P., Parsons, M. B., & Reid, D. H. (2008). Simulation training of community job skills for adults with autism: A further analysis. *Behavior Analysis in Practice, 1*, 24–29. https://doi.org/10.1007/bf03391717

Lever, A. G., & Geurts, H. M. (2016). Psychiatric co-occurring symptoms and disorders in young, middle-aged, and older adults with autism spectrum disorder. *Journal of Autism and Developmental Disorders, 46*(6), 1916–1930.
Lindsay, C. J., Moore, D. W., Anderson, a., & Dillenburger, K. (2013). The role of imitation in video-based interventions for children with autism. *Developmental Neurorehabilitation, 16*, 283–289. https://doi.org/10.3109/17518423.2012.758185
Lloyd, J., Riley, G. A., & Powell, T. E. (2009). Errorless learning of novel routes through a virtual town in people with acquired brain injury. *Neuropsychological Rehabilitation, 19*(1), 98–109. https://doi.org/10.1080/09602010802117392
Love, J. R., Carr, J. E., Almason, S. M., & Petursdottir, A. I. (2009). Early and intensive behavioral intervention for autism: A survey of clinical practices. *Research in Autism Spectrum Disorders, 3*(2), 421–428. https://doi.org/10.1016/j.rasd.2008.08.008
Luce, S. C., Green, G., & Maurice, C. (1996). *Behavioral intervention for young children with autism*. Retrieved February 4, 2015, from http://www.amazon.co.uk/Behavioral-Intervention-Young-Children-Autism/dp/0890796831
Luiselli, J. K., St. Amand, C., MaGee, C., & Sperry, J. M. (2008). Group training of applied behavior analysis (ABA) knowledge competencies to community-based service providers for adults with developmental disabilities. *International Journal of Behavioral Consultation and Therapy, 4*(1), 41–47. https://doi.org/10.1037/h0100830
Marshall, S. L., Parker, P. D., Ciarrochi, J., & Heaven, P. C. L. (2014). Is self-esteem a cause or consequence of social support? A 4-year longitudinal study. *Child Development, 85*(3), 1275–1291. https://doi.org/10.1111/cdev.12176
Martin, C., & Dillenburger, K. (2019). Behavioural water safety and autism: A systematic review of interventions. *Review Journal of Autism and Developmental Disorders, 6*, 356–366. https://doi.org/10.1007/s40489-019-00166-x
McCarton, C., Weiss, M. J., Feldman, I., & Hickie, J. (2009). *Improving the generalization of skills in learners with autism*. Retrieved November 13, 2020, from https://autismspectrumnews.org/improving-thegeneralization-of-skills-in-learners-with-autism/
McCoy, J. F., Epstein, L. H., Parker, F. C., Brush, M. E., & Stephens, R. M. (1977). Effective components of contingency contracts with academic behaviors of college students. *Journal of Experimental Education, 46*(1), 26–33. https://doi.org/10.1080/00220973.1977.11011606
McGrath, C., McCourt, C., Corry, A., Dounavi, K., Dillenburger, K., & Gormley, G. (2018). The use of "Precision Teaching" in enhancing medical students' dermatological diagnostic skills. *MedEdPublish, 7*(2). https://doi.org/10.15694/mep.2018.0000091.1
McGreevy, P. (2016). *Errorless teaching*. https://s3.amazonaws.com/poacwebsite/wpcontent/uploads/2016/06/04185727/Errorless-Teaching.pdf
Miltenberger, R. G. (2012). *Behavior modification: Principles and procedures* (5th edn.).
Miltenberger, R. G., Zerger, H. M., Novotny, M., & Livingston, C. (2017). Behavioral skills training to promote social behavior of individuals with autism. In J. Leaf (Ed.), *Handbook of social skills and autism Spectrum disorder* (pp. 325–342). Springer International Publishing. https://doi.org/10.1007/978-3-319-62995-7_19
Mitchell, J. (2019). *The danger of 'neurodiversity.'* Retrieved November 13, 2020, from https://www.spectator.co.uk/article/the-danger-of-neurodiversity
Munteanu, C., & Dillenburger, K. (2009). Family functioning during the diagnosis process in families with children on the autism spectrum. *Terapia Sistemica / Systemic Therapy, 3*, 1–17. Retrieved from http://www.ceeol.com/aspx/issuedetails.aspx?issueid=10a16024-7678-4fad-bf4c-db02ff3f4ded&articleId=b2ddd12a-d33b-49dc-ad9d-59e57776951d
Murphy, C. M., Wilson, C. E., Robertson, D. M., Ecker, C., Daly, E. M., Hammond, N., Galanopoulos, A., Dud, I., Murphy, D. G., & McAlonan, G. M. (2016). Autism spectrum disorder in adults: Diagnosis, management, and health services development. *Neuropsychiatric Disease and Treatment, 12*, 1669–1686. https://doi.org/10.2147/NDT.S65455
Myers, S. M., & Johnson, C. P. (2007). Management of children with autism spectrum disorders. *Pediatrics, 120*(5), 1162–1182. https://doi.org/10.1542/peds.2007-2362

NICE. (2012). *Autism: recognition, referral, diagnosis and management of adults on the autism spectrum: Guidance and guidelines*. Retrieved January 14, 2015, from https://www.nice.org.uk/guidance/CG142/resources

NICE. (2014). *Challenging behaviour and learning disabilities: Prevention and interventions for people with learning disabilities whose behaviour challenges (Consultation document)*. Retrieved December 29, 2014, from https://www.nice.org.uk/guidance/gid-cgwave0654/documents/challenging-behaviour-and-learning-disabilities-draft-nice-guideline2

Nicolosi, M., & Dillenburger, K. (2024). The effect of phonics skills intervention on early reading comprehension in an adolescent with autism: A longitudinal study. *Behavioral Interventions, 39*(2). https://doi.org/10.1002/bin.2007

Nikopoulos, C., & Keenan, M. (2006). *Video modelling and behaviour analysis: A guide for teaching social skills to children with autism*. Jessica Kingsley Publishers.

Nuernberger, J. E., Ringdahl, J. E., Vargo, K. K., Crumpecker, A. C., & Gunnarsson, K. F. (2013). Using a behavioral skills training package to teach conversation skills to young adults with autism spectrum disorders. *Research in Autism Spectrum Disorders, 7*(2), 411–417. https://doi.org/10.1016/j.rasd.2012.09.004

OAR. (2015). *Lack of services and research to support adults with autism*. Retrieved November 18, 2020, from https://researchautism.org/lack-of-services-and-research-to-support-adults-with-autism/

Orinstein, A. J., Helt, M., Troyb, E., Tyson, K. E., Barton, M. L., Eigsti, I.-M., & Fein, D. A. (2014). Intervention for optimal outcome in children and adolescents with a history of autism. *Journal of Developmental and Behavioral Pediatrics, 35*(4), 247–256. https://doi.org/10.1097/DBP.0000000000000037

Pace, G. M., Iwata, B. A., Cowdery, G. E., Andree, P. J., & McIntyre, T. (1993). Stimulus (instructional) fading during extinction of self-injurious escape behavior. *Journal of Applied Behavior Analysis, 26*(2), 205–212. https://doi.org/10.1901/jaba.1993.26-205

Partington, J. W., & Mueller, M. M. (2012). The assessment of functional living skills guide - Essential skills for independence at home, school and in the community. *Behaviour Analysts, Inc*. https://partingtonbehavioranalysts.com/products/afls/afls-samples/

PEAT. (2020). *Road safety videos*. Retrieved November 16, 2020, from http://www.peatni.org/road

Pohl, A. L., Crockford, S. K., Blakemore, M., & Baron-Cohen, S. (2020). A comparative study of autistic and nonautistic women's experience of motherhood. *Molecular Autism, 11*(3), 1–12. https://doi.org/10.1186/s13229-019-0304-2

Rausa, V. C., Moore, D. W., & Anderson, A. (2016). Use of video modelling to teach complex and meaningful job skills to an adult with autism spectrum disorder. *Developmental Neurorehabilitation, 19*(4). https://doi.org/10.3109/17518423.2015.1008150

Reinecke, D. R., Krokowski, A., & Newman, B. (2016). Self-management for building independence: Research and future directions. *International Journal of Educational Research, 87*, 119–126. https://doi.org/10.1016/j.ijer.2016.08.006

Rizzi, D., & Dibari, A. (2019). Using behavior skills training and other environmental manipulations to teach safety skills to adolescents with ASD. *Autism and Developmental Disorders, 17*(3), 12–28. https://doi.org/10.17759/autdd.2019170302. (In Russ., abstr. in Engl.).

Roberts, K., DeQuinzio, J. A., Taylor, B. A., & Petroski, J. (2020). Using behavioral skills training to teach interview skills to young adults with autism. *Journal of Behavioral Education*. https://doi.org/10.1007/s10864-020-09389-z

Rosenblatt, M. (2008). *I Exist: the message from adults with autism in England*. Retrieved July 18, 2014, from http://www.autism.org.uk/get-involved/campaign-for-change/learn-more/our-campaigns/past-campaigns/i-exist.aspx

Rosenwasser, B., & Axelrod, S. (2001). The contributions of applied behavior analysis to the education of people with autism. *Behavior Modification, 25*(5), 671–677. https://doi.org/10.1177/0145445501255001

Rossi, M. R., Vladescu, J. C., Reeve, K. F., & Gross, A. C. (2017). Teaching safety responding to children with autism spectrum disorder. *Education and Treatment of Children, 40*(2), 187–208. https://doi.org/10.1353/etc.2017.0009

Ruddy, L., Booth, N., Gaw, M., Liao, Y., Dounavi, K., & Dillenburger, K. (2015). Autism in the air: Using point-of-view video-priming and natural environment teaching to help children with autism travel by plane. *Good Autism Practice, 16*, 25–32.
Russell, G. (2020). Critiques of the neurodiversity movement. In *Autistic Community and the Neurodiversity Movement*. https://doi.org/10.1007/978-981-13-8437-0_21.
Schaafsma, D., Kok, G., Stoffelen, J. M. T., & Curfs, L. M. G. (2017). People with intellectual disabilities talk about sexuality: Implications for the development of sex education. *Sexuality and Disability, 35*, 21–38. https://doi.org/10.1007/s11195-016-9466-4
Shattuck, P. T., Narendorf, S. C., Cooper, B., Sterzing, P. R., Wagner, M., & Taylor, J. L. (2012). Postsecondary education and employment among youth with an autism spectrum disorder. *Pediatrics, 129*(6), 1042–1049. https://doi.org/10.1542/peds.2011-2864
Sidman, M. (1989). Avoidance at Columbia. *The Behavior Analyst, 12*(2), 191–195. https://doi.org/10.1007/BF03392496
Simonoff, E., Pickles, A., Charman, T., Chandler, S., Loucas, T., & Baird, G. (2008). Psychiatric disorders in children with autism spectrum disorders: Prevalence, comorbidity, and associated factors in a population-derived sample. *Journal of the American Academy of Child and Adolescent Psychiatry, 47*(8), 921–929. https://doi.org/10.1097/CHI.0b013e318179964f
Singer, J. (1998). NeuroDiversity: The birth of an idea. In *Disability discourse* (2nd ed., p. 64). Amazon Media EU: Kindle Edition.
Stedman, A., Taylor, B., Erard, M., Peura, C., & Siegel, M. (2019). Are children severely affected by Autism Spectrum Disorder underrepresented in treatment studies? An analysis of the literature. *Journal of Autism and Developmental Disorders, 49*(4), 1378–1390. https://doi.org/10.1007/s10803-018-3844-y
Stein, S., & Dillenburger, K. (2017). Ethics in sexual behavior assessment and support for people with intellectual disability. *International Journal on Disability and Human Development, 16*(1). https://doi.org/10.1515/ijdhd-2016-0023
Stein, S., Kohut, T., & Dillenburger, K. (2017). The importance of sexuality education for children with and without intellectual disabilities: What parents think. *Sexuality and Disability*. https://doi.org/10.1007/s11195-017-9513-9
Stokes, T. F., & Baer, D. M. (1977). An implicit technology of generalization. *Journal of Applied Behavior Analysis, 10*(2), 349–367. https://doi.org/10.1901/jaba.1977.10-349
Summers, J., Tarbox, J., Findel-Pyles, R. S., Wilke, A. E., Bergstrom, R., & Williams, W. L. (2011). Teaching two household safety skills to children with autism. *Research in Autism Spectrum Disorders, 5*, 629–632.
Surgeon General. (1999). *Mental Health: A Report of the Surgeon General*. Retrieved July 21, 2014, from http://profiles.nlm.nih.gov/ps/retrieve/ResourceMetadata/NNBBHS
Taylor, B. A., Hughes, C. E., Richard, E., Hoch, H., & Coello, A. R. (2004). Teaching teenagers with autism to seek assistance when lost. *Journal of Applied Behavior Analysis, 37*, 79–82. https://doi.org/10.1901/jaba.2004.37-79
Test, D. W., Fowler, C. H., Wood, W. M., Brewer, D. M., & Eddy, S. (2005). A conceptual framework of selfadvocacy for students with disabilities. *Remedial and Special Education, 26*(1), 43–54. https://doi.org/10.1177/07419325050260010601
Travers, J. C., & Whitby, P. (2014). Sexuality and relationships for individuals with autism spectrum disorders. In M. Tincani & A. Bondy (Eds.), *Autism spectrum disorders in adolescents and adults: Evidence-based and promising interventions* (pp. 182–207). Guilford.
UNCRC. (2001). United Nations convention on the rights of the child. *Right to Education*. Retrieved June 17, 2020, from https://www.refworld.org/docid/4538834d2.html
UNCRPD. (2006). *United Nations Convention on the Rights of Persons with Disabilities*. Retrieved October 13, 2014, from http://www.un.org/disabilities/convention/conventionfull.shtml
Van Bourgondien, M. E., & Woods, A. V. (1992). Vocational possibilities for high-functioning adults with autism. In E. Schopler & G. B. Mesibov (Eds.), *High-functioning individuals with autism* (pp. 227–239). Springer. https://doi.org/10.1007/978-1-4899-2456-8_12

Virués-Ortega, J. (2010). Applied behavior analytic intervention for autism in early childhood: Meta-analysis, meta-regression and dose-response meta-analysis of multiple outcomes. *Clinical Psychology Review, 30*(4), 387–399. https://doi.org/10.1016/j.cpr.2010.01.008

Warren, Z., McPheeters, M. L., Sathe, N., Foss-Feig, J. H., Glasser, A., & Veenstra-Vanderweele, J. (2011). A systematic review of early intensive intervention for autism spectrum disorders. *Pediatrics, 127*(5), e1303–e1311. https://doi.org/10.1542/peds.2011-0426

Warrier, V., Greenberg, D. M., Weir, E., Buckingham, C., Smith, P., Lai, M.-C., & Baron-Cohen, S. (2020). Elevated rates of autism, other neurodevelopmental and psychiatric diagnoses, and autistic traits in transgender and gender-diverse individuals. *Nature Communications, 11*, 3959.

WHO. (2020). *The ICD-11: International Classification of Mental and Behavioural Disorders.* https://doi.org/10.1002/1520-6505(2000)9:5<201::AID-EVAN2>3.3.CO;2-P

Wing, L., & Gould, J. (1979). Severe impairments of social interaction and associated abnormalities in children: Epidemiology and classification. *Journal of Autism and Developmental Disorders, 9*, 11–29. https://doi.org/10.1007/BF01531288

Wolf, M. M. (1978). Social validity: The case for subjective measurement or how applied behavior analysis is finding its heart. *Journal of Applied Behavior Analysis, 11*(2), 203–214. https://doi.org/10.1901/jaba.1978.11-203

Wright, C. S., & Vollmer, T. R. (2002). Evallluation of a treatment package to reduce rapid eating. *Journal of Applied Behavior Analysis, 35*(1), 89–93. https://doi.org/10.1901/jaba.2002.35-89

York State Department of Health, N. (2011). *Clinical Practice Guidelines: Quick reference guide for parents and professionals. Autism/Pervasive Development Disorders. Assessment and Intervention for Young Children (age 0–3 years).* New York: http://www.health.ny.gov/publications/4216.pdf. Retrieved from http://www.health.ny.gov/publications/4216.pdf

Chapter 4
Reducing the Risk of Rights Restrictions for Autistic People Experiencing Behaviours of Concern

Alan Tennyson and Ciara Maye

Abstract This chapter explores the risk to the human rights of autistic people, specifically those experiencing concerning behaviours and in receipt of professional support. We will see how human rights happen in the 'small places', in the everyday decisions regarding how people are supported. Autistic people experiencing concerning behaviours are at risk of having their rights arbitrarily restricted, without the due process available to the general population. Emphasising consent and an individual's will and preferences expressed through their assent, we show how behaviour analysis can provide assent-based methods that meet a person's needs. We propose that behaviour analytic supports are reasonable accommodations that identify and seek to remove barriers to inclusion. While acknowledging the reality that people with significant support needs face restrictions due to balancing their rights with the rights of others, we explore how human rights-based due process can be embedded in organisational and policy frameworks. Arguing that while this is good practice in the short term, people experiencing these concerns need access to justice on an equal basis with others and, therefore, any process that restricts rights should become statutory. Behaviour analysis is uniquely positioned to provide robust outcome measures to inform due process. This approach underscores the necessity of realising equality before the law for all people regardless of their support needs.

Keywords Reasonable Accommodations · Human Rights · Consent and assent · Intellectual disabilities · Autism

A. Tennyson (✉)
Irish Society for Behaviour Analysis, Dublin, Ireland
e-mail: alan@isba.ie

C. Maye
Brothers of Charity Services Ireland, Southern Region, Galway, Ireland
e-mail: ciara.maye@bocsi.ie

S. Halder et al. (eds.), *Applied Behavior Analysis-Based Interventions for Autism Spectrum Disorder*, https://doi.org/10.1007/978-981-95-2889-9_4

4.1 The Historic Context of Human Rights

Human rights refer to a set of fundamental principles that recognise the equal entitlement of all people, regardless of their identity, background, or circumstances, to basic rights and freedoms. These rights are considered inalienable, universal, and indivisible, and are protected through various mechanisms at the national, European, and international levels, including the Universal Declaration of Human Rights (UDHR) (United Nations General Assembly, 1948) and the Convention against Torture and Other Cruel, Inhuman or Degrading Treatment (United Nations, 1984). In the European Union, people can seek legal recourse through the European Court of Human Rights.

The UN Convention on the Rights of Persons with Disabilities (UNCRPD) (United Nations, 2006) offers a structure to safeguard and promote human rights for all people with disabilities, including autistic people experiencing concerning behaviours.

As behaviour analysts, we understand that each person's phylogenetic and ontogenic provenance is unique and that operant responding exists in complex cultural contexts. Behaviour analysis, as a scientific approach, is grounded in nature. It recognises the reality of physical differences and the social construction of such differences. This scientific reality provides an expansive view of the emergence and maintenance of concerning behaviour. It also offers insights into the occurrence of individual and systematic contingencies which deny or restrict human rights.

Behaviour analysts can provide empirical outcomes to inform due process and demonstrate what works to preserve and restore human rights. Behaviour support plans can identify and remove environmental barriers and support the participation of people experiencing concerning behaviour in their communities.

4.2 Concerning Behaviour and Restrictive Practice

Concerning behaviour can be defined as behaviour that is so intense, frequent or lasts so long that it threatens the quality of life or the physical safety of the person or others; and is likely to lead to responses that are restrictive, aversive, or result in exclusion (National Collaborating Centre for Mental Health, 2020). Examples of behaviours which can cause concern are self-injurious behaviours such as head-banging, behaviours which impact on others such as kicking or hitting, destructive behaviours, and non-consensual or public sexual behaviours. It is now commonly understood that such behaviour is influenced by the interaction between a person and environment, and so changing the environment so that it can support an individual's needs is key to reducing behaviour of concern and improving quality of life.

Definitions of restrictive practice and subtypes of restrictions provided in law or by service providers and professional bodies vary at different times and according to each body's purpose (see Sturmey, 2015 for a detailed discussion). However restrictive practices are broadly understood as limits placed on a person's voluntary movement or behaviour, and therefore restrictive practices are necessarily rights restrictions. They are generally considered according to a range of categories including physical restraint (i.e. physically holding a person against their will), mechanical restraint (e.g. a helmet which a person cannot remove), environmental restraint (e.g. locked doors), seclusion, and pharmacological or chemical restraint.

4.3 Emancipatory Values and Behaviour Analysis

The UN High Commissioner for Human Rights and the World Health Organisation, in the document *Mental Health, Human Rights and Legislation: Guidance and Practice* (World Health Organisation & United Nations High Commissioner for Human Rights, 2023), have called on state parties to legislate "to end all forms of coercion and to develop non-coercive responses that respect the rights of service users" (p. 27). This goal aligns with values expressed by pioneers of behavioural science. Baer et al. (1968), Skinner (1971), Goldiamond (1974), LaVigna and Donnellan (1986) and Sidman (1989) all set out ways to counteract societal practices of coercion and control which were seen as an affront to human freedom and dignity.

These early writers envisaged a world in which individuals with disabilities and mental health concerns would be free from institutional coercion. With rigorous measurement of behavioural change, behaviour analysts could pinpoint the environmental contexts in which distress was alleviated, the change in behaviour that signalled such relief, and the environmental contingencies that led to improvements. By following the data and implementing evidence-based interventions, the aspiration was to reduce distress, eliminate coercion, and enhance the quality of life (Sidman, 1989; Delprato, 1995). Why then, have practitioners of applied behaviour analysis not realised these aspirations more widely?

4.4 The Evolution of Care and Obliteration of Personal Autonomy

As with other scientific disciplines, the practice of behaviour analysis is shaped by societal values in ways which have resulted in both harm and benefits. As society evolves, so does the practice of behaviour analysis. Just as corporal punishment is no longer acceptable as a mainstream cultural practice, it is equally unacceptable as a behavioural intervention. In a society which seeks to celebrate difference, an autistic child being 'indistinguishable from their peers' (Lovaas, 1987) would no longer be lauded as a positive outcome, particularly if that outcome compromised the child's emotional well-being.

Models of care and support for the vulnerable in society have developed considerably. Historically, mass care provision was designed by states or religious organisations to meet basic survival needs. For example, asylums evolved in the early 1800s, based on the 'workhouse' model of providing for society's destitute (Kelly, 2019). In these institutions, which housed hundreds or thousands of people, personal autonomy was automatically limited or removed completely (Goffman, 1961; Curry, 2013).

The focus shifted gradually towards the categorisation of disability and in turn the medicalisation of support (Kelly, 2019). Institutions evolved away from their original purpose into mechanisms of social control and a means of containment of various sections of the population. The delivery of services based on the category of disability continues in current service delivery. While support for a wide range of needs now generally takes place in much smaller service settings, cultural legacy, academic and institutional, can still influence 'how things are done around here'. This is what Professors Julie Beadle-Brown and Jim Mansell have referred to as 'institutional legacy' (Beadle-Brown et al., 2007).

The harms caused by institutionalisation are widely acknowledged and a commitment to community living has developed. However, while the old system is dying, the new has yet to be born, and societies continue to grapple with how to evolve practices to be consistent with human rights, prevent further damage, and secure justice for those harmed by past practices (Punzi & Steele, 2024). By advancing evidence-based policy, behaviour analysis can inform this transition and progress towards realising the original vision of a society free from coercion.

4.5 Multilevel Contingencies that Influence Cultural and Institutional Practices

It is important for all behaviour analysts to maintain an awareness of the broader contingencies influencing service provision so that they can positively influence the context they operate within.

While policies and legislation for service providers are increasingly aligning with human rights frameworks, a gap can exist between policy aspirations and the actual support delivered. Scholars in cultural and behavioural evolution, such as Henrich (2020) and Wilson (2019), describe the multilevel contingencies influencing cultural and institutional practices. They note that institutional practices resist change without a concurrent transformation in the underlying contingencies. Behaviour analysts operate within broad cultural and organisational contexts encompassing various parties, including social care staff, educators, multidisciplinary teams, managers, funders, policymakers, civil services, governments and the person's community and family life.

It is crucial for behaviour analysts and others who wish to inspire change, to recognise the complex layers of contingencies that perpetuate institutional legacies. Behaviour analysts alone neither created this legacy nor can be held solely accountable for its continued existence. Awareness of this is necessary so that effective strategies for transformational change in human rights preservation and restoration can be collectively designed. For instance, multilevel contingencies affecting service providers', including behaviour analysts' ability to improve individual lives might involve the following:

1. Contingencies within organisations and wider systems that influence underreporting of concerning behaviours and related restrictions. This can affect the validity of functional behavioural assessment and plan implementation. Identifying and removing restrictions requires a transparent and assertive outreach to identify concerning behaviours and restrictions in use.
2. Regulatory compliance may act as a motivating operation for organisations and may impact their responses to individuals' needs post reaching the minimum standard for compliance.
3. There may be insufficient attention to contingencies present for those delivering direct support.
4. In inpatient settings, Quinn et al. (2023) have noted that individuals, particularly those with autism or intellectual disabilities, face risks such as inappropriate psychotropic medication, physical restraint, seclusion, and, in some cases, long-term segregation, iatrogenic deprivation, and trauma (Care Quality Commission, 2019, 2021; Hubert, 2006 in Quinn et al., 2023). A reason for delayed discharge from segregated settings can be the absence of adequate community-based social care and housing, another multilevel contingency impacting on the lives of people supported.
5. Reluctance to seek additional resources is likely due to aversive responses from service commissioners who are responsible for controlling budgets.
6. Rigid funding models can confine individuals at risk of concerning behaviours to standardised group education and living arrangements.
7. The political context and the broader understanding of behaviour analysis at national and regional levels can affect the use of evidence-based support. For example, in Ireland, public discourse, including on social media, about early behaviour analysis practices, and practices in other countries, has negatively impacted the perception of behaviour analysis in Ireland. This necessitates that behaviour analysts provide clear examples of their current positive impact in line with human rights to foster a constructive view of applied behaviour analysis.

To affect changes within these extensive systems, behaviour analysts must hold positions organisations which enable them to influence multilevel contingencies.

4.6 Human Rights and Restrictive Practices

Although focusing on human rights has the potential to reduce coercion, it does not guarantee its elimination without recognition of the contingencies that maintain the existing practices. The UNCRPD places significant responsibility on individual clinicians without adequately addressing the broader nature and availability of services within which clinicians operate. However, it can be argued that politicians and service managers have a greater influence on the rights to treatment and support than individual clinicians, whose options may be limited in specific care situations (Kelly, 2023). Implementing human rights-based reform requires modifying the legislation that governs the contingencies directing service design, resource allocation, professional training, and rules that affect rights in different settings. Legal responsibility for human rights preservation and restoration must be distributed more clearly and appropriately. In other words, there is a need to identify the rights-holders and duty-bearers in this context.

Before examining how autistic individuals' human rights can be violated in service settings, it should be noted that it can be necessary to balance the rights of autistic people with the rights of others when providing health and social care. Debates about human rights sometimes conflate human rights issues with restrictive measures. However, such measures are not inherently abusive. There are situations where people without disabilities have their actions restricted or face consequences, such as when breaking traffic laws they may have their driving licence revoked. Other restrictive measures may be necessary to ensure equity for individuals with disabilities and may not be discriminatory, e.g. using a restrictive harness for transportation to enable a person with a disability to participate in community activities. Additionally, organisations have a legal duty of care to ensure reasonable safety for the people they support and their staff, which requires a balanced approach considering the preferences of individuals being supported, the rights of all parties, and the assessed risks (Brothers of Charity Southern Services, 2024).

The pressing issue demanding substantial change involves the heightened risk faced by autistic individuals, particularly those who do not communicate verbally and exhibit behaviours of concern, of having their individuality pathologised and their rights arbitrarily restricted. To counteract this risk, service providers, including behaviour analysts must actively contribute to the development of a society that:

(1) Embraces behaviours that do not infringe on the rights of others
(2) Employs effective, non-traumatising behaviour support strategies
(3) Advocates for the rights of disabled people
(4) Ensures the solicitation of consent and assent from individuals who may struggle with communication
(5) Promotes adherence to ethical and legal processes when there are indications that rights may be infringed upon

The ultimate aim is to reduce and eliminate arbitrary restrictions on rights.

4.7 Human Rights Vignettes

The ability of a person to exercise their autonomy can be influenced by their diagnosis and the form of support or care they receive. To illustrate this consider the vignettes below describing John and Jack. Both men face similar challenges, but their differing diagnoses and support arrangements lead to distinct differences in terms of their human rights.

John Struggles with Depression, But His Human Rights Are Not Affected

John is a 28-year-old self-employed computer programmer with a history of depression, which emerged in his mid-teens, following the loss of his mother; he does not have a diagnosis of autism though he does describe himself as having 'autistic traits'. John has left his parent's home and found a room in a shared apartment. John has a number of 'bad habits'. He does not wash very much during winter, considering it 'hibernating season'. Flatmates who have a problem with his hygiene either persuade him to shower for their sake or they move out. John vapes and drinks a lot of energy and fizzy drinks. His diet leans towards frozen pizza and chocolate. As a consequence of his lifestyle, John is quite overweight, his doctor recommends that he lose weight or he may develop Type 2 diabetes. A blood test is recommended. John has a needle phobia and refuses the test.

John's history of depression does not affect his ability to make his own decisions, his decision-making capacity is not in question. While his doctor provides advice, he cannot force the issue, John maintains his autonomy and continues to live a life of his choosing.

Now let us consider Jack. There are some similarities with John's story initially, but then their paths diverge.

4.8 Jack Is Autistic and Accesses Services, his Rights Are At Increased Risk

The following story relates to the progress of Jack's care, and rights violations which emerge during care. Although service providers, including behaviour analysts are obligated to safeguard clients' rights, there are often situations where rights have been infringed upon prior to intervention and instances where the protection of rights is difficult within the wider service system without clear frameworks for doing so.

Jack is a 28-year-old autistic man. Jack's mother is critically ill and his father's early onset dementia is advancing. Since he was a teenager Jack has accessed respite care, which he enjoyed. He has always had a lot of energy and has been very vocal about his special interests (steam engines). One weekend when Jack was at the respite house, his Mum died. His Dad was not in a position to look after Jack. Due to the emergency need for care provision, a vacancy in a 24-hour staffed group home an hour away from his Dad was provided. Jack is very distressed by the loss of his mother and not being at home. Jack has to share the home with two other people, one person sings a lot and the other cries often, two sounds that Jack finds hard to tolerate. Jack is frequently upset and responds to the sounds of the other men by cursing, pacing and banging on doors. The waiting list for another accommodation is five years.

Jack's situation has failed to take account of the UNCRPD Article 19: "Persons with disabilities have the opportunity to choose their place of residence and where and with whom they live on an equal basis with others and are not obliged to live in a particular living arrangement". Jack is removed from his own home without due regard for the continuity of family life.

Jack likes to drink a lot of cola and eat chocolate, he is overweight. His doctor has recommended blood tests and that he lose weight. Jack avoids the nurse's efforts to draw blood. The nurse is under pressure and responds with more tension to Jack frequently getting in and out of the seat. Jack refuses to go back to the doctor's clinic for the next six months. When Jack returns to the clinic, the nurse on duty and a colleague use a clinical hold against Jack's will to take blood. Blood results indicate Jack is at high risk of Type 2 diabetes.

Taking blood in this way is against Jack's will. It contravenes his autonomy, as articulated in Article 17 of the UNCRPD, and is an infringement on his right to reasonable accommodations to support access to health services.

Feeling a duty of care, the staff restrict Jack's diet. Jack strikes staff if they refuse his requests for cola and chocolate, he starts to pick at his skin when stressed, causing a surface injury. When the team try to direct Jack to shower regularly he starts to hit or kick others to get staff to leave him alone.

Here, there is a violation of the general principles of respect for individual autonomy and the freedom to make one's own choices. It could also be argued that Jack has not had access to a range of "in-home, residential and other community support services, including personal assistance necessary to support living and inclusion in the community, and to prevent isolation or segregation from the community" (Article 19, UNCRPD).

Jack is referred to a psychiatrist who prescribes antipsychotic medication to reduce agitation. A side effect of the medication is increased appetite. Jack puts on more weight and grabs others' food in public. The team becomes reluctant to bring Jack out. The decrease in trips out leads to boredom and frustration.

Over the year since admission to the placement, Jack's stress level has increased and his behaviour has deteriorated, his distress becoming particularly acute when his father passes away. He begins to lash out at his peers. Physical restraint is used when Jack is considered a risk to other service users. Jack is removed to his bedroom and the door is locked when he lashes out.

The use of physical restraint and confinement to his room challenges Jack's right to liberty and security of person, as per Article 14. In neglecting to provide appropriate support, Jack's right to "enjoy the highest attainable standard of physical and mental health" (Article 25) (United Nations, 2006) is violated. Article 15 on "freedom from torture or cruel, inhuman or degrading treatment or punishment" may also be called into question here.

The team feel that Jack is experiencing a mental health breakdown and that his residential service can no longer accommodate him due to the risk to himself, other service users and staff. Jack is transferred to an Assessment and Treatment Facility four hours away for six weeks. His behaviour further escalates in the new setting. Jack's original service provider asserts the organisation is not in a position to take him back and he stays in the new setting without a concrete discharge plan for several years. This inappropriate placement is provided at a high financial cost to the public health service. Jack's extended family are not in contact with him.

Jack's involuntary transfer to an assessment and treatment facility disregards his right to "live in the community and not to be obliged to live in a particular living arrangement", isolated and segregated from the community, as emphasised in Article 19 of the UNCRPD. This vignette shows that Jack's rights to habilitation and rehabilitation (Article 26 UNCRPD) are neglected.

4.9 Paternalism and Human Rights Restrictions and Their Effects

In Jack's case paternalism, where actions are taken which are expected to help or benefit a person's welfare but not necessarily with their consent, has interfered with Jack's autonomy and liberty in several ways. The support systems in place for him failed to safeguard his rights or provide him with due process. When his rights were violated, he was not provided with access to the justice necessary to rectify these infringements. This experience echoes that of others who rely on social care, whose experience can be marked by intersectional and compounding forms of discrimination, abuse, and marginalisation within their social and systemic interactions (Didi et al., 2018).

A growing body of research highlights the detrimental consequences of restrictive practices on individuals with disabilities (Advonet & Change, 2023). Such practices have been associated with traumatic experiences, feelings of abandonment, fear, distress, disempowerment, and learned helplessness. They can erode trust in current staff relationships and impede the formation of trust in future staff. Individuals may respond to these restrictions with anger, fear, or frustration, potentially increasing their likelihood of further restrictions being imposed.

4.10 Supporting Jack with Multi-Element Behaviour Support

To mediate against these restrictions and related risks, it is imperative to adopt trauma-informed frameworks of care provision, such as the Multi-Element Behaviour Support paradigm (LaVigna et al., 2022), when working with individuals who have experienced adverse consequences stemming from traumatic experiences. An essential aspect of this support approach is actively preventing re-traumatisation, which means avoiding continued restrictions that may exacerbate past trauma.

By proactively applying the Multi-Element Behaviour Support (MEBS) paradigm to Jack's story from the beginning, we can explore ways to provide comprehensive support that respects his autonomy, supports his needs, and maintains or restores his rights (Doody, 2009). The MEBS model of behaviour support uses a combined linear and nonlinear approach to functional behavioural assessment (Layng, 2009) which considers a person's uniqueness, support needs and interactions with the environment (Liberman & LaVigna, 2016). MEBS was founded on the assumption that behavioural support should be non-aversive.

We will retell Jack's story, highlighting where MEBS intervention features can be used in italics and brackets.

Knowing of Jack's parents' ill health, his social worker has been supporting Jack and his family to make plans for the future (*positive futures planning*) including where he will live. Since there is a query regarding Jack's capacity to consent to this decision, Jack's social worker arranged an assessment of his capacity to consent. Jack's Uncle Eoin is close to Jack and his parents and a co-decision-making agreement is made. Jack's Uncle Eoin becomes Jack's co-decision maker (a defined role in Irish law) in relation to his personal welfare, property and affairs. When Jack's Mum dies there is a crisis period where Jack moves into a group home temporarily while Jack's social worker support him to secure an individualised budget (Pike et al., 2016). When Jack becomes increasingly upset in the group home, a behaviour support practitioner is recruited to help understand why. Jack is supported to withdraw and play computer games with headphones when it is to noise (functionally related and coping skills and situational management). Jack is supported to go out to the movies twice a week to reduce his exposure (prevention) and to work in local garden centre. His work, laundry and food preparation are worked on through tasks analyses (skills teaching and prevention). A low-arousal non-aversive approach is used when Jack is stressed (changes in environment and situational management). It is recognised that Jack could live in his original family home with staff support during the day and a nightwatch service.

Pictures are used to support Jack to understand that staying clean can make his body 'ping!', and 'not pong!'. Jack thinks this is hilarious and it is connected to 'being ready for the working day'. Jack becomes more motivated to shower, though only on a Saturday, the busiest day in the garden centre (*daily living skills teaching*).

Visuals are used to support Jack's understanding of too much sugar leading to headaches (*education/skills teaching*). He is offered a taste test of 100% cola, or cola with 95% cola and 5% water diluted (*prevention*), as well as a variety of other drinks. He accepts the diluted version, gradually accepts less and less in his glass and chooses less cola with extra popcorn.

With a trusting relationship with staff, Jack is motivated to move gradually towards healthier foods (*using stimulus fading, and prevention*).

After three years of doing the walk around the local soccer pitch, the groundskeeper is on friendly terms with Jack. Jack's relationships are beginning to expand beyond his staff and his Uncle Eoin.

4.11 RIGHTS-Based Model of Positive Behaviour Support

Given all there is to consider in designing and implementing behavioural supports, behaviour analysts will benefit from Leif et al.'s (2023) clear articulation of a RIGHTS-based model of positive behaviour support. Similarly, Cianci and Sevon (2023) have produced a range of prompts for behaviour analysts to consider

Table 4.1 RIGHTS-based model related to the UN Convention of Rights of People with Disabilities (CRPD)

Component of RIGHTS-based model of PBS	Alignment with specific CRPD articles	Practical recommendations for behaviour support practitioners
Respect the person's dignity and self-worth	Article 3: General principles	1. Communicate with the PWD in ways that enable their understanding and participation
	Article 16: Freedom from exploitation, violence, and abuse	2. Enable the PWD to make choices and express their preferences throughout all phases of behaviour support
	Article 17: Protecting the integrity of the person	3. Support the person to identify and report occurrences of exploitation, violence, and abuse
Include the person in decisions that are about them	Article 3: General principles	1. Use a supported decision-making framework into practice to help the PWD make their own decisions
	Article 12: Equal recognition before the law	2. Individualise the supported decision-making approach for the PWD
	Article 21: Freedom of expression and opinion, and access to information	3. Identify trusted people who can support the PWD to make decisions
Get to know the person and their family	Article 3: General principles	1. Build a strong therapeutic alliance with the PWD and their family
	Article 26: Habilitation and rehabilitation	2. Use person-centred planning during and after the functional behaviour assessment to co-design the behaviour support plan with the PWD and their family and support team members
		3. Listen and encourage the PWD to express their wants and needs
Take a holistic approach when supporting the person	Article 19: Living independently and being included in the community	1. Conduct a comprehensive assessment of the environment around the PWD as part of the functional behaviour assessment and address environments of concern as part of the provision of support
	Article 24: Education	2. Identify if the PWD is facing hardships in areas of safety, housing, relationships, or other lifestyle areas, and, if so, take steps to connect the family with social support services or other community-based supports
	Article 25: Health	3. Ensure the PWD's medical and health needs are addressed. Identify the last time the PWD was able to visit the doctor and dentist. Support the PWD to maintain regular contact with their healthcare providers
	Article 27: Work and employment	
	Article 28: Adequate standard of living and social protection	
	Article 30: Participation in cultural life, recreation, leisure, and sport	

(continued)

Table 4.1 (continued)

Component of RIGHTS-based model of PBS	Alignment with specific CRPD articles	Practical recommendations for behaviour support practitioners
Teach and tell others about human rights	Article 4: General obligations	1. Provide information about human rights to the PWD and their family in easy-read formats
	Article 8: Awareness raising	2. Develop organisational policies that describe how the human rights of PWD who receive services will be protected and upheld in service delivery
		3. Ensure all staff receive regular training on the human rights of PWD, ways to protect and uphold human rights in practice, and what to do if they encounter practices that may conflict with human rights
Support the person to achieve their goals and live a good life	Article 15: Freedom from torture or cruel, inhuman, or degrading treatment or punishment	1. Use safe, evidence-informed behaviour support strategies that support people to learn new skills
		2. Develop behaviour support plans that incorporate the least restrictive practices
	Article 26: Habilitation and rehabilitation	3. Support the implementation of behaviour support strategies that help the PWD experience enhanced quality of life, community presence, choice, and control

[a]Reproduced from Leif et al. (2023). "I Look at Their Rights First": Strategies Used by Australian Behaviour Support Practitioners' to Protect and Uphold the Rights of People with Disabilities. Advances in Neurodevelopmental Disorders. http://creativecommons.org/licenses/by/4.0/
[b]Person with a disability

specifically in relation to children's rights. Leif et al. (ibid) use the word RIGHTS as an acronym with the following explanation:

R = **Respect** the person's dignity and self-worth
I = **Include** the person in decisions that are about them
G = **Get to know** the person and their family
H = Take a **holistic** approach when supporting the person
T = **Teach and tell** others about human rights
S = **Support** the person to achieve their goals and live a good life

Leif et al. have produced a table for behaviour support practitioners to reference in the design of behavioural supports consistent with protecting and upholding a person's rights. Table 4.1 shows how each element of the RIGHTS-based model relates to specific articles from the UN Convention of Rights of People with Disabilities (CRPD) together with practical actions behaviour support practitioners can take to protect and uphold a person's rights.

4.12 Behavioural Health, Behavioural Health Integration, Rights, Reasonable Accommodations, and Behaviour Support Plans

The implementation of the Multi-Element Behaviour Support Plan is not necessarily an easy process and there are barriers to implementation. However, it can represent the integration of a number of concepts which can relate to the preservation and restoration of human rights in the context of concerning behaviour.

4.12.1 Behavioural Health Integration and the Right to Habilitation and Rehabilitation

Behavioural health can be defined as 'care that addresses mental health … life stressors and crises, and stress-related physical symptoms' (American Medical Association, 2021 p.6). Jack's story, in the second iteration, is an example of 'behavioural health integration' in action, i.e. 'the result of primary care (or other care settings) and behavioural health clinicians, working together with patients and families, using a systematic approach to provide patient-centred care' (American Medical Association, 2021; Levey et al., 2012). Gaining the necessary support for behavioural health can be seen as relating to Jack's right to habilitation and rehabilitation (Article 26, UNCRPD). This right includes the right of persons with disabilities to*:*

> "attain and maintain maximum independence, full physical, mental, social and vocational ability, and full inclusion and participation in all aspects of life," through "services and programmes, particularly in the areas of health, employment, education and social services, in such a way that these services and programmes:

(a) Begin at the earliest possible stage, and are based on the multidisciplinary assessment of individual needs and strengths;
(b) Support participation and inclusion in the community and all aspects of society, are voluntary, and are available to persons with disabilities as close as possible to their communities, including in rural areas".

4.12.2 Discrimination, Reasonable Accommodations, and Behaviour Support Plans

Discrimination on the basis of disability is defined as: "any distinction, exclusion or restriction on the basis of disability which has the purpose or effect of impairing or nullifying the recognition, enjoyment or exercise, on an equal basis with others, of all human rights and fundamental freedoms in the political, economic, social, cultural, civil or any other field. It includes all forms of discrimination, including denial of reasonable accommodation" (ibid UNCRPD).

Some people with disabilities need individualised support to access their communities, their health services or public and private amenities. In order to access services, accommodations may be required. A *reasonable* accommodation is defined as: "necessary and appropriate modification and adjustments not imposing a disproportionate or unduc burden, where needed in a particular case, to ensure to persons with disabilities the enjoyment or exercise on an equal basis with others of all human rights and fundamental freedoms" (Article 2 of UNCRPD). Reasonable accommodation is intrinsic to the duty of non-discrimination. The term "reasonable" refers to the relevance, appropriateness and effectiveness of the accommodation. A reasonable accommodation must achieve the purpose (or purposes) for which it is being made, and be tailored to meet the requirements of the individual. Furthermore, the concept of "disproportionate or undue burden" sets a limit to what a third party must do to provide an accommodation; an accommodation should not pose a possible excessive or unjustifiable burden on the accommodating party (World Health Organisation & United Nations High Commissioner for Human Rights, 2023).

Accommodations are justifiable by their effective outcomes. It follows that in health and social care, evidence-based support which can be shown to enable the participation of people with disabilities, can be viewed as a reasonable accommodation. The provision of behavioural support in the community for people experiencing behaviour of concern is associated with lower costs and better outcomes for both the person supported and the people supporting them (Beadle-Brown et al., 2007; Felce, 2017; Emerson, 2009; Mansell & Beadle-Brown, 2009). In this context, we assert that Behaviour Support Plans are reasonable accommodations in the context of people experiencing concerning behaviour, in the same way that wheelchair ramps are reasonable accommodations for people with limited mobility.

4.13 Legal Autonomy, Capacity, Consent, Assent, and the Functional Approach

To robustly pursue a rights-based approach, behaviour analysts should have a foundational understanding of autonomy and legal capacity as it relates to their state or country's laws, while also adhering to relevant ethical codes. Autonomy comes from the Greek 'auto'/self and 'nómos'/law, meaning the ability to make independent decisions and pursue desired actions (Taylor 2005). Autonomy establishes the basis for Western legal systems' approach to decision-making, rights, and responsibilities (Flynn & Arstein-Kerslake, 2014).

Historically, the ability to verbally demonstrate cognition and rationality was a marker for differentiating between those who are deemed eligible for 'legal personhood' or *'legal capacity'* and those who are not. When a person is deemed to have legal capacity this means they are recognised as having legal rights, as well as the power to exercise those rights and associated responsibilities. Legal capacity is demonstrated in a person's ability to understand the facts involved in a choice, apply the facts to a situation, weigh up the pros and cons, and choose consistently. In practical terms, recognition that a person has legal capacity validates a person's choices. Before the advancement of capacity assessment, legal systems typically deployed blanket, all-or-nothing approaches when determining the capacity of people with neurological disabilities or differences to consent. Contemporary approaches presume the capacity to provide consent. If there is reason to doubt that a person has the capacity to make a specific decision then, in Ireland, a 'functional assessment of capacity' process must be engaged, i.e. an assessment of the capacity to make a particular decision. This assessment considers a person's will and preference. Specific professional disciplines have the authority to legally conduct capacity assessments.

In the context of engaging with health professionals in Ireland, consent is defined as "the giving of permission or agreement for treatment, investigation, receipt or use of a service or participation in research or teaching (intervention). It involves a process of communication about the proposed intervention in which the person has received sufficient information to enable them to understand the nature, potential risks and benefits of the proposed intervention" (*Health Service Executive*, 2022). Assent is "an expression of willingness or affirmative agreement to an intervention given by a young person/adult who cannot provide legally valid consent. The assent procedure should reflect all practicable efforts to support the young person/adult to understand and communicate what their agreement would involve" (*Health Service Executive*, 2022). The absence of disagreement does not indicate assent. Rather it is considered an affirmative agreement, a response to a choice offered, such as a person responding to the question 'Would you like to come with me?' by moving along with you willingly. If a person demonstrates assent, this can be taken as an expression of legal will and preference.

Communication difficulties can make it challenging to express choice and consent. Furthermore, people may not have learned how to choose, not been given the opportunity to choose, had their choices invalidated, or felt overwhelmed by choice. Choosing and decision-making are sometimes skills that need to be taught and practised (Breaux & Smith, 2023). Hanley (2010) and Gover et al. (2023) have demonstrated practical methods for incorporating assent into behaviour-support procedures. For example, Hanley has highlighted concurrent chain schedules for assessing children's preferences and evaluating treatment effectiveness. This approach allows students to choose among cues linked to distinct teaching interventions, emphasising individualised approaches. Hanley has emphasised the role of assent in assessing social validation and enhancing satisfaction with behaviour-change procedures, and the importance of assent as a practical means to respect individuals' preferences and the right to opt out. This area of assent-based treatment is gaining traction in behavioural analytic research (Rajaraman et al., 2023).

Functional capacity assessments (distinct from functional behavioural assessments) evaluate an individual's decision-making capacity on a decision-by-decision basis, considering unique contexts and the person's abilities. This approach recognises that capacity is not an all-or-nothing concept, but exists on a continuum. The UN Special Rapporteur on the Rights of Persons with Disabilities emphasises the importance of consent in our daily and significant life decisions (Kurki, 2019). Therefore, the commencement of the Assisted Decision-Making (Capacity) Act (2015) has been a very important development in Ireland and should support autistic people's access to justice on an equal basis with others.

4.14 Legislation, Restrictive Practice, and Current Good Practice

In Australia, the Disability Act of 2006 mandates that the Office of the Senior Practitioner oversees the balance between individual freedom and public safety. This includes registering any restrictive practices used with individuals with disabilities with the office (Disability Act (Vic), 2006). In Ireland, there is no specific legislation governing the use of restrictive practices due to disability. Instead, restraint is considered within the broader framework of rights enshrined in the Irish Constitution (Oifig an tSoláthair, 1937) and the European Convention on Human Rights (Council of Europe, 1950). The use of restraint on a person without consent is currently unlawful, and any planned intervention must align with the person's consent and adhere to relevant legislation and policies. Decision-making regarding restrictive practices must align with the individual's will and preference when they lack the capacity to make a specific decision. However, limited interference with a person's bodily integrity or personal liberty may be justified in certain circumstances to protect the individual or others from imminent harm. The extent of restraint used must be proportionate to the risk of harm, and the least restrictive measure and the shortest possible duration must be considered (Assisted Decision-Making [Capacity] Act, 2015; Health Service Executive Consent Policy, 2022). Equal legal recognition for persons with disabilities is central to the human rights discourse, which includes providing reasonable accommodations. Statutory mechanisms in health and social care are necessary to maintain equality. These mechanisms should harmonise rights and duties, formal decision-making, and sanctioning processes while incorporating an individual's voice or assent.

Good practice relating to restrictive practice is currently represented within organisational policies in Ireland (e.g. Brothers of Charity Southern Services 2024). It involves a focus on the creation of capable environments (McGill et al., 2020) addressing the underlying causes of behaviour of concern and best practice approaches to behaviour support. Support for decision-making should occur as close to the area of impact as possible. Access to independent advocacy must be supported where required. Formal processes are engaged around identifying restrictions that may be in place, and preventing, sanctioning, reducing, and ultimately eliminating them, all under independent oversight. Accountability and transparency are vital and are achieved through documentation, collection and analysis of data to support the reduction and elimination of restrictions, oversight, audit, and evaluation. If a restriction is deemed necessary, thorough planning and staff training specific to that restriction should precede its implementation.

Where consent for restrictive practice is not obtained or the individual's will and preference does not support the implementation of a restrictive practice, good organisational practice indicates that the sanctioning process cannot continue at a local level, and the proposed restriction should be reviewed by more senior clinicians and managers in the context of the person's rights, will and preference of the person supported, the rights of others impacted, and the level of risk. At this level, the practice must be robustly challenged and examined for alignment with good practice. The work can be overseen by a rights committee which includes members independent of the organisation. Any person supported, their family/guardians or other advocates (including staff) have the right to appeal decisions in relation to sanctioning of restrictive practices. Any appeal which cannot be resolved at the first senior level will automatically be referred to the rights committee, the function of which is to ensure fair and proportionate treatment by providing a transparent and independent review.

These processes, perhaps among the best possible in the current service landscape, continue to place decision-making in the hands of the organisation prescribing the restriction, where a power imbalance exists. In this context, access to statutory and independent processes that balance a person's rights with those of others is needed to rectify the power imbalance. Central to the human rights discourse is ensuring that there is equal legal recognition for persons with disabilities. In health and social care contexts, statutory mechanisms are essential to uphold this equality before the law. Which must include the provision of reasonable accommodations to avoid, reduce or remove restrictions.

4.15 Conclusion

In this chapter, we have illustrated how Multi-Element Behaviour Support Plans take account of will and preference, and function as reasonable accommodations which minimise the risk of coercive or restrictive practices. They foster an environment where differences are not only accepted but celebrated, and where every individual, regardless of their difference, is treated with the dignity their humanity demands. The evidence-based nature of Multi-Element Behaviour Support Plan underscores its reasonableness as an accommodation to ensure persons with disabilities the enjoyment or exercise on an equal basis with others of all human rights and fundamental freedoms. Behaviour Support Plans can also provide empirical outcome measures to evaluate the effectiveness of support at an individual level and inform due process. Multi-element Behaviour Support Plans represent a convergence of scientific rigour and compassionate, person-centred human rights-based behavioural health and social care. Implementing evidence-based support signifies a commitment to creating an inclusive society that recognises and accommodates diverse needs, and takes effective action to achieve this goal. By acknowledging and addressing the specific needs and contributions of individuals, communities can move beyond traditional norms, ensuring equitable access to essential services and fostering a culture of genuine inclusion. In this way the community as a whole can grow in its compassion and diversity, ultimately embodying the essence of a rights-based and inclusive society.

To deliver equality, people with disabilities must have access to protections which are comparable to people without disabilities, particularly when they face rights restrictions. This necessitates the involvement of independent statutory authorities to balance power between support providers and recipients, ensuring that support is rights-based, and take remedial action where it is not. This approach underscores our societal commitment to upholding the dignity and rights of all individuals, ensuring that those experiencing concerning behaviours are treated with the respect they deserve within a framework that mirrors the rights and protections afforded to those without disabilities.

Future research should continue to extend Doody's work (2009) in providing examples of behaviour analysis applications that explicitly focus on preserving and restoring human rights. Additionally, it is important to explore ways to incorporate qualitative methods to assess social validity (Burney et al., 2023; Wolf, 1978) and enable an open science-based approach to progress (Keenan & Dillenburger, 2023). By focusing on rigorous outcome measures behaviour analysis can play a crucial role in advancing this ongoing endeavour.

References

American Medical Association. (2021). *Behavioral Health Integration Compendium*. https://www.ama-assn.org/delivering-care/public-health/compendium-behavioral-health-integration-resources-physician

Assisted Decision-Making (Capacity) Act 2015. (2015). https://www.irishstatutebook.ie/eli/2015/act/64

Baer, D. M., Wolf, M. M., & Risley, T. R. (1968). Some current dimensions of applied behavior analysis. *Journal of Applied Behavior Analysis, 1*(1), 91–97. https://doi.org/10.1901/jaba.1968.1-91

Beadle-Brown, J., Mansell, J., & Kozma, A. (2007). Deinstitutionalization in intellectual disabilities. *Current Opinion in Psychiatry, 20*(5), 437–442. https://doi.org/10.1097/YCO.0b013e32827b14ab

Breaux, C. A., & Smith, K. (2023). Assent in applied behaviour analysis and positive behaviour support: Ethical considerations and practical recommendations. *International Journal of Developmental Disabilities, 69*(1), 111–121. https://doi.org/10.1080/20473869.2022.2144969

Brothers of Charity Services Ireland Southern Region. (2024). *Fuller Lives/Safer Lives - Policy on Restrictive Practices*. Brothers of Charity Services Ireland, Southern Region.

Burney, V., Arnold-Saritepe, A., & McCann, C. M. (2023). Rethinking the place of qualitative methods in behavior analysis. *Perspectives on Behavior Science, 46*(1), 185–200. https://doi.org/10.1007/s40614-022-00362-x

Cianci, R. A., & Sevon, M. A. (2023). An introduction to a child's rights approach to applied behavior analysis. *Behavior Analysis in Practice*. https://doi.org/10.1007/s40617-023-00867-0

Council of Europe. (1950). *Convention for the protection of human rights and fundamental freedoms*. https://www.coe.int/en/web/conventions/full-list

Curry, K. (2013). The Sunland Training Centers: Florida's institutes for children with intellectual disabilities. *Florida Public Health Review, 10*, 14–24.

Delprato, D. J. (1995). Beyond Murray Sidman's coercion and its fallout. *The Psychological Record, 45*(3), 339–347. https://doi.org/10.1007/BF03395146

Didi, A., Dowse, L., & Smith, L. (2018). Intellectual disability and complex support needs: Human rights perspective for policy and practice. *The International Journal of Human Rights, 22*(8), 989–1006. https://doi.org/10.1080/13642987.2018.1485653

Disability Act (Vic), Pub. L. No. 23/2006 (2006). https://www.legislation.vic.gov.au/in-force/acts/disability-act-2006/048

Doody, C. (2009). Multi-element behaviour support as a model for the delivery of a human rights based approach for working with people with intellectual disabilities and behaviours that challenge. *British Journal of Learning Disabilities, 37*(4), 293–299. https://doi.org/10.1111/j.1468-3156.2009.00585.x

Emerson, E. (2009). *Quality and costs of residential supports for people with learning disabilities: A comparative analysis of quality and costs in village communities, residential campuses and dispersed housing schemes*. Hester Adrian Research Centre, University of Manchester. https://eprints.lancs.ac.uk/id/eprint/26190/

Felce, D. (2017). Community living for adults with intellectual disabilities: Unraveling the cost effectiveness discourse. *Journal of Policy and Practice in Intellectual Disabilities, 14*(3), 187–197. https://doi.org/10.1111/jppi.12180

Flynn, E., & Arstein-Kerslake, A. (2014). Legislating personhood: Realising the right to support in exercising legal capacity. *International Journal of Law in Context, 10*(1), 81–104. https://doi.org/10.1017/S1744552313000384

Goffman, E. (1961). *Asylums: Essays on the social situation of mental patients and other inmates* (1. Anchor Books ed). Anchor Books.

Goldiamond, I. (1974). Toward a constructional approach to social problems: Ethical and constitutional issues raised by applied behavior analysis. *Behaviorism, 2*(1), 1–84.

Gover, H. C., Hanley, G. P., Ruppel, K. W., Landa, R. K., & Marcus, J. (2023). Prioritizing choice and assent in the assessment and treatment of food selectivity. *International Journal of Developmental Disabilities, 69*(1), 53–65. https://doi.org/10.1080/20473869.2022.2123196

Hanley, G. P. (2010). Toward effective and preferred programming: A case for the objective measurement of social validity with recipients of behavior-change programs. *Behavior Analysis in Practice, 3*(1), 13–21. https://doi.org/10.1007/BF03391754

Health Service Executive. (2022). *National Consent Policy*. Health Service Executive. https://assets.hse.ie/media/documents/ncr/hse-national-consent-policy.pdf

Henrich, J. P. (2020). *The WEIRDest people in the world: How the West Became Psychologically Peculiar and Particularly Prosperous* (1st ed.). Farrar, Straus and Giroux.

Keenan, M., & Dillenburger, K. (2023). Advocacy and open science in the UK: Case studies in the Autism Wars. *Behavior Analysis in Practice*. https://doi.org/10.1007/s40617-023-00881-2

Kelly, B. D. (2019). *HEARING VOICES: The history of psychiatry in Ireland*. IRISH ACADEMIC.

Kelly, B. (2023). *Asylum: Inside Grangegorman*. Royal Irish Academy, Dub.

Kurki, V. A. J. (2019). A theory of legal personhood. In I. V. A. Kurki (Ed.), *A theory of legal personhood* (1st ed., p. 1-C0.P110). Oxford University Press. https://doi.org/10.1093/oso/9780198844037.003.0001

LaVigna, G. W., & Donnellan, A. M. (1986). *Alternatives to punishment: Solving behavior problems with non-aversive strategies*. Irvington Publishers.

LaVigna, G. W., Hughes, E. C., Potter, G., Spicer, M., Hume, L., Willis, T. J., & Huerta, E. (2022). Needed independent and dependent variables in multi-element behavior support plans addressing severe behavior problems. *Perspectives on Behavior Science, 45*(2), 421–444. https://doi.org/10.1007/s40614-022-00331-4

Layng, T. V. J. (2009). The search for an effective clinical behavior analysis: The nonlinear thinking of Israel Goldiamond. *The Behavior Analyst, 32*(1), 163–184. https://doi.org/10.1007/BF03392181

Leif, E. S., Subban, P., Sharma, U., & Fox, R. (2023). "I Look at Their Rights First": Strategies used by Australian behaviour support practitioners' to protect and uphold the rights of people with disabilities. *Advances in Neurodevelopmental Disorders*. https://doi.org/10.1007/s41252-023-00355-0

Levey, S. M. B., Miller, B. F., & deGruy, F. V. (2012). Behavioral health integration: An essential element of population-based healthcare redesign. *Translational Behavioral Medicine, 2*(3), 364–371. https://doi.org/10.1007/s13142-012-0152-5

Liberman, R. P., & LaVigna, G. W. (Eds.). (2016). *New directions in the treatment of aggressive behavior for persons with mental and developmental disabilities*. Nova Publishers.

Lovaas, O. I. (1987). Behavioral treatment and normal educational and intellectual functioning in young autistic children. *Journal of Consulting and Clinical Psychology, 55*(1), 3–9. https://doi.org/10.1037/0022-006X.55.1.3

Mansell, J., & Beadle-Brown, J. (2009). Dispersed or clustered housing for adults with intellectual disability: A systematic review. *Journal of Intellectual & Developmental Disability, 34*(4), 313–323. https://doi.org/10.3109/13668250903310701

McGill, P., Bradshaw, J., Smyth, G., Hurman, M., & Roy, A. (2020). Capable environments. *Tizard Learning Disability Review, 25*(3), 109–116. https://doi.org/10.1108/TLDR-05-2020-0007

National Collaborating Centre for Mental Health. (2020). *Challenging Behaviour and Learning Disabilities: Prevention and interventions for people with learning disabilities whose behaviour challenges NICE guideline 11 Methods, evidence and recommendations*. National Institute for Health and Care Excellence.

Oifig an tSoláthair, electronic I. S. (1937). *CONSTITUTION OF IRELAND*. Office of the Attorney General. https://www.irishstatutebook.ie/eli/cons/en/html

Pike, B., O'Nolan, G., & Farragher, L. (2016). *Individualised budgeting for social care services for people with a disability: International approaches and evidence on financial sustainability*. Health Research Board.

Punzi, E., & Steele, L. (Eds.). (2024). *Sites of conscience: Place, memory, and the project of deinstitutionalization*. UBC Press.

Quinn, A., Wood, A., Lodge, K.-M., & Hollins, S. (2023). Listening to the experts: Person-centred approaches to supporting autistic people and people with an intellectual disability in the mental health system. *BJPsych Advances, 29*(5), 308–317. https://doi.org/10.1192/bja.2023.31

Rajaraman, A., Austin, J. L., & Gover, H. C. (2023). A practitioner's guide to emphasizing choice-making opportunities in behavioral services provided to individuals with intellectual and developmental disabilities. *International Journal of Developmental Disabilities, 69*(1), 101–110. https://doi.org/10.1080/20473869.2022.2117911

Sidman, M. (1989). *Coercion and its fallout* (Rev. ed). Authors Cooperative.

Skinner, B. F. (1971). *Beyond freedom & dignity*. Hackett Pub.

Sturmey, P. (2015). *Reducing Restraint and Restrictive Behavior Management Practices*. Springer International Publishing. https://doi.org/10.1007/978-3-319-17569-0

Taylor, J. S. (2005). Introduction. In J. S. Taylor (Ed.), *Personal Autonomy* (1st ed., pp. 1–30). Cambridge University Press. https://doi.org/10.1017/CBO9780511614194.001

United Nations. (1984). *Convention against Torture and Other Cruel, Inhuman or Degrading Treatment or Punishment*. United Nations, Treaty Series, vol. 1465, p. 85. https://www.refworld.org/docid/3ae6b3a94.html

United Nations. (2006). *Convention on the Rights of Persons with Disabilities*. OHCHR. https://www.ohchr.org/en/instruments-mechanisms/instruments/convention-rights-persons-disabilities

United Nations General Assembly. (1948). *Universal Declaration of Human Rights.* https://www.un.org/en/about-us/universal-declaration-of-human-rights

Wilson, D. S. (2019). *This view of life: Completing the Darwinian revolution* (1st ed.). Pantheon Books.

Wolf, M. M. (1978). Social validity: The case for subjective measurement or how applied behavior analysis is finding its heart. *Journal of Applied Behavior Analysis, 11*(2), 203–214. https://doi.org/10.1901/jaba.1978.11-203

World Health Organisation, & United Nations High Commissioner for Human Rights. (2023). *Mental Health, Human Rights and Legistation. Guidance and Practice*. World Health Organisation. https://www.ohchr.org/en/publications/policy-and-methodological-publications/mental-health-human-rights-and-legislation

Part II
Interventions and Innovations in ABA

Chapter 5
The Impact of Changing Social Systems on Behavior Analytic Practice: Overcoming Barriers to Providing Socially Valid Behavioral Interventions

Traci M. Cihon

Abstract The rise in popularity of interventions based on behavior analytic principles for individuals with autism/autistic individuals has changed the contingencies for applied behavior analysis and practice. Systems-level practices and/or regulations have been established or have evolved by a variety of governing organizations (e.g., licensing boards and certifying organizations, university-based training programs in behavior analysis) and social systems (e.g., economic, education, health care). Many practices and/or regulations have been established or have evolved due to the need to serve increasing numbers of clients and those providing/coordinating the provision of services. These practices and/or regulations serve several functions—strengthening, evocative, and selective. They set the occasion for individual behaviors to be reinforced or punished, they restrict or expand the repertoire of potential responses that are likely to be emitted, and they condition or make different classes of reinforcers available. Practitioners, scientist-practitioners, students, researchers, and professors should be engaging in the complex contingency analyses that elucidate how these practices and/or regulations affect our contributions to the science, discipline, research, practice, and to the education and training of behavior analysts to ensure that we are engaging in a scientific approach to socially valid behavior change.

Keywords Autism · Behaviorally based interventions · Contingency analysis · Social validity

---

Portions of this manuscript were presented at the 2019 Association for Behavior Analysis International Autism conference. Please address all correspondence to traci.cihon@wmich.edu.

T. M. Cihon (✉)
Western Michigan University,
Kalamazoo, MI, USA

S. Halder et al. (eds.), *Applied Behavior Analysis-Based Interventions for Autism Spectrum Disorder*, https://doi.org/10.1007/978-981-95-2889-9_5

5.1 The Impact of Changing Social Systems on Behavior Analytic Practice: Overcoming Barriers to Providing Socially Valid Behavioral Interventions

I found my way to behavior analysis/behavior science (cf. Hantula, 2018) through its applications to enhance the lives of individuals with autism/autistic individuals and their families over 20 years ago.[1] My recent work in the area of autism intervention has been as the faculty advisor for a university-based initiative to support adults with autism, leading teams of graduate students to support an adolescent with autism in a home- and community-based program, serving as a resource and advocate for another young teenager with autism and his family, and a 15-year collaboration with the Università di Parma and Centro TICE to support their efforts in providing behavioral interventions for children and adolescents with and without disabilities in Italy. However, for the last several years, I have concentrated more on applications of behavior science to the education and training of behavior scientists and in promoting more socially-, economically-, and environmentally-just communities. Much of this work has been conducted from the lens of a recently defined and developing concentration area in behavior science—culturo-behavior science (CBS; cf. Cihon et al., 2021; Cihon & Mattaini, 2020).

From very early on in my career I knew that behavior science had broader applications and implications than autism interventions, and I was intrigued by the science—by the generality of the basic principles and by the potential for the natural science of behavior to "save the world" through its application to broader societal issues (e.g., Chance, 2007; Cihon & Mattaini, 2020; Dixon et al., 2018; Leigland, 2011; Mattaini, 2019; Rumph et al., 2005; Skinner, 1987). Nevertheless, supporting children with autism was the impetus for me to learn about behavior science. I also firmly believe that we need more broadly and comprehensively trained behavior analysts to serve individuals with autism and their families. Given the increasing prevalence of autism spectrum disorders and the growing interest from aspiring behavior analysts to engage this work, I often feel conflicted about shifting my professional activities. In fact, I still say yes to some opportunities to provide support for individuals with autism and their families or for students and colleagues. This chapter is one example.

In thinking about how to organize this chapter and what I could contribute to readers,[2] I reflected on my history in behavior science. Specifically, I recalled my early experiences entering into the field in through its application to autism service provision (see for example, Cihon et al., 2016 and Cihon et al., 2025), and later as a behavior scientist as I worked in different applications of the science (cf. Cihon,

[1] Different members of the neurodiverse population have different preferences for the use of person-first or identify-first language (cf. Devault, 2023). For brevity, this author has adopted the use of person-first language.

[2] This chapter is loosely based off an invited presentation from the Association for Behavior Analysis International (ABAI) Autism Conference in 2019.

2023a). I also reflected on how much the profession and practice of behavior analysis has changed and how quickly these changes have come about. My work in CBS led me to further ponder the impact these changes have had on what it means to be a behavior analyst/behavior scientist today, and more specifically on what it means to be practicing behavior analysis in the area of autism intervention today.

Sidman's (1998) talk for the Society for the Quantitative Analysis of Behavior entitled "The Scientist/Practitioner in Behavior Analysis: A Case Study" served as an additional inspiration for this chapter. Sidman reflects on his experiences moving from the nonhuman, basic operant lab to the clinical setting, working with individuals who had been institutionalized because of disability or mental illness and who had otherwise been considered unable to learn (see also Sidman, 2011). There were no programs, rules, instructions, or textbooks in applied behavior analysis at this time. There were no task analyses that described how to establish a previously neutral stimulus as a conditioned reinforcer, how to set up a system of token reward and exchange, or how to apply the basic principles of behavior analysis in a setting less controlled than the nonhuman operant lab, though more controlled than the community itself. One point that Sidman made resonated. He commented that, "...a number of the so called 'standard practices' are rarely practiced..." (Sidman, 1998, 4:10). Sidman is not the only scholar who has commented as to how changing contingencies have affected our science and practice and have led to changes in the repertoires of applied behavior analysts (e.g., Cihon, 2022; Cihon et al., 2025; Keenan et al., 2023; Keenan et al., 2010; Leaf et al., 2022; Leaf et al., 2016). Even though Sidman's comments focused on the contingencies operating on his behaviors and those of his team at the inception of applied behavior analysis, similar sentiments about behavior analysts—particularly about practitioners—from both inside and outside (e.g., Ram, 2020) of the discipline have persisted.

Given the longstanding, and perhaps increasing concerns (e.g., Bascom, 2014; Devita-Raeburn, 2016; Latimer, 2019; Lynch, 2019; Ram, 2020) that have proliferated the practice of behavior analysis and its applications with individuals with autism, I began to question why we, as an organized group of scientists and scientist-practitioners, have not taken a closer look at our behavior, analyzing the networks of contingencies embedded in the systems, practices, and regulations for our science, discipline, and practice, and especially how they have controlled and shaped our behavior and the cultural practices of our profession. Could we be making clearer predictions as to how different social systems, practices, and regulations might continue to shift, and how they might affect our behavior? Might we be able to shift our teaching, supervision, and mentoring practices proactively—preparing future generations of behavior analysts/behavior scientists to employ more socially valid interventions, despite the barriers to doing so? It seems, that as behavior scientists, we should know enough about behavior-environment relations that we could arrange the environment in such a way that we can reliably produce and foster the behavioral repertoires that continue to advance the science and the practice in ethical and socially valid ways. Is it not our responsibility, and perhaps even our moral imperative, to ensure that future generations of behavior analysts are taught to engage in the 'standard practices' and to arrange the environment and the networks of contingencies supporting our cultural practices such that we are engaging in a scientific approach to socially valid behavior change?

In considering these ideas, three questions emerged that became the focus of this chapter. First, what are some of the systems-level practices and/or regulations that have changed the contingencies for behavior analytic practice in autism intervention? Second, what have the effects of these practices and/or regulations been on our behaviors and practices, and how have they shifted the science, discipline, research, practice, and the education and training of behavior analysts/behavior scientists? Finally, how might we adjust our research, practice, and teaching to overcome the unwelcome or unintended effects (i.e., barriers) these practices and or regulations have had or might continue to have such that we can provide more socially valid behavioral interventions?

5.2 Personal and Historical Reflections on Changing Contingencies

I entered the field in 1998, at a moment when the power of behavior analysis to change the trajectory of a child with autism's life and that of their family was evident. The University of California-Los Angeles, Princeton, Rutgers, Emory, and others were leading behavior analysts in promoting a scientific approach to socially valid behavior change with individuals with autism (e.g., Harris & Weiss, 1998; McClannahan & Krantz, 1997; McGee et al., 1999; Smith & Lovaas, 1998). Behavior analytic interventions for children with autism were on the rise (e.g., Lovaas, 1987; Maurice, 1993). Although I was not early enough to see the pioneering work in the field, I was fortunate to have had the opportunity to learn from many who were.

As I was entering the field, parents of children with autism were suing school districts on the premise that instruction grounded in the principles of behavior analysis was the free and appropriate education that their children deserved (e.g., Wrightslaw, 1998). Consulting agencies were being established around the world to meet the growing need for qualified professionals to provide services. High school and university students across the USA were getting jobs as what we now call Registered Behavior Technicians (RBTs). There were already 40 years of the *Journal of the Experimental Analysis of Behavior* and 30 years of the *Journal of Applied Behavior Analysis* that I had not yet read. *The Analysis of Verbal Behavior* had also published years of research and theory regarding the environmental controlling variables for verbal behavior and successful applications to help individuals learn to talk, read, write, and sign that I needed to study.

There were some behavioral technologies available. Princeton Childhood Development Institute had published about using activity schedules to teach children with autism leisure skills and activities of daily living (e.g., McClannahan & Krantz, 1999). Iwata and colleagues (e.g., 1982/1994) had published numerous papers about their emerging technology to identify the controlling variables for severe problem behavior. Carr and Durand's (1985) functional communication training procedures were standard practice. And, we were all fairly certain that given the right conditions we could toilet train a child in just a day (cf. Azrin & Foxx, 1989).

Many early intensive behavioral intervention programs were heavily grounded in discrete trial training (e.g., Smith, 2001). It was already easier to train high schoolers and college students to deliver an instruction and a prompt, to wait for a response, and then provide a consequence of "no let's try again" or an edible or tangible stimulus paired with social praise than it was to teach them how to use shaping to establish a behavior not previously in the child's repertoire, or to organize the environment to create teaching opportunities as one might do with naturalistic behavioral interventions (e.g., Schreibman et al., 2015) or incidental teaching (e.g., McGee et al., 1999). Mand, tact, and intraverbal were not tossed around in our casual conversations.

Those who entered the discipline before me will recall changes in the contingencies for applied behavior analysts long before I came onto the scene, just as I am now for those just entering the field. Figure 5.1 shows a sample of some of the seminal events in the history of applied behavior analysis and its increasing adoption by caregivers and families of children with autism and their service providers. Within 10 years of the publication of Lovaas' (1987) seminal study, full degree programs in behavior analysis were starting to meet Association for Behavior Analysis International (ABAI) accreditation requirements (ABAI Accreditation Board, 2023), board certification for behavior analysts moved from individual US states to an international scope, and certification requirements were already shifting in an effort to increase the quality certified practitioners (cf. Johnston et al., 2017). Shortly thereafter, online education became more popular, skyrocketing in 2012 and again during and following the COVID-19 pandemic (cf. Hamilton, 2023). The prevalence of autism was (and is) on the rise (CDC, 2023), and states in the US moved forward approving insurance coverage for behavioral interventions for autism (see Callaghan & Sylvester, 2019). In just under 30 years, we saw behavior analysts struggle with what it means for a science to mature, tackling issues such as establishing criteria for minimum competence for practicing behavior analysts, establishing a certifying body tasked with developing criteria to evaluate and verify course sequences, organizing supervised practical experience standards, and developing an ethical and compliance code specific to behavior analysis (cf. Johnston et al., 2017; Sellers et al., 2023).

We have also seen a growing interest in behavior analysis from consumers and families affected by autism (BACB, 2023) as the prevalence of autism increases (CDC, 2023). Combined with increased funding opportunities in the USA for behaviorally based autism interventions due to insurance mandates (Callaghan & Sylvester, 2019), there has been a growing interest in studying behavior analysis and becoming certified, as evident in the increasing numbers of RBTs, Board Certified Assistant Behavior Analysts (BCaBAs), and Board Certified Behavior Analysts (BCBAs; BACB, n.d.).

- **1968:** First issue of the *Journal of Applied Behavior Analysis*.
- **1983:** Formation of the Florida Certification Board of ABA.
- **1987:** Publication of Lovaas' study.
- **1993:** First ABAI accredited program.
- **1994:** First Behavior Analyst Certification Board (BACB) Task List.
- **1998:** Second BACB Task List.
- **2001:** Indiana is the first state with insurance coverage for ABA.
- **2002:** Third BACB Task List.
- **2004-2009:** Incidence of autism is 1 in 166; rise of online education; first state introduces licensure for ABA; establishment of the Association of Professional Behavior Analysts; first issue of *Behavior Analysis in Practice*
- **2010:** Fourth BACB Task List; incidence of autism is 1 in 110.
- **2014-2016:** Incidence of autism is1 in 68.
- **2017:** Fifth BACB Task List.
- **2018:** Incidence of autism is 1 in 44.
- **2019:** BACB announces a shift away from an international focus.
- **2020:** Introduction of ABAI's Tiered Model of Education; incidence of autism is 1 in 36; initiation of the EuroABA Project.
- **2023:** Draft of APBA Accreditation Standards.

Fig. 5.1 Milestones in applied behavior analysis and behaviorally based interventions for individuals with autism

5.3 Unintended Consequences

The confluence of these variables has placed more demands and restrictions on faculty and university-based behavior analysis training programs to meet the increasing numbers of students and increasing demands of supervision requirements (cf. Dubuque & Dubuque, 2018; Sellers et al., 2019). This occurred in the context of changing university systems, asking faculty to do more with fewer resources and to navigate the nuances of teaching individuals how to change contingencies to promote desirable behavior without directly interacting with them given the increasing focus on online courses. Simultaneously, faculty members were balancing the need to advance a young science and to conduct higher rates of more innovative research with fewer resources and to publish in more prestigious journals to meet promotion and tenure contingencies at their respective institutions (see Cihon, 2023a; Cihon et al., 2023; Millem et al., 2000).

The professionalization of behavior analysis, particularly in its applications to autism intervention, and the increasing market demand further increased the need to establish of a number of systems-level practices and/or regulations, a variety of governing organizations (ABAI, 2023; APBA, n.d.; Johnston et al., 2017; Shook et al., 2002), and an influx of university-based training programs or course sequences in behavior analysis (see Dubuque & Dubuque, 2018; Garner et al., 2022; Silbaugh & El Fattal, 2022). Behavior analysts also found themselves interacting with different social systems than before—economic (cf. Broderick & Roscigno, 2021; Garner et al.; Keenan et al., 2010; Summers, 2021), education (e.g., Cihon et al., 2023; Heward et al., 1995; Vargas, 2020), and health care (cf. Garner et al.)—all of which further changed and intertwined the systems-level contingencies operating on our individual behaviors and organizational practices. Further, these changed contingencies created the need for more actors, sectors, and organizations to become involved in the training and supervision of behavior analysts as well as in service provision for individuals with autism. What was once comprised of interactions among ABAI, faculty members; students; consumers or clients; families; and an organization, home, or community-based organization has now more than doubled (e.g., universities, BACB, APBA, affiliate chapters of ABAI, insurance companies, private equity, BCBA supervisors, and more) who might be involved in regulating the profession, advancing the science, training and mentoring behavior analysts, providing and/or funding services, and more. This increase in the number of key actors and sectors involved has increased the complexity of the system and presented challenges with respect to the quality and consistency with which our science is applied.

Moreover, each of the actors, sectors, and organizations often faced and imposed competing contingencies between and among each other, sharing few goals or reinforcers. For example, the BACB could not increase the requirements to obtain credentials as a minimally competent behavior analyst fast enough. Struggling with the competing contingencies in effect from consumer demand and the needs of the science, which was also quickly becoming a profession, they gradually increased coursework and supervision requirements for those seeking certification while maximizing the number of certificants (cf. Johnston et al., 2017). University-based behavior analysis training programs and course sequences adjusted to increasing numbers of students, influenced by market demand, combined with pressure from college administrators to increase enrollment, build online programs, and do more with less (cf. Garner et al. 2022). Simultaneously, the BACB was asking faculty to do more individualized instruction with each university student (cf. Johnston et al., 2017). The contingencies were in direct competition with one another, creating positive feedback loops that accelerated the problems, and faculty faced impossible situations such as moving content online and sacrificing the junior colleague model (e.g., Heward et al., 1995; see the section entitled "Supervision") that had been employed for decades in the preparation of scientist-practitioners (cf. Dorsey & Harper, 2018).

Those who kept in-person courses tried to meet the increasing supervision requirements imposed by the BACB were doing so in a system that did not value and/or recognize low student-faculty ratios. Many faculty started to arrange practicum experiences outside of the university setting, with master's level practicing behavior analysts rather than doctoral level faculty advisors, as the doctoral level credential was no longer necessary for practice or supervision. Moreover, many of those providing supervision had been certified when the benchmarks for meeting the minimum competence were less stringent than what they were being asked to provide their mentees (e.g., attending a weekend workshop on behavior analysis was sufficient to sit for the certification exam).

Many students began to enter behavior analysis training programs because it led to a job in high demand or because it led to more favorable salaries than available in other helping professions (Burning Glass Technologies, 2015), rather than with an interest in the science itself or in advancing the science and broadening its applications. Often, we see students who apply to graduate training programs based on their stated desire to become a BCBA, as if checking this box is the penultimate goal rather than developing the repertoire necessary to be a skilled and compassionate behavior scientist. With the increasing costs of higher education in the USA, these students seek (and find) programs with the fewest number of courses (and lowest tuition) such that they can be eligible to sit for the certification exam as quickly as possible. These factors are often in direct competition with finding ABAI accredited programs that emphasize developing a full understanding of the relevance of basic principles in applied interventions and understanding how one person's behavior affects another person's behavior which is critical in being responsive to noticing how the contingencies they have arranged produce a significant change in their client's behavior (cf. Cihon et al., 2025; Leaf et al., 2016). This shift has permeated into our applied practice; and in some instances, has left profound impacts on the recipients of services.

One might conclude then, that not only are the so-called 'standard practices' Sidman (1998) referred to not being practiced, the standard practices are changing. The changed practices are also being practiced by greater numbers of behavior analysts. Graduates of behavior analytic training programs are going into the community with little knowledge of the basic principles or an understanding of why they are engaging in certain practices. We have fewer problem solving or analytical skills (cf. Kieta et al., 2019). And, we are providing behaviorally based interventions based on following procedures or rules that often impede sensitivity to the direct acting contingencies (cf. Cihon et al., 2025; Leaf et al., 2016), and the contingencies that can be discovered from an analysis of the relevant environmental controlling variables.

The problems we are facing as a science and as a profession are problems that few fully understand. In fact, many may not even see that there are problems. However, those who do see the problems, and recognize the depth and scope of the problems, are coming into contact with them more frequently. Perhaps it is by chance alone that I started to "notice" the problems and to see them more often. It is more likely, however, that it is because I was trained by those who saw the science and the practice when it was different. They showed me how to engage in a scientific approach to socially valid behavior change, and arranged the conditions such that I could differentiate between what applied behavior analysis was and what applied behavior analysis is now. Nevertheless, the problems are severe enough and frequent enough now that they are evoking my "noticing" on more occasions. Many other scientists, professionals, and community members have also "noticed" many of the same emerging problems.

For example, we have practitioners who are unable to identify which environmental variables need to be arranged in order to produce a more desirable repertoire than the one maintained by current contingencies without a written program or protocol or rule. At present, the field has researchers conducting studies that are simply demonstrations that reinforcement works under different conditions or with different populations and that we can bring different topographies of responses under stimulus control. Although this work has made some noted impacts, some might argue that different questions need to be asked to advance our science, improve our practice, or give practitioners empirically based techniques to help us solve some the more pragmatic problems. These limitations can be seen in the practices of insurance companies who provide only 8 hours to conduct an assessment for a new case or dictate the need to decrease direct service hours while still meeting certain goals or that reviewing graphs and updating treatment plans are not billable services. Practices we have simply accepted rather than collecting the evidence needed to show what we need to actualize the quality of intervention programs we once produced more reliably. We have faculty who are no longer providing supervised experiences for students because they cannot meet the demands of the faculty position along with the demands of the BACB. Even worse, we have clients whose repertoires are taught under the wrong stimulus control and whose repertoires are maintained under the wrong reinforcer control (Ala'i-Rosales et al., 2018). The result—79,544 BCBAs and 232,792 RBTs (BACB, n.d.) engaging in macrobehaviors, established, taught, and reinforced across generations of members of our own cultural system of behavior analysis who have produced and who are producing a cumulative effect, the effects of which are additive, and that have greatly shifted the direction of our science (see Glenn et al., 2016 for a further explanation of cumulative effects and culture-behavioral lineages).

5.4 Overcoming Barriers

Exploring some of the reasons for the aforementioned unintended consequences and why we have not yet overcome them could be instructional. For instance, building from what we have studied with respect to CBS and especially Behavioral Systems Analysis (BSA; cf. Houmanfar et al., 2021) and Cultural Systems Analysis (CSA; cf. Mattaini, 2019, 2020), we have considered each system, sector, or actor predominately in isolation rather than considering the interdependencies (e.g., Biglan, 1995; Mattaini, 2013) between and among the actors, sectors, and organizations involved in setting the standards for competent applied behavior analysts and for our practice and the networks of contingencies that support, maintain, or challenge the current cultural practices of our science (also see Cihon, 2023b). We overlook the interdependencies between and among the various actors, sectors, and organizations that are part of the cultural system that promote and perpetuate the macrobehaviors that contribute to the problems we are facing. M. Malott (2003) notes that in attempts to produce organizational change,

> we seem more comfortable if the department, process, or activity we want to change exists in isolation…[we] bypass the complexity caused by interacting with other departments, processes, or activities…we place walls where there were none…and create an illusion of simplicity and permanent results. (p. 23)

In examining the changing contingencies of our science and of our practice there are few intentionally designed interdependencies between and among the various sectors—the BACB increases supervision requirements without considering the impact on faculty work load, faculty design courses in response to the BACB task list without engaging with clinical service providers to determine the skill sets they seek in their employees, and clinical service providers create new practice standards without consulting with researchers or considering the basic science (see also Cihon, 2023b). There is a lack of shared purpose and shared reinforcers across the relevant sectors, organizations, and actors. Different stakeholders have moved forward, independent of one another, trying in our own ways to respond to the changing needs of the communities we serve producing an example of what M. Malott (2003) calls an organizational myopia, "to produce without realizing the purpose" as our organizations continued to change "without understanding its macrosystem and ultimate mission" (p. 48). For instance, we have blamed lazy or disinterested students (cf. R. Malott, 2005), noting that changing systems and organizational regulations and requirements have been imposed on us. We have blamed others for engaging in the behaviors that we have set the occasion for; the courses, training, and mentoring programs that *we* designed, and that are maintained by the systems-level practices and regulations that *we* established. We say, like Keller, that the student is always right but we do not behave accordingly. Each of us—practitioner, student, faculty member, supervisor, researcher—is responding to the contingencies that *we* have arranged or permitted to be arranged on our behalf.

Reflecting on the reasons we are facing these problems, one can see that designing a different path forward requires an examination of the evocative and selective effects of these systems-level practices and regulations, governing organizations, controlling agencies, and the how the changes to the education and training of behavior analysts have changed our repertoires. In doing so, we might find better ways to design our courses; improve instructional, supervision and mentoring practices; and enhance practice. We might be able to change the practices in ways that better meet the growing demand for our science and its applications while creating a future generation of behavior analysts/scientists whose practices are informed by the basic science, who are reinforced by advances in their consumers' repertoires and in advances in the science, and who are good stewards and representatives of both the science and its application.

5.4.1 Entry Points

One starting point is to examine the contingencies under which early behavior analysts came into contact with behavior analysis and consider how they are different than those operating on students who are now coming into contact with behavior analysis. Historically, we did not come into degree programs with an eye toward majoring in behavior analysis or the goal of obtaining a job as a BCBA. Instead, we took a course that happened to have a rat lab or we said yes to an opportunity to get a volunteer or paid position working with children with autism. Some of us were told that behaviorism was dead; some of us were fortunate enough to be at a university that employed a significant number of behaviorally inclined faculty. Many of us were *not* told that behavior analysis was something we could study. Behavior analysis did not have a prescribed academic program of study nor a streamlined career path.

Now, however, many students *know* about behavior analysis before they enroll in classes. They find universities with degree programs with a verified course sequenced or master's program in behavior analysis. They have worked as RBTs or know someone who has, and they aspire to be a BCBA not a behavior analyst let alone a behavior scientist. Academic advisors suggest behavior analysis courses to students with an interest in working with certain populations, and dissuade them if they have other interests (e.g., cultural and community applications of behavior science). Students have already declared a major/minor in behavior analysis or are considering switching majors or minors when they enroll in courses. Of course, not all of the students who come into our courses *know* something about behavior analysis. There is still a subset of students who find us serendipitously; who took the course because it filled a general education requirement, sounded interesting, or fit their schedule; and there are others who took the course because they thought it was like the behavioral analysis unit in Criminal Minds or the Irrational. Nonetheless, one development of systems-level changes like the professionalization, credentialing, and greater demand for the application of behavior analysis to early intensive intervention programs for individuals with autism, has been to forge a clear path toward employment as a BCBA. This, in turn, has changed how we teach behavior analysis.

5.4.2 Coursework

Another area for consideration is that our course content is more rigidly established and market-driven. A research methods course, for example, must cover specific experimental designs *in addition to* baseline logic. The same course may or may not cover how to create an experimental design less often or never before used that is based on the experimental question one wants to answer rather than teaching students to fit one's research question into an existing experimental design (Sidman, 1960). A verbal behavior course must cover conditioned motivating operations but does not necessarily have to cover potentiating variables; it must teach the mand, tact, intraverbal, and echoic but not necessarily transcription, the textual, the codic, the duplic, the sequelic, or the autoclitic. The course goals may have shifted from emphasizing the conceptual and theoretical underpinnings of Skinner's (1957) verbal behavior and/or Hayes et al.' (2001) Relational Frame Theory to the pragmatics of conducting commercially available assessments and designing teaching protocols around establishing less developed verbal repertoires, bringing different forms of responses under their respective stimulus controls. The changing systems-level practices and regulations have restricted the potential responses that might be emitted by faculty which in turn restricts the repertoires that are likely to be emitted by aspiring behavior analysts post-graduation.

5.4.3 *Clinical Practice*

Turning toward clinical practice, one issue we know is that there are not enough behavior analysts to meet the current demand. Alongside the insurance mandates in many states in the USA, behavior analysts can make a lot of money. One does not have to be an economist to see that given the demand exceeds the supply, nor does one have to be superlative in their duties do to get a good paying job. Comparing the average salaries for special educators with those for BCBAs illustrates this point. In 2023, the median salary for a special education teacher in the USA was $62,130 (range, $48,978 to $81,367; https://www1.salary.com/Special-Education-Teacher-Salary.html) while the average base salary for a BCBA was $85,571 (range, $70,000 to $89,500 with the potential to earn as much as $151,000; https://www.appliedbehavioranalysisedu.org/salaries).[3] For practicing behavior analysts, even those who did not enter into the science with money as their primary motivator, many fall prey to the financial contingencies that are now in effect.

Thus, the changing systems-level practices and regulations have made different classes of stimuli available as reinforcers. These reinforcers, in turn, have selective effects—money is contingent upon billable hours provided, not on client success, on advances to the science, or on effective supervision and mentoring practices. Given the choice between professions with fairly equivalent degree and training requirements, many choose behavior analysis over special education as their career choice, often based on access to a particular population or salary, not on the process distinctions or worldview that comes with behavior analysis (see also Keenan et al., 2010).

[3] It is not clear if these data included the same variables in their calculations such as benefits or lack thereof, if the salaries were pre- or post-tax, etc.

5.4.4 Supervision

Supervision practices have changed and may have exacerbated the problems. The junior colleague model has been powerfully effective in producing motivated, innovative, and conceptually strong repertoires for behavior scientists. Students worked closely with doctoral level faculty on research, teaching, and service/practice activities, developing as closely as possible the repertoire of their faculty advisor, and further extending that repertoire as it recombined with the skills and knowledge of other faculty members, interactions with students in their classes, and their own individual histories and experiences. Students took courses, some more and some less, but most of their training occurred in lab-based and experiential learning activities such as conducting research, providing clinical services to community partners, and serving as teaching or research assistants. In general, students of behavior analysis would receive the majority of their supervision from their doctoral level faculty advisor.

The establishment of certification for behavior analysts brought with it the need to indicate a particular number of courses and a specific number of supervised experience hours to determine when would be exam takers had met the minimum requirements to be eligible to apply to sit for the exam. These regulations, in addition to the market demand and the changing university contingencies, resulted in the adoption of new systems-level practices related to the supervision of aspiring behavior analysts (e.g., LeBlanc & Luiselli, 2016). Many faculty members stopped providing individual supervision that counted toward the BACB requirements as the response effort, financial costs, and time needed to maintain supervisor qualifications, meet the minimum number of hours and student-supervisor ratios, and paperwork requirements became too high in comparison to the credit they received from their respective institutions for providing supervision. Others standardized the supervised practicum experiences such that all students would go through the same experiences regardless of baseline repertoires, diverse learning histories, individual interests and skills, or areas in need of improvement. Still other training programs hired "Practicum Coordinators" or outsourced the supervision requirement for the BACB altogether.

Another consequence then of the changing systems-level practices and regulations is that more master's level behavior analysts, rather than doctoral level behavior analysts, came to supervise more aspiring behavior analysts. The changing supervision practices now closely parallel the supervised experience models adopted by special education programs (cf. Dubuque & Dubuque, 2018). This model, often referred to as the "student teaching triad" involves three people—the student teacher, a university supervisor, and a mentor teacher (e.g., Veal & Rikard, 1998). The university supervisor places the student teacher with a mentor teacher. The university supervisor and the student teacher meet on several occasions throughout the semester but the university supervisor and the mentor teacher rarely interact. The student teacher and the mentor teacher engage more regularly as they are in the same classroom. Mentor teachers are provided with some training or support for how to arrange the student teaching experience but more often they are left on their own. The student teaching supervision triad does not work very well according to data collected largely via qualitative research (cf. Lawson et al., 2015), with each member often responding to different and only infrequently interlocked behavioral contingencies. Behavior analysts are quick to point out the weaknesses, touting the sophistication and differential effectiveness of behavior analysis while our teaching and supervision processes become more similar—content rather than process focused (cf. Glenn & Malagodi, 1991)—despite the limitations of the supervision models.

5.5 Changing the Contingencies

The context and contingencies under which we study, teach, practice, supervise, and research behavior analysis have changed. These modifications have also changed our repertoires, sensitivity to reinforcers, and access to information and resources. We have changed the way we study, teach, and practice behavior analysis and the ways in which we supervise behavior analysts. These changes have produced unintended consequences, some that strengthen concerns related to the advancement of the science, the composition and outcomes of our graduate training programs, and our practice and service provision for individuals with autism.

Nevertheless, the networks of contingencies that comprise the different social systems, practices and regulations that govern our behavior (see Fig. 5.2) are in effect because of *our* behavior. Each of us are part of the complex social environments and the contingencies highlighted thus far. Moreover, it is *our* behavior that has produced these networks of contingencies. While it is often easier to remove oneself from the situation, to absolve oneself of having entered into any of the contingencies that are acting upon our behavior at this very moment, that have acted upon our behavior in the past, or that may act on our behavior in the future, and to think that *we* are not part of the problem or that there is not a problem at all; however, we have an ethical and moral responsibility to do better. Day (1977) wrote that, "if behaviorists are not now used to an examination of the contingencies governing their own behavior, *to an examination of their own motives,* as they say, then they should get used to it" (p. 19). As we consider how to move forward as a science, discipline, and field, we must act strategically to overcome the barriers to providing socially valid behavioral interventions. In doing so, we should look no further than the contingencies. Once we have acknowledged that *each one of us* are creating the problems facing our science and practice (see also Cihon, 2023b), we can start to apply our science to shift these contingencies to increase the probability that we continue to improve our science and practice, and promote more socially valid behavioral interventions.

Perhaps the most readily available place to start is to examine the contingencies surrounding the behavior of those currently practicing behavior analysis—the 79,544 BCBAs and 232,792 RBTs. Starting with a full recognition that these are

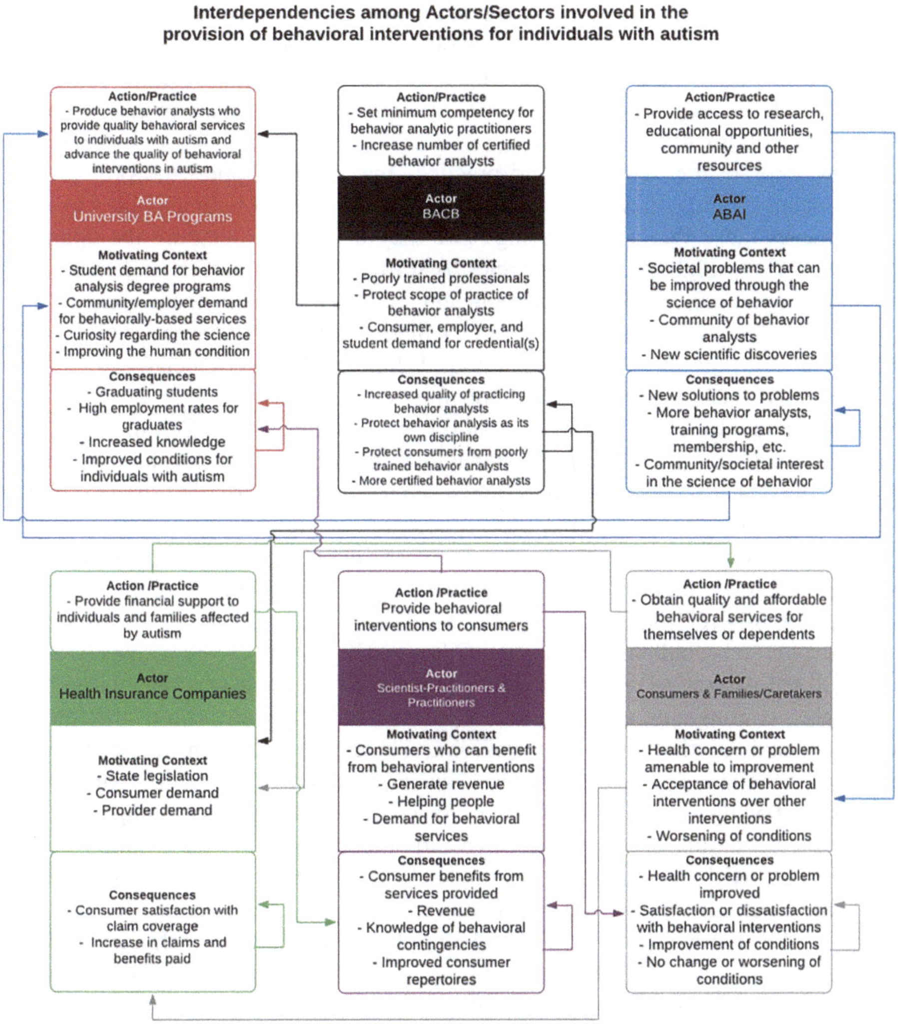

Fig. 5.2 Matrix analysis depicting key actors and sectors involved in the provision of behavioral interventions for individuals with autism, their behaviors and practices, motivating conditions, and consequences for the behaviors and practices, as well as some of the interlocking behavioral contingencies and interdependencies between and among them. For a copy of the matrix with print that can be enlarged, please reach out to traci.cihon@wmich.edu

often social contingencies (cf. Skinner, 1953), meaning that other key actors/sectors' behaviors and practices provide the antecedents and consequences for other key actors/sectors' behaviors; current practitioners can start by identifying the relevant actors and sectors, including themselves, that participate in what they do. Who is involved? Parents? Siblings? Administrators? What organizations? The BACB? Insurance companies? What are the macrosystems? Healthcare? Education?

Next, determine the behaviors and practices of the key actors/sectors before capturing the contingencies that promote, evoke, and sustain these behaviors and practices. Similar to the functional assessments conducted in clinical practice, what are the antecedents, motivating conditions, and consequences that operate on these behaviors and practices?

Now, explore the behaviors and practices that might support the provision of more socially valid behavioral interventions for individuals with autism. Are these the same as those that are occurring? Are they different? What are the opposing practices? How might the contingencies be shifted to encourage and select the supporting practices and to disrupt the opposing practices? What is the evidence?

Finally, identify any interactions, or lack thereof between and among the sector(s) needed to promote more effective action? What are the interdependencies? What contingencies may need to shift and how might one begin?

A matrix analysis (see Fig. 5.2; Biglan, 1995; Mattaini, 2013; Cihon, 2023b) can be used to create a plan to improve behavior analytic practice. Consider your reinforcers. It is ok if they are not the same as others or if they are not selfless, but it is not suitable to not know what they are and how they control your behavior. Contingencies affect behavior whether they are noticed or not; yet, being aware of the contingencies can provide information as to how one can organize their environment differently (cf. Skinner, 1974).

What we do is challenging (also see Cihon, 2022). There are no recipes or books that will tell us how to respond to every client in every situation. We rely on basic principles, contingency analyses, and data to guide the application of the science. How we navigate the barriers to providing a scientific approach to socially valid behavior change is up to us *and* it may have a profound effect on the future of our science and on the future of our practice. As we move forward, expanding the scope, reach, and versatility of our own science and practice, we must have humility (e.g., Cihon, 2022; Kirby et al., 2022; Neuringer, 1991). We have a powerful technology for behavior change but we are still a young science, an even younger practice, and there is a lot that we do not know including how we might fit within other disciplines, contexts, and service provision (e.g., geriatrics, home-health care, reducing youth violence, public policy, and more).

Be humble. Identify what you know but also recognize what you do not know. Engage in philosophic doubt. Question everything you think you know and find ways to keep learning. Identify a mentor. Build a community of practice. Partner with a university or a clinical service provider. Many of us were trained, supervised, mentored, or taught when the contingencies operating on the education and training of behavior scientist were different (cf. Cihon et al., 2025). We were exposed to different aspects of the science, when there were fewer restrictions in place, when the practice was younger and it was more closely tied to the science (see Sidman, 2011). The majority of the current practitioners, however, were trained after the contingencies had shifted to produce only minimally competent practitioners. For those readers, it may be even more important to doubt the things you think you know. The contingencies related to the education and training of behavior analysts have changed.

Our science is not going to save itself; the supply may soon exceed the demand and the demand may move toward less expensive and equally (or even less) effective interventions and supportsfor individuals with autism. It is long past time for us to examine the contingencies governing our own behavior. Perhaps even more importantly, it is time for us to take action. We can and *we must* do better.

References

ABAI Accreditation Board. (2023). *About the Association for Behavior Analysis International Accreditation Board.* https://accreditation.abainternational.org/about.aspx#:~:text=1993%3A%20ABAI%20accredited%20its%20first,for%20graduate%2Dlevel%20training%20programs

Ala'i-Rosales, S., Cihon, J. H., Currier, T. D. R., Ferguson, J. L., Leaf, J. B., Leaf, R., McEachin, J., & Weinkauf, S. M. (2018). The Big Four: Functional assessment research informs preventative behavior analysis. *Behavior Analysis in Practice, 12*(1), 222–234. https://doi.org/10.1007/s40617-018-00291-9

Association for Professional Behavior Analysts (APBA) (n.d.). *About us.* https://www.apbahome.net/page/About

Azrin, N., & Foxx, R. (1989). *Toilet training in less than a day*. Mass Market.

Bascom, J. (2014, March 24). *Quiet hands.* http://neuroqueer.blogspot.com/2014/03/quiet-hands-by-julia-bascom.html

Behavior Analyst Certification Board. (n.d). *BACB certificant data.* https://www.bacb.com/bacb-certificant-data/#demographic_data.

Behavior Analyst Certification Board (BACB). (2023). *US employment demand for behavior analysts: 2010–2022.* Author.

Biglan, A. (1995). *Changing cultural practices: A contextualist framework for intervention research.* Context Press.

Broderick, A. A., & Roscigno, R. (2021). Autism, Inc.: The autism industrial complex. *Journal of Disability Studies in Education, 2*(1), 77–101. https://doi.org/10.1163/25888803-bja10008

Burning Glass Technologies. (2015). *US behavior analyst workforce: Understanding the national demand for behavior analysts*. http://bacb.com/workforce-demand-report/.

Callaghan, T., & Sylvester, S. (2019). Autism spectrum disorder, politics, and the generosity of insurance mandates in the United States. *PLoS One, 14*(5), e0217064. https://doi.org/10.1371/journal.pone.0217064

Carr, E. G., & Durand, V. M. (1985). Reducing behavior problems through functional communication training. *Journal of Applied Behavior Analysis, 18*(2), 111–126. https://doi.org/10.1901/jaba.1985.18-111

Centers for Disease Control and Prevention (CDC). (2023, April 4). *Data & statistics on autism spectrum disorder.* https://www.cdc.gov/ncbddd/autism/data.html

Chance, P. (2007). The ultimate challenge: Prove B. F. Skinner wrong. *The Behavior Analyst, 30*(2), 153–160. https://doi.org/10.1007/bf03392152

Cihon, T. M. (2022). Editorial: Expanding our scientific lens in the search for humility and advancing a Culturo-Behavior Systems Science. *Behavior and Social Issues, 31*, 1–10. https://doi.org/10.1007/s42822-022-00112-3

Cihon, T. M. (2023a). Expanding. In R. A. Rehfeldt, T. M. Cihon, & E. Rasmussen (Eds.), *Women in behavior science – Observations on life inside and outside of the academy. Association for behavior analysis international book series: Behavior science: Theory, research, and practice.* Routledge.

Cihon, T. M. (2023b). Advancing research and practice in culturo-behavior science: A call to action. *Behavior and Social Issues, 32,* 39–359. https://doi.org/10.1007/s42822-023-00146-1

Cihon, T. M., Bedient, G. M., & Cihon, J. H. (2025). Developing and integrating a common vocabulary into staff training practices. In J. H. Cihon (Ed.), *Clinical handbook of autism intervention training* (pp. 107–134). Springer.

Cihon, T. M., Borba, A., Benvenuti, M., & Sandaker, I. (2021). Research and training in culturo-behavior science. *Behavior and Social Issues, 30*, 237–275. https://doi.org/10.1007/s42822-021-00076-w

Cihon, T. M., Cihon, J. H., & Bedient, G. M. (2016). Establishing a common vocabulary of key concepts for the effective implementation of applied behavior analysis. *International Electronic Journal of Elementary Education (Special Issue), 9*(2), 337–348.

Cihon, T. M., Kim, B. A., & Eshleman, J. W. (2023). Applied behavior analysis and college teaching. In J. Luiselli (Ed.), *Applied behavior analysis advanced guidebook: A manual for professional practice* (2nd ed.). Elsevier.

Cihon, T. M., & Mattaini, M. A. (Eds.) (2020). *Behavior science perspectives on culture and community*. Association for Behavior Analysis International book series: Behavior Science: Theory, Research, and Practice. Springer.

Day, W. (1977). Ethical philosophy and the thought of B. In F. Skinner, I. J. E. Krapfl, & E. A. Vargas (Eds.), *Behaviorism and ethics* (pp. 7–23). Behaviordelia, Inc.

Devault, N. (2023, Jan 18). "Autistic" vs. "Person with Autism": Let's Talk about Disability Language. *Ameridisability.* https://www.ameridisability.com/autistic-vs-person-with-autism-lets-talk-about-disability-language/

Devita-Raeburn, E. (2016, August 11). *Is the most common therapy for autism cruel?* https://www.theatlantic.com/health/archive/2016/08/aba-autism-controversy/495272/

Dixon, M. R., Belisle, J., Rehfeldt, R. A., & Root, W. B. (2018). Why we are still not acting to save the world: The upward challenge of a post-Skinnerian behavior science. *Perspectives on Behavior Science, 41*(1), 241–267. https://doi.org/10.1007/s40614-018-0162-9

Dorsey, M. F., & Harper, J. M. (2018). The application of the scientist-practitioner model in educating applied behavior analysts to meet the needs of children [Special Issue]. *Education and Treatment of Children, 41*(3).

Dubuque, E. M., & Dubuque, M. L. (2018). Guidelines for the establishment of a university-based practical training system. *Behavior Analysis in Practice, 11*, 51–61. https://doi.org/10.1007/s40617-016-0154-8

Garner, J., Peal, A., Klapatch-Totsch, J., & Gamba, J. (2022). Exploitation, freedom, and coercion: The integration of applied behavior analysis in a capitalist system. *Behavior and Social Issues, 31*, 174–189. https://doi.org/10.1007/s42822-022-00100-7

Glenn, S. S., & Malagodi, E. F. (1991). Process and content in behavioral and cultural phenomena. *Behavior and Social Issues, 1*, 1–14. https://doi.org/10.5210/bsi.v1i2.163

Glenn, S. S., Malott, M. E., Andery Benvenuti, M., Houmanfar, R., Sandaker, I., Todorov, J. C., Tourinho, E. Z., & Vasconcelos, L. (2016). Toward consistent terminology in a behaviorist approach to cultural analysis. *Behavior and Social Issues, 25*, 11–27. https://doi.org/10.5210/bsi.v25i0.6634

Hamilton, I. (2023, May 24). By the numbers: The rise of online learning in the U.S. *Forbes Advisor.* https://www.forbes.com/advisor/education/online-learning-stats/

Hantula, D. A. (2018). Behavior science emerges. *Perspectives on Behavior Science, 41*, 1–6. https://doi.org/10.1007/s40614-018-0163-8

Harris, S. L., & Weiss, M. J. (1998). *Right from the start: Behavioral intervention for young children with autism.* Woodbine House.

Hayes, S. C., Barnes-Holmes, D., & Roche, B. (Eds.). (2001). *Relational frame theory: A post-Skinnerian account of human language and cognition.* Kluwer Academic/Plenum Press.

Heward, W. L., Cooper, J. O., Heron, T. E., Gardner, R., & Sainato, D. M. (1995). Preparing research leaders for special education: A Ph.D. program with an emphasis in Applied Behavior Analysis. *Teacher Education and Special Education, 18*(3), 192–204. https://doi.org/10.1177/088840649501800307

Houmanfar, R. A., Fryling, M., & Alavosius, M. P. (Eds.). (2021). *Applied Behavior Science in organizations: Consilience of historical and emerging trends in organizational behavior management* (1st ed.). Routledge. https://doi.org/10.4324/9781003198949

Iwata, B. A., Dorsey, M. F., Slifer, K. J., Bauman, K. E., & Richman, G. S. (1982). Toward a functional analysis of self-injury. *Analysis & Intervention in Developmental Disabilities, 2*(1), 3–20. https://doi.org/10.1016/0270-4684(82)90003-9

Johnston, J. M., Carr, J. E., & Mellichamp, F. H. (2017). A history of the professional credentialing of applied behavior analysts. *The Behavior Analyst, 40*(2), 523–538. https://doi.org/10.1007/s40614-017-0106-9

Keenan, M., Dillenburger, K., Konrad, M. H., Debetencourt, N., Vuksan, R., Kourea, L., et al. (2023). Professional development of behavior analysts in Europe: A snapshot for 21 countries. *Behavior Analysis in Practice, 16*(3), 709–729. https://doi.org/10.1007/s40617-022-00754-0

Keenan, M., Dillenburger, K., Moderato, P., & Röttgers, H. R. (2010). Science for sale: But at what price? *Behavior & Social Issues, 19*, 126–143. https://doi.org/10.5210/bsi.v19i0.2879

Kieta, A. R., Cihon, T. M., & Abdel-Jalil, A. (2019). Problem solving from a behavior analytic perspective: Implications for educators. *Journal of Behavioral Education, 28*(2), 275–300. https://doi.org/10.1007/s10864-018-9296-9

Kirby, M. S., Spencer, T. D., & Spiker, S. T. (2022). Humble behaviorism redux. *Behavior and Social Issues, 31*, 133–158. https://doi.org/10.1007/s42822-022-00092-4

Latimer, O. (2019, August 31). *International day of protest against ABA: Gentle ABA is still abuse.* https://www.asparenting.com/international-day-of-protest-against-aba-gentle-aba-is-stillabuse/?fbclid= IwAR20N45D5RE0B6vD6GjWIQGJP8ulSMPCfPCu9q9NBaqEHQTjQAVSXJAAJ4I

Lawson, T., Çakmak, M., Gündüz, M., & Busher, H. (2015). Research on teaching practicum – A systematic review. *European Journal of Teacher Education, 38*(3), 392–407. https://doi.org/10.1080/02619768.2014.994060

Leaf, J. B., Cihon, J. H., Leaf, R., McEachin, J., Liu, N., Russell, N., Unumb, L., Shapiro, S., & Khosrowshah, D. (2022). Concerns about ABA-based intervention: An evaluation and recommendations. *Journal of Autism and Developmental Disorders, 52*, 2838–2853. https://doi.org/10.1007/s10803-021-05137-y

Leaf, J. B., Leaf, R., McEachin, J., Taubman, M., Ala'i-Rosales, S., Ross, R. K., Smith, T., & Weiss, M. J. (2016). Applied behavior analysis is a science and, therefore, progressive. *Journal of Autism and Developmental Disorders, 46*, 720–731. https://doi.org/10.1007/s10803-015-2591-6

LeBlanc, L. A., & Luiselli, J. K. (2016). Supervision practices [Special Section]. *Behavior Analysis and Practice, 9*(4), 271–348.

Leigland, S. (2011). Beyond freedom and dignity at 40: Comments on behavioral science, the future, and Chance (2007). *The Behavior Analyst, 34*(2), 283–295. https://doi.org/10.1007/bf03392258

Lovaas, O. I. (1987). Behavioral treatment and normal educational and intellectual functioning in young autistic children. *Journal of Xonsulting and Clinical Psychology, 55*(1), 3–9. https://psycnet.apa.org/doi/10.1037/0022-006X.55.1.3

Lynch, C. L. (2019, March 28). *Invisible abuse: ABA and the things only autistic people can see.* https://neuroclastic.com/2019/03/28/invisible-abuse-aba-and-the-things-only-autistic-people-can-see/

Malott, M. E. (2003). *Paradox of organizational change: Engineering organizations with behavioral systems analysis.* Context Press.

Malott, R. (2005). Behavioral systems analysis and higher education. In W. L. Heward, T. E. Heron, N. A. Neef, S. M. Peterson, D. M. Sainato, G. Cartledge, R. Gardner, L. D. Peterson, S. B. Hersh, & J. C. Dardig (Eds.), *Focus on behavior analysis in education: Achievements, challenges, & opportunities* (pp. 211–236) Merrill Prentice Hall.

Mattaini, M. A. (2013). *Strategic nonviolent power: The science of Satyagraha.* Athabasca University Press.

Mattaini, M. A. (2019). Out of the lab: Shaping an ecological and constructional cultural systems science. *Perspectives on Behavior Science, 42*(4), 713–731. https://doi.org/10.1007/s40614-019-00208-z

Mattaini, M. A. (2020). Cultural systems analysis: An emerging science. In T. M. Cihon & M. A. Mattaini (Eds.), *Behavior science perspectives on culture and community* (pp. 43–65). Springer.

Maurice, C. (1993). *Let me hear your voice*. Knopf.

McClannahan, L. E., & Krantz, P. J. (1997). Princeton child development institute. *Behavior and Social Issues, 7*, 65–68. https://doi.org/10.5210/bsi.v7i1.301

McClannahan, L. E., & Krantz, P. J. (1999). *Activity schedules for children with autism: Teaching independent behavior*. Woodbine House.

McGee, G. G., Morrier, M. J., & Daly, T. (1999). An incidental teaching approach to early intervention for toddlers with autism. *Journal of the Association for Persons with Severe Handicaps, 24*(3), 133–146. https://doi.org/10.2511/rpsd.24.3.133

Millem, J. F., Berger, J. B., & Dey, E. L. (2000). Faculty time allocation. *The Journal of Higher Education, 71*(4), 454–475. https://doi.org/10.1080/00221546.2000.11778845

Neuringer, A. (1991). Humble behaviorism. *The Behavior Analyst, 14*(1), 1–13. https://doi.org/10.1007/BF03392543

Ram, J. (2020, June 2). *I am a disillusioned BCBA: Autistics are right about ABA*. https://neuroclastic.com/2020/06/02/i-am-a-disillusioned-bcba-autistics-are-right-about-aba/

Rumph, R., Ninness, C., McCuller, G., & Ninness, S. K. (2005). Guest editorial: Twenty years later, commentary on Skinner's "Why we are not acting to save the world". *Behavior and Social Issues, 14*(1), 1–6. https://doi.org/10.5210/bsi.v14i1.117

Schreibman, L., Dawson, G., Stahmer, A. C., Landa, R., Rogers, S. J., McGee, G. G., Kasari, C., Ingersoll, B., Kaiser, A. P., Bruinsma, Y., McNerney, E., Wetherby, A., & Halladay, A. (2015). Naturalistic developmental behavioral interventions: Empirically validated treatments for autism spectrum disorder. *Journal of Autism and Developmental Disorders, 45*(8), 2411–2428. https://doi.org/10.1007/s10803-015-2407-8

Sellers, T. P., Seniuk, H. A., Lichtenberger, S. N., & Carr, J. E. (2023). The history of the behavior analyst certification board's ethics codes. *Behavior Analysis in Practice.* https://doi.org/10.1007/s40617-023-00803-2

Sellers, T. P., Valentino, A. L., Landon, T. J., & Aiello, S. (2019). Board Certified Behavior Analysts' supervisory practices of trainees: Survey results and recommendations. *Behavior Analysis in Practice, 12*(3), 536–546. https://doi.org/10.1007/s40617-019-00367-0

Shook, G. L., Ala'i-Rosales, S., & Glenn, S. S. (2002). Training and certifying behavior analysts. *Behavior Modification, 26*(1), 27–48. https://doi.org/10.1177/0145445502026001003

Sidman, M. (1960). *Tactics of scientific research: Evaluating experimental data in psychology*. Basic Books.

Sidman, M. (1998). *The scientist/practitioner in Behavior Analysis: A case study* [Video]. YouTube. https://www.youtube.com/watch?v=n6YxnRsU4Bs

Sidman, M. (2011). Can an understanding of basic research facilitate the effectiveness of practitioners? Reflections and personal perspectives. *Journal of Applied Behavior Analysis, 44*(4), 973–991. https://doi.org/10.1901/jaba.2011.44-973

Silbaugh, B. C., & El Fattal, R. (2022). Exploring quality in the applied behavior analysis service delivery industry. *Behavior Analysis in Practice, 15*, 571–590. https://doi.org/10.1007/s40617-021-00627-y

Skinner, B. F. (1953). *Science and human behavior*. Macmillan.

Skinner, B. F. (1974). *About behaviorism*. Vintage books.

Skinner, B. F. (1987). Why we are not acting to save the world. In *Upon further reflection* (pp. 1–14). Prentice Hall.

Smith, T. (2001). Discrete trial training in the treatment of autism. *Focus on Autism and Other Developmental Disabilities, 16*(2), 86–92. https://doi.org/10.1177/108835760101600204

Smith, T., & Lovaas, I. O. (1998). Intensive and early behavioral intervention with autism: the UCLA Young Autism Project. *Infants & Young Children, 10*(3), 67–78.

Summers, J. (2021, April 2). As private equity comes to dominate autism services… it's time to ask ourselves how long we want to keep rewarding bad behavior. *The Nation.* https://www.thenation.com/article/society/private-equity-autism-aba/

Vargas, J. S. (2020). *Behavior analysis for effective teaching* (3rd ed.). Routledge.

Veal, M. L., & Rikard, L. (1998). Cooperating teachers' perspectives on the student teaching triad. *Journal of Teacher Education, 49*(2), 108–119. https://doi.org/10.1177/0022487198049002004

Wrightslaw (1998, May 22). *The Special School District and the parents of a child with autism have agreed to a $133,000 settlement of the parents' case against the district* [Press Release]. https://www.wrightslaw.com/advoc/articles/news_asbury_lovaas_pressrelease_980713.html

Chapter 6
ABA-Based Intervention in Addressing the Challenging Behavior in Children with Autism

Santoshi Halder

Abstract The effectiveness and importance of functional analyses in identifying the cause or source of challenging behavior cannot be overstated. Although standard functional analyses are effective, they tend to be time-consuming and resource-intensive. Additionally, research shows that functional analyses are rarely conducted in early childhood education settings. Therefore, there is a critical need to explore alternative methods that can provide the same effectiveness as standard functional analyses while requiring less time and resources. Functional analyses play a crucial role in identifying the causes of problem behavior. While standard functional analyses are effective, they are often time-consuming and resource-intensive, and research shows they are rarely used in early childhood education settings. Thus, there is a need for alternative methods that maintain this effectiveness but require fewer resources. In this context, the study investigates the effectiveness of functional analyses to determine the function of challenging behavior in a child with autism within a classroom setting. The findings indicate that this approach is effective in identifying the function of head hitting. The study endorses the effectiveness of a trial-based identification of the challenging behavior and the design and implementation of a function-based intervention to successfully reduce the challenging behavior in the child with autism.

Keywords Functional analyses · Child with autism · Problem behavior · Head hitting · Challenging behavior

---

S. Halder (✉)
Department of Education, University of Calcutta, Kolkata, West Bengal, India

S. Halder et al. (eds.), *Applied Behavior Analysis-Based Interventions for Autism Spectrum Disorder*, https://doi.org/10.1007/978-981-95-2889-9_6

6.1 Background Literature

People with special needs often display disruptive behavior that impacts. More than 6.9% of children in special needs education engage in severe to moderate challenging behavior, impacting their teaching-learning, socialization, interpersonal relationships, social interactions. Many researchers reported existing interventions to be ineffective and time-consuming, primarily due to the interventions being designed without exploring the function or the source of the challenging behavior. Identifying the source of such behavior before designing an intervention can significantly enhance its effectiveness, allowing the educators to mediate the antecedents and consequences that contribute to enhancing their behavior responses (Iwata & Dozier, 2008). A thorough literature review shows that functional analysis (FA), an ABA (Applied Behavior Analysis) technique, is an effective method for determining the function source of behavior (Wilder et al., 2007). The traditional functional analysis is also limited in certain ways, leading researchers to explore alternative methods. While the effectiveness of standard FA has been confirmed in numerous studies, experts recommend modifying FA to be executed in the classroom or natural settings, which could be beneficial. Research indicates that the trial-based functional analyses, which may be considered a shorter version of the standard functional analysis (FA) can help identify the factors maintaining challenging behavior (Rispoli et al., 2014). A review of studies revealed an increasing need for and application of FA in naturalistic environments, such as homes and schools (Iwata & Dozier, 2008). Conducting the intervention execution in a child's natural, regular environment has its advantages and disadvantages that need more exploration (Kodak et al., 2013).

6.2 Functional Behavior Analyses (FBA)

The development of functional analysis (FA) by Iwata et al. (1982/1994) marked a significant milestone in applied behavior analysis (ABA). Before the introduction of FA, individuals often had to attempt multiple behavioral interventions before finding an effective one. Research indicates that both appropriate and inappropriate behaviors are conditioned or learned in an environment and maintained through behavior-environment interactions with social and physical environments categorized as reinforcement contingencies.

Functional behavior analysis (FBA) is used to identify the nature and sources of reinforcement of challenging behaviors. This thorough, systematic assessment serves as the foundation for ameliorating or designing an effective intervention strategy for reducing the targeted behaviors. The main goal of functional analysis (FA) is to pinpoint reinforcement contingencies so that effective interventions can be developed to decrease challenging behavior while promoting adaptive behavior. This can be achieved through three systematic strategies: (a) altering or changing the antecedent variables, (b) modifying the consequences, and (c) learning alternative behaviors (Cooper et al., 2007). FA is recognized as a "gold standard" for identifying the function of challenging behavior (Mace, 1994). FA explores the functional relationships between the challenging behavior and the environmental contingencies. During an FA, potential antecedents and consequences of the challenging behavior are organized through an experimental condition, allowing for the observation and measurement of their individual effects on the individual behavior (Cooper et al., 2007).

One of the most pertinent advantages of functional analysis (FA) is its ability to demonstrate the variables associated with problem behavior. However, conducting a traditional FA has several limitations. Though there is ample evidence of the effectiveness and reliability of the FA procedure (Iwata et al., 1982/1994) but achieving controlled environments in educational settings can be challenging. Research has found that traditional FA assessments may temporarily strengthen or reinforce the challenging behavior during the experimental sessions (Carr et al., 2009). Additionally, some behaviors may be less suitable for implementing FA if they occur infrequently (Kelly et al., 2003). Furthermore, FAs conducted in contrived settings may disregard factors that increase the likelihood of challenging behavior in natural environments (Lang et al., 2008). Moreover, Lang et al. (2008) noted that as FAs are not conducted in naturalistic settings, an individual's behavior may appear atypical until they have adjusted to the conditions. Given these limitations, researchers have speculated about alternatives that can maintain the same effectiveness as traditional FA. Research shows that a brief trial-based FBA can effectively identify the maintaining contingencies of a disruptive behavior (Wilder et al., 2006).

6.3 Trial-Based Functional Analysis

Trial-based FBA (Bloom et al., 2011) is a shorter version of the traditional FA method designed to bridge the gap between research and practice in a regular natural setting. Trial-based FA is conducted through brief trials during an individual's regular routine in their natural setting. Findings on the accuracy of trial-based FA indicate a 60% accuracy in identifying the functions as the standard FA. This suggests that trial-based FA may serve as a suitable alternative when the standard functional analysis cannot be conducted or is not feasible (Bloom et al., 2011).

6.4 Literature Review

Hanley et al. (2003) conducted a thorough literature review of 5 years of data from 1961 to 2000 and found a steep increase in FA, indicating the popularity of the use of FA strategies over the years for assessing the function of the targeted behavior with various types and natures of disabilities (Baker et al., 2006; Dwyer-Moore & Dixon, 2007). It was also found that the self-injurious behavior (SIB) was reported to be the most frequently reported by Hanley et al. (2003). The importance and generality of functional analysis procedures established in numerous studies suggest that assessment based on an FA might be useful in identifying the source of reinforcement for self-injurious behavior (SIB) and subsequently, in designing more effective interventions to eliminate or alter the contingency maintaining the challenging behavior.

The primary advantage of functional analysis (FA) is its ability to demonstrate the variables associated with the challenging behavior. However, conducting a traditional FA has several limitations, as achieving controlled environments in educational settings can be challenging (Iwata et al., 1982/1994). Traditional FA assessments may temporarily strengthen or reinforce problem behavior during the sessions (Carr et al., 2009). FAs conducted in contrived settings may overlook factors that increase the likelihood of challenging behavior in natural environments (Lang et al., 2008). Finally, Lang et al. (2008) noted that an individual's behavior may appear atypical until they have adjusted to the conditions due to the lack of natural or environmental settings. Given these limitations of traditional FA, researchers have speculated about possible alternatives that can maintain the same effectiveness. While the utility of the standard FA is well-documented in numerous studies, there is a growing interest in modifying it to be used in classrooms or natural settings with familiar individuals serving as therapists. Research indicates that brief trial-based functional analyses can be effectively used to identify the maintaining variables for identifying the challenging behavior (Wilder et al., 2006).

6.5 Trial-Based Functional Behavior Analysis

Trial-based functional analysis (Bloom et al., 2011) is a newly developed method designed to bridge the gap between research and practical application in educational settings. Sigafoos and Saggers (1995), in their study, used a discrete trial format in classroom settings for identifying whether the aggressive behavior served an attention or escape function, by conducting the trial-based functional analysis during a child's natural, regular environment. Although many studies explore the utility of FA, there is very little work on early childhood or preschool children. While Iwata and Dozier (2008) reported that FAs conducted outside of natural settings can effectively identify the functions of behavior for treatment development, critics argue that controlled environments may lack the stimuli present in natural settings, potentially leading to inaccurate results (Lang et al., 2008). Lambert and Bloom (2012) conducted trial-based FAs to identify the functions of challenging behavior in early childhood special needs education. All trial-based FAs successfully identified the function of the behavior and the subsequent functional communication training (FCT), resulting in reductions in problem behavior and increases in communication skills. Bloom et al. (2011) conducted a functional analysis in classroom settings involving ten students with challenging behavior, who were assessed through a series of trials interspersed throughout the school day. Results suggest that trial-based functional analysis may be an appropriate assessment method when the resources required for a standard functional analysis are limited or unavailable. Hence, the trial-based functional analyses of challenging behavior represent a variation of traditional functional analyses and have gained importance in empirical research for their numerous advantages (Rispoli et al., 2014). Regardless of the type of FA employed, assessing behavior in naturalistic settings presents potential advantages and disadvantages (Kodak et al., 2013). Therefore, further research extending FA into children's natural settings is crucial for addressing the limitations of standard FA.

6.6 Methodology

6.6.1 Objectives of the Study

- Identify the function of the targeted head-hitting behavior through trial-based functional analysis (FA), in a regular classroom setting.
- Effectiveness of the trial-based functional analysis by a suitable function-based intervention.

6.6.2 Participant

A 7-year-old child with autism from a special school was identified for the study on self-injurious behavior, specifically head hitting. The child had no verbal communication skills.

6.6.3 Setting for the Research

All the FA sessions were conducted in the child's natural classroom setting.

6.6.4 Response Measurement

The researcher collected data on the occurrence of head hitting during both control and trial segments.

6.6.5 Self-Injurious Behavior

Head-hitting behavior is operationally defined as the child hitting his head against his own body, another person, or a solid object.

6.6.6 Research Design

A multi-element design trial-based functional assessment was used for the implementation of the trial-based functional analysis. A changing criterion design was used for the function-based intervention.

6.6.7 Duration of Research

The study was completed in Forty-five days (approximately).

6.6.8 Potential Hazards/Risks

Conducting a functional assessment (FA) may temporarily increase the frequency or intensity of behaviors, which poses a potential risk. Parents were informed of this risk, and any threatening situations during the assessment led to immediate session termination for safety.

6.6.9 *Experimental Method*

6.6.9.1 Trial-Based Functional Analysis (FA)

The trial-based functional analysis (FA) consists of four conditions: Attention, Demand, Alone, and Tangible, conducted over sessions. Each trial lasted for 4 minutes, with 2 minutes dedicated to a control condition and 2 minutes for the test condition. A total of ten sessions were conducted for each condition across five days.

The four conditions of the FA are (a) *Attention Condition:* Control segment; the teacher interacted with the child and a moderately preferred item was available. During the test segment, the teacher turned away and stated she had work to do. (b) *Demand Condition:* Control segment; the child was seated without any preferred items & if the child exhibited challenging behavior, the trial was terminated without any consequences. Test segment: The teacher presented tasks, and the trial was terminated if any challenging behavior occurred. (c) *Tangible Condition:* Control segment; the teacher is present with the child with a preferred item. Test segment: The teacher removed the preferred item for 2 minutes, returning it immediately if any challenging behavior was observed. (d) *Alone Condition:* The child is left alone for two consecutive 2-minute segments, without any items or activities. Challenging behavior had no consequences and did not lead to the termination of the trial.

6.7 Function-Based Intervention

Once the function of the targeted behavior is identified, an intervention based on the function of the behavior is designed based on the FA. This intervention adhered to the evidence-based practices outlined by Tiger et al. (2008). The intervention lasted for 2 hours, over 3–4 weeks. They were conducted in a designated area of the school during various activities, such as free play, ensuring that motivating operations were in place. Treatment sessions continued until stable behavior was observed, allowing for an assessment of the intervention's effectiveness. If a decrease in the targeted challenging behavior was noted, it indicated that the trial-based FA had correctly identified the source or function of the behavior. A function-based intervention was designed following the identification that included various ABA components/strategies: (a) Functional Communication Training (FCT), (b) Differential Reinforcement of Alternative Behavior (DRA), and (c) Extinction (EXT), organized into different phases to promote effective implementation. The same researcher conducted both the FA and the function-based intervention sessions with the child. Baseline data were collected until a stable baseline was reached and noted. The antecedents and consequences used during the baseline period were consistent with those in the test segment of the FA associated with the highest level of responding. During the baseline, no FCT responses were observed from the participant.

6.8 Intervention for Tangible Function

6.8.1 Setting/Environment

The intervention was primarily conducted in a designated place with the child having access to various preferred items and activities. Efforts were made to eliminate all escape-motivating operations (MOs) and any stimuli that could provoke disruptive behavior. No demands other than those directly related to the intervention were placed on the child. The setting or the environment was enriched with a variety of highly preferred reinforcers based on systematic reinforcer assessment. The goal was to provide the child with more alternative options or choices in the environment.

6.8.2 Functional Communication Training (FCT)

Functional communication training (FCT) is one of the most widely used effective differential reinforcement strategies recognized in the literature (Lambert & Bloom, 2012; Wacker et al., 2011). FCT is a differential reinforcement strategy where the child learns an alternative response resulting in the same reinforcer as maintaining the challenged behavior while the challenging behavior is placed on extinction (meaning it is no longer reinforced). The FCT intervention was carried out in three stages. First, a functional analysis was performed to find the environmental circumstances that reinforce the challenging behavior and the conditions that trigger it, followed by a physical prompt with a progressive delay to teach a socially appropriate alternative communicative response. The child is reinforced with the same reinforcer that maintained the problem behavior. The child learned to request functional reinforcers using the alternative communication method. The ultimate goal was to generalize the learnt alternative functional communication across various settings. Whenever the child engaged in head-hitting behavior, he was redirected and taught to use manual signs to request what they wanted. This process continued until the child could independently use appropriate requests (mands) without resorting to head hitting. The child learned various mands for things like "swing" and "push" through manual signs, receiving immediate reinforcement for each successful communicative response.

6.8.3 Differential Reinforcement of Alternative Behavior (DRA)

This intervention reinforces desirable behaviors that serve as alternatives to targeted behaviors for reduction, while withholding reinforcement for the challenging behavior (Cooper et al., 2007). The child was instructed to put their "hands in pockets," followed by a reinforcer. In differential reinforcement of alternative behavior (DRA), trainers reinforce acceptable alternative behaviors, even if they are not incompatible with the challenging behavior (Cooper et al., 2007). The child was prompted every 2 min to exhibit the alternative behavior, receiving immediate reinforcement with the same rewards used for the problem behavior. Mastery criteria required the child to independently engage in positive, socially acceptable behaviors. The child was prompted to exhibit this alternative behavior ("hands in pockets") every 2 min and was immediately reinforced with the same reinforcer that maintained the targeting challenging behavior. Continuous reinforcement was provided for the alternative behavior. Mastery criteria required that the child independently engage in positive, socially acceptable behaviors (such as appropriate mands) instead of head-hitting behavior (self-injurious behavior).

6.8.4 *Extinction*

This intervention involves stopping the reinforcement of previously reinforced behaviors (Cooper et al., 2007). In this case, the child was ignored and turned away from when they engaged in self-injurious behavior (SIB), while appropriate behaviors were reinforced. Consequently, terminating reinforcement during head-hitting behavior contributed to its maintenance. In severe cases, physical blocking was used to prevent the behavior.

6.8.5 *Reinforcement Schedule*

The intervention began with a dense reinforcement schedule and gradually shifted to an intermittent reinforcement schedule. In the first phase, functional communication training (FCT) was reinforced at a fixed ratio (FR) of 1, and differential reinforcement of alternative behaviors (DRA) at a fixed interval (FI) of 5 s. This changed to an FR of 10 and an FI of 10 s in the second phase, and the third phase, to an FR of 30 and an FI of 30 s. During the second phase, the child learned to "wait" and was encouraged to keep their hands in their pockets while being reinforced for independent responses. The goal was to increase the duration for which the child kept their hands in their pockets while managing problematic behavior. The reinforcement schedule was further thinned in the third phase.

6.8.6 Inter-Observer Agreement (IOA)

IOA was conducted according to guidelines from the Behavior Analyst Certification Board (BCBA). Two experienced observers collected data during 100% of trial-based functional analysis (FA) sessions, achieving 100% IOA. For the function-based intervention, IOA recorded 70% of sessions, ranging from 95% to 100%. Data were reliable with at least 80% agreement, and IOA for all assessments ranged from 90% to 100%, indicating strong reliability (see Appendix C for the IOA data sheet). An independent observer, trained by the researcher, recorded data for 30% of trial-based functional analyses (FAs) to assess whether problem behavior led to the premature discontinuation of segments based on control and test conditions. Treatment integrity for these FAs ranged from 95% to 100%.

For function-based intervention sessions, treatment integrity data were collected during 40% of the sessions to determine if alternate behaviors effectively produced breaks or attention. When problem behaviors occurred, the researcher implemented extinction by terminating reinforcement. The treatment integrity for the function-based interventions ranged from 80% to 90%. The IOA was calculated by the following formulae:

6.9 Results & Interpretation

Figure 6.1 displays the functional communication training (FCT) results for the participant. Analysis revealed that, apart from the ignore condition, challenging behavior was more frequent during test segments. High and stable levels of problem behavior occurred in the demand and tangible conditions, with none observed in the alone and attention conditions. This suggests the behavior was reinforced by access to preferred items or escape from tasks or demands. The child showed head-hitting behavior at its highest level (100%) during the test segment of the tangible condition and also displayed behaviors during the test (36.36%) and control (18%) segments of the demand trials. Figure 6.2 shows that during the intervention, the participant successfully learned FCT responses and received reinforcement for alternative behaviors, resulting in a significant decrease in head-hitting occurrences from 161 during baseline to an average of 5 per hour.

This study emphasizes the effectiveness of trial-based functional analysis (FA) in identifying the reasons behind head-hitting behavior in a child with Autism in a classroom environment (Bloom et al., 2011). Trial-based FA is particularly beneficial in early childhood stages because it allows for brief assessments during a natural, regular classroom environment (Sigafoos & Saggers, 1995). By clarifying the functions of problematic behaviors, interventionists can effectively implement differential reinforcement strategies (Pelios et al., 1999). Conducting a functional analysis followed by functional communication training has been found to be highly effective in reducing problem behaviors (Asmus et al., 2001; Kurtz et al., 2003;

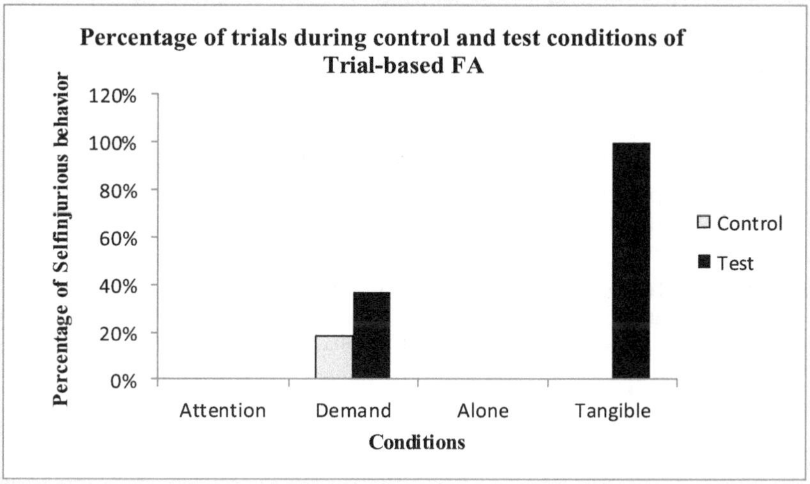

Fig. 6.1 The results of trial-based functional analysis of the participant

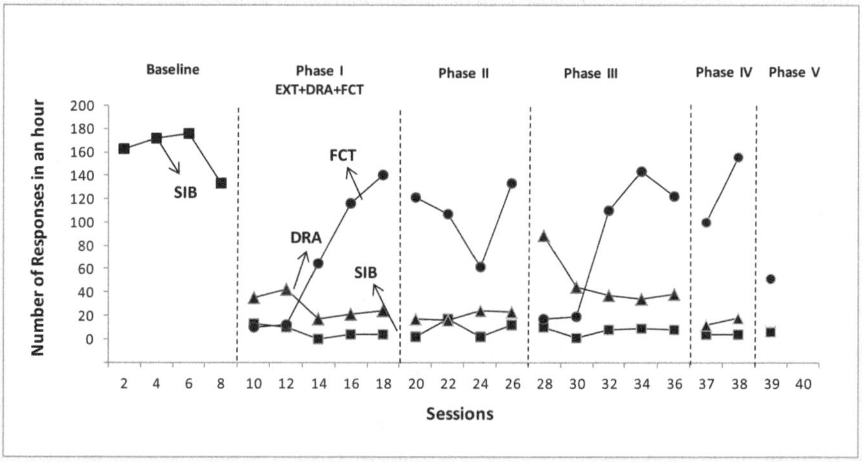

Fig. 6.2 Function-based intervention of the participants during baseline & intervention sessions (*FCT* Functional Communication Training, *EXT* Extinction)

Wacker et al., 1998). The findings support the use of function-based interventions in classrooms, providing educators with a solid basis for applying trial-based FA over more traditional methods. The study successfully identified two functions of the problem behavior and implemented an effective intervention plan. This demonstrates that trial-based FAs can enhance functional communication while reducing problem behaviors. This method can also be applied in various natural settings, warranting further research (Wacker et al., 2005).

6.9.1 Delimitations of the Study

While the researcher effectively addressed all functions with follow-up support, these results are not detailed due to time constraints. The study was limited to a classroom setting and did not extend to home environments, which could yield additional insights and challenges. Thus, results should be replicated in different settings and with other populations. The demand function of the target behavior is also not reported due to limited time.

Acknowledgment The work was carried on at Amrit Somani Autism Center, ASMC, Kolkata, West Bengal, India. I acknowledge the support and assistance provided by Namita Somani, ASMC, and Julianne Bell, BCBA, Former Director, ASMC, Kolkata, West Bengal, India

References

Asmus, J. M., Ringdahl, J. E., Sellers, J. A., Call, N. A., Andelman, M. S., & Wacker, D. P. (2001). Use of a short-term inpatient model to evaluate aberrant behavior: Outcome data summaries from 1996 to 2001. *Journal of Applied Behavior Analysis, 37*, 283–304.

Baker, J. C., Hanley, G. P., & Mathews, R. M. (2006). Staff-administered functional analysis and treatment of aggression by an elder with dementia. *Journal of Applied Behavior Analysis, 36*, 469–474.

Bloom, S. E., Iwata, B. A., Fritz, J. N., Roscoe, E. M., & Carreau, A. B. (2011). Classroom application of a trial-based functional analysis. *Journal of Applied Behavior Analysis, 44*(1), 19–31.

Carr, J. E., LeBlanc, L. A., & Love, J. R. (2009). Experimental functional analysis of problem behavior. In W. T. O'Donohue & J. E. Fisher (Eds.), *Cognitive behaviour therapy: Applying empirically supported techniques in your practice* (2nd ed., pp. 211–221). Wiley.

Cooper, J. O., Heron, T. E., & Heward, W. L. (2007). *Applied behavior analysis* (2nd ed.). Pearson Education.

Dwyer-Moore, K., & Dixon, M. (2007). Functional analysis and treatment of problem behavior of elderly adults in long-term care. *Journal of Applied Behavior Analysis, 40*, 679–683.

Hanley, G. P., Iwata, B. A., & McCord, B. E. (2003). Functional analysis of problem behavior: A review. *Journal of Applied Behavior Analysis, 36*, 147–185.

Iwata, B. A., Dorsey, M. F., Slifer, K. J., Bauman, K. E., & Richman, G. S. (1982/1994). Towards a functional analysis of self-injury. *Journal of Applied Behavior Analysis, 27*, 197–209.

Iwata, B. A., & Dozier, C. (2008). Clinical application of functional analysis methodology. *Behavior Analysis in Practice, 1*, 1–9. 35.

Kelly, M., Reitman, D., & Noell, G. R. (2003). *Practitioners guide to empirically based measures of school behavior*. Kluwer Academic and Plenum Press.

Kodak, T., Fisher, W. W., Paden, A., & Nitasha Dickes, N. (2013). Evaluation of the utility of a discrete-trial functional analysis in early intervention classrooms. *Journal of Applied Behavior Analysis, 46*(1), 301–306.

Kurtz, P. F., Chin, M. D., Huete, J. M., Tarbox, R. S. F., O'Connor, J. T., Paclawskyj, T. R., & Rush, K. S. (2003). Functional analysis and treatment of self-injurious behavior in young children: A summary of 30 cases. *Journal of Applied Behavior Analysis, 36*, 205–219.

Lambert, J. M., & Bloom, S. E. (2012). Trial-based functional analysis and functional communication training in an early childhood setting. *Journal of Applied Behavior Analysis, 45*(3), 579–584.

Lang, R., O'Reilly, M. F., Lancioni, G., Machalicek, W., Rispoli, M., & Chan, J. (2008). A comparison of functional analysis results when conducted in contrived versus naturalistic settings. *Journal of Applied Behavior Analysis, 41*, 441–445.

Mace, F. C. (1994). The significance and future of functional analysis methodologies. *Journal of Applied Behavior Analysis, 27*, 385–392.36

Pelios, L., Morren, J., Tesch, D., & Axelrod, S. (1999). The impact of functional analysis methodology on treatment choice for self-injurious and aggressive behavior. *Journal of Applied Behavior Analysis, 32*, 185–195.

Rispoli, M., Ninci, J., Neeli, L., & Jaini, S. (2014). A systematic review of trial-based functional analyses of challenging behaviour. *Journal of Physical Developmental Disabilities, 26*, 271–283.

Sigafoos, J., & Saggers, E. (1995). A discrete-trial approach to the functional analysis of aggressive behavior in two boys with autism. *Australia & New Zealand Journal of Developmental Disabilities, 20*, 287–297.

Tiger, J. H., Hanley, G. P., & Bruzek, J. (2008). Functional communication training: A review and practical guide. *Behavior Analysis in Practice, 1*, 16–23.

Wacker, D. P., Berg, W. K., Harding, J. W., Barretto, A., Rankin, B., & Ganzer, J. (2005). Treatment effectiveness, stimulus generalization, and acceptability to parents of functional communication training. *Educational Psychology, 25*(2–3, 233), –256.

Wacker, D. P., Berg, W. K., Harding, J. W., Derby, K. M., Asmus, J. M., & Healy, A. (1998). Evaluation and long-term treatment of aberrant behavior displayed by young children with disabilities. *Journal of Developmental and Behavioral Pediatrics, 19*, 260–266.

Wacker, D. P., Harding, J. W., Berg, W. K., Lee, J. F., Schieltz, K. M., Padilla, Y. C., Nevin, J. A., & Shahan, T. A. (2011). An evaluation of persistence of treatment effects during long-term treatment of destructive behavior. *Journal of the Experimental Analysis of Behavior, 96*, 261–282.

Wilder, D. A., Chen, L., Atwell, J., Pritchard, J., & Weinstein, P. (2006). Brief functional analysis and treatment of tantrums associated with transitions in preschool children. *Journal of Applied Behavior Analysis, 39*, 103–107.

Wilder, D. A., Harris, C., Reagan, R., & Rasey, A. (2007). Functional analysis and treatment of noncompliance by preschool children. *Journal of Applied Behavior Analysis, 40*, 173–177.

Chapter 7
Innovative Interventions for Common Behaviors Utilizing a New Competing Pathways Chart

Laura A. Riffel and Karen L. Gischlar

Abstract This chapter utilizes an approach to the development of behavior support plans that is based upon the competing pathways model often used in applied behavior analysis. Our framework, the Triple T-Triple R, simplifies the competing pathways method with use of more accessible language and an easier to use graphic. The new chart is demonstrated through the use of case studies from the authors' work to provide real-world applications. The chapter explains the necessity of determining the function, or why, of a behavior and how to teach a functionally equivalent replacement behavior. Finally, the chapter explains how to structure environments for student success through manipulating antecedents (in our model "triggers") and applying reinforcement (or, impacTs in our revised pathways model). We provide examples and resources that should render our model readily accessible to teachers, service providers, and parents alike.

Keywords Autism · Competing pathways chart · Behavioral interventions · Proactive strategies

Students with Autism Spectrum Disorder (ASD), and other behavior disorders, should be educated with typically developing peers to the maximum extent possible to meet the Least Restrictive Environment (LRE) criterion under the Individuals with Disabilities Education Improvement Act (IDEIA; § 1412 (a)(5) of U.S. Code Title 20). The proficiency of special and general education teachers, paired with collaboration with families, will maximize the success of students with ASD and/or

L. A. Riffel (✉)
Behavior Doctor Seminars, University of Kansas, Lawrence, KS, USA

K. L. Gischlar
Rider University, Lawrenceville, NJ, USA
e-mail: kgischlar@rider.edu

S. Halder et al. (eds.), *Applied Behavior Analysis-Based Interventions for Autism Spectrum Disorder*, https://doi.org/10.1007/978-981-95-2889-9_7

problematic behaviors in the inclusive setting. However, many general and special education teachers report little to no training in evidence-based practices, particularly those anchored in Applied Behavior Analysis, or ABA (Lauderdale-Littin & Brennan, 2018). Years of research support ABA as a best practice for students with and without disabilities (Trump et al., 2018), and its principles are widely recommended for teaching individuals with ASD (Donaldson & Stahmer, 2014). Nevertheless, despite myriad research supporting the behavior reinforcement and reduction strategies associated with ABA, reviews of teacher training programs evidence scant coursework in behavior support and emphasis on reactive, rather than preventive, strategies in managing problem behaviors in the classroom (Flower et al., 2017). This leaves educators seeking quick-fix answers to problematic behaviors, rather than understanding the complexities behind those behaviors.

Concisely, the principles of ABA suggest that supporting a student with ASD, and/or behavioral challenges, in the classroom requires the teacher first to hypothesize the function, or purpose, of a student's problematic behavior(s), and then to teach and reinforce more desirable replacement behaviors that meet the same function (Oakes et al., 2018). Behavioral function is typically hypothesized through observing the environmental conditions that elicit, or trigger, the behavior (antecedents) and those that reinforce (consequences) the behavior. When a teacher is able to identify the antecedents (A) and consequences (C) surrounding a challenging behavior (B), she can structure the environment to minimize triggering events (A) and instruct more appropriate behaviors (B) that result in "pay-off" for the student (C). In other words, the replacement behaviors must meet the same behavioral function as the problem behaviors to evoke behavioral change (Lloyd et al., 2017). Along with the functional hypothesis, ABA calls for the collection of quantitative data on the behavior, including frequency, duration, and/or latency, depending on topography. Baseline data are collected prior to the implementation of an intervention to determine levels of the problematic—or desirable—behavior and to provide a comparison to eventual intervention data to measure the effectiveness of the plan. Typically, these data are graphed to enable visual analysis of the student's progress in the treatment and to promote informed decision-making for programming (Trump et al., 2018).

When ABA practices are implemented properly, students with ASD and/or problematic behaviors receive instruction and intervention tailored to their unique needs, which promotes student success (Trump et al., 2018). As more children diagnosed on the spectrum, or with other mental health challenges, are entering our nation's classrooms (Flower et al., 2017; von der Embse et al., 2018), we contend that all teachers require training in behavioral tenets to equip them with the necessary knowledge and skills to manage behavior effectively and efficiently. This chapter presents a framework, the Triple T-Triple R Competing Pathways Model, which was developed by the first author, a nationally renowned behavioral trainer, in response to anecdotal observations she made regarding the accessibility of ABA terminology to teachers during her trainings. Triple T-Triple R is grounded in ABA principles and simplifies the competing pathways chart frequently utilized by behaviorists. We believe that this version of the competing pathways chart makes the process of behavioral change easier to understand and, thus, readily accessible to teachers, especially those in general education classrooms, who might not have the previous training and/or experience with application of behavioral tenets (Gischlar & Riffel, 2020). In the following sections of this chapter, we define and explain the components of the Triple T-Triple R Competing Pathways Model and demonstrate its application through case studies.

7.1 The Triple T-Triple R Competing Pathways Model

The starting point of the Triple T-Triple R model is the operationalization of behaviors targeted for intervention. The operational definition should include examples demonstrating the presence and absence of the behavior (i.e., positive and negative, or non-, examples) to promote consistency and reliability among observers (Alberto et al., 2022; Hojonski et al., 2009). Once a clear behavioral definition has been derived, observation of environmental conditions and data collection can begin. The teacher will want to record quantitative data (i.e., frequency, duration, and/or latency) and information regarding the environment, as described in the following sections.

7.1.1 Triple T: Trigger, Target, ImpacT

Determining behavioral function is the primary purpose of the Triple T component of our model. As noted, the function relates to the effect that a behavior has on the environment or, in other words, the purpose that it serves for the individual. Function refers to the relationship between two variables, an environmental event, and a behavior, in which one varies given the presence or absence of the other (Hanley et al., 2003). In our model, the teacher should consider the following three questions: (a) What started or elicited the behavior? (Trigger); (b) What is the behavior we want to change? (Target); and (c) What is the student trying to get, or get out of, by engaging in this behavior? (ImpacT). Once the three T questions have been answered, a summary statement is formed: When this happens.... (Trigger) the student does this.... (Target) to get, or get out of, this.... (impacT). The three Ts lead us to a functional hypothesis (Gischlar & Riffel, 2020).

It is important to note that there may be other triggers for behaviors that are more distal in time, termed setting events. A setting event can occur at a time removed from the behavior by hours or days that sets the sequence or chain in motion (Iovannone et al., 2017). Examples of setting events include changes to the family structure, such as the birth of a new sibling, an early morning argument with a parent, or illness. Setting events are important to understand when hypothesizing function, as they can affect a student's behavior in the classroom, despite being "outside" events. Finally, it is important for the teacher to recognize that problematic behaviors can be classified into two primary categories—externalizing and internalizing. Externalizing behaviors are those that are readily observable, such as aggression, rule-breaking, and cursing. Conversely, internalizing behaviors are directed inward and are often characterized by symptoms of depression and anxiety (Fomby & Mollborn, 2017). Whether a behavior is deemed externalizing or internalizing, it is important to operationalize its definition in specific, observable, and measurable terms (Hojonski et al., 2009) and to consider the three Ts when analyzing it (Gischlar & Riffel, 2020).

7.1.2 Triple R: Revise, Replace, Reframe

Once the final T, impacT, or function, of the behavior has been hypothesized, the teacher can proceed to the next step in our model, the three Rs: (a) Revise the environment; (b) Replace the target behavior with one that is more acceptable for the setting and meets the hypothesized function; and (c) Reframe the response (Gischlar & Riffel, 2020). In revising the environment, our first R, the teacher implements strategies designed to prevent the problem behavior from occurring; this is akin to antecedent manipulation in ABA (Johnston et al., 2006). For example, if a student engages in problematic behaviors as a means to escape from, or avoid, a lengthy math worksheet, the teacher can "chunk" the problems to enable the student to take a break between sets. This should reduce the need for problem behaviors because the teacher is revising the student's environment to include breaks, thereby allowing him to avoid for brief periods.

Our second R, Replace, pertains to teaching the student a new behavior that is functionally equivalent to the problematic target behavior. The replacement behavior should be of similar effort to the problem and be effective in achieving the same function, or impacT (Gischlar & Riffel, 2020). Referring to our previous example, the teacher could model, prompt, and reinforce the student for requesting a break, rather than engaging in problematic behaviors. Paramount to the Replace step in our model is the identification of a behavior that is functionally equivalent to the problem, lest the student revert to the target behavior, which resulted in the desired impacT. To help teachers remember the steps in identifying and teaching an alternative replacement behavior, we devised the acronym "TIPP It." TIPP It stands for: (a) Teach the replacement behavior; (b) Imprint by modeling it; (c) Practice the behavior across settings; and (d) Praise the replacement behavior when it occurs (Gischlar & Riffel, 2020).

Finally, our third R, Reframing the response, is relative to impacT (Gischlar & Riffel, 2020). In ABA, this step entails the functional consequence (e.g., attention, avoidance, tangible, sensory) previously associated with the problematic target behavior being applied to the replacement behavior. The goal is to withhold reinforcement for the problematic target behavior and apply it upon production of the desired replacement behavior (Hieneman, 2015). In the previous example, the teacher should grant a break contingent upon the production of work and/or an appropriate request.

7.2 Utilizing the Triple T-Triple R Competing Pathways Model

7.2.1 Example 1: Josh McKinley

7.2.1.1 History

Josh was an 11-year-old male who had been identified with autism at the age of 3 years, and later identified with bipolar disorder and intellectual disabilities. He had been attending a special school for children with disabilities since the age of 3 years. He displayed tantrum behaviors daily, and the school's primary response had been to send Josh home at the end of the tantrum. His tantrums lasted up to 4 hours per day, and the end of the tantrum almost always resulted in him biting someone. Josh's mother had lost her job numerous times due to the constant calls from the school to retrieve him. She was a single mother and the only financial support for the family.

His mother was considering institutionalization because the school suggested this as a viable alternative to her. The Behavioral Intervention Program team asked for parental permission to take Josh to the day clinic for evaluation. The Behavioral Intervention Day Program stipulated that the school district would hire a teacher and a paraprofessional to be trained in positive behavior support and functional assessments. The school district and mother agreed to this intervention rather than institutionalization. Once Josh was stable, he would be returned to his home school from the Day Program and, once acclimated, other students would be integrated into his classroom.

7.2.1.2 Operational Definition of Tantrum Behavior

The first task undertaken by the team was the operationalization of the term "tantrum" to ensure that all professionals would collect data in a consistent manner. The following table includes the operationalized definition, with examples and non-examples (Table 7.1).

7.2.1.3 Analysis of the Behavior

Because Josh was nonverbal upon entrance to the Behavioral Intervention Program Day Clinic, the team conducted a functional analysis using Iwata's Four Conditions (Iwata, 2008). It was determined that Josh needed a way to communicate his wants and needs as he usually began exhibiting problematic behaviors when he wanted to communicate; his previous school had not provided him any means of communicating. Their basic intervention had been to give him a spoon to use in a self-stimulatory, or stereotypical, manner when he entered the classroom in the morning. Much of his

Table 7.1 Josh's operationalized behavioral definition

Target	Operational definition	Possible examples	Possible non-examples
Tantrum	Being so upset that he is unable to interact with his surroundings and the people around him	Jumping up and down paired with screaming Pacing back and forth with a pained look on his face while crying Biting the nearest person at the end of his tantrum Engaging in self-injurious behaviors (biting, scratching, and slapping) Not responding to any adult attempting to engage with him	Making noises such as throat-clearing Pacing back and forth with a smile on his face while engaging with an adult in an academic task Screaming and crying when injured or sick

Table 7.2 Josh's triple T summary statement

Trigger	Target	ImpacT
Inability to communicate effectively	Being so upset that he is unable to interact with his surroundings or the people around him	To gain access to his wants and needs

new intervention package would revolve around teaching him how to communicate, and training staff, family, and daycare how to interpret his communication.

Josh's mother was assured that she would not be called to retrieve her son and that she could seek employment. A daycare that utilized a sliding scale and provided once-a-month weekend respite for families was enlisted. Daycare staff agreed to be trained by the Behavioral Intervention Program Day Clinic staff (Table 7.2).

Due to Josh's lack of verbal communication skills, he engaged in other behaviors to communicate his wants and needs until he became so upset that his behavior escalated, and he would be sent home where his mother would meet his wants and needs (Table 7.3).

The following sections provide evidence for the strategies employed in Josh's BSP.

7.2.1.4 Amygdala Recalibration Station

The amygdala recalibration station, like a calming corner, is a safe space in the classroom free from judgment or distractions where students can use tools they have been taught to self-regulate. This helps learners by meeting their social and

Table 7.3 Josh's triple R behavior support plan (BSP)

Trigger	Target	ImpacT
Unable to communicate wants and needs	Being so upset that he is unable to interact with his surroundings or the people around him	To gain access to his wants and needs
Revise	**Replace**	**Reframe**
Revise the Environment	Replace the Behavior	Reframe the Response
• Set up an amygdala recalibration station at home, school, and daycare (see description in Fig. 7.1) • Have PECS cards available so Josh can indicate his desires • Have 60 bpm music playing in the area • Have nature pictures for Josh to see in the area	• Make a video of Josh showing signs of being mad and going to the amygdala recalibration station and choosing PECS cards to illustrate his desires • Build in praise in the video for his choices (This is done through editing and all non-desired behaviors are deleted, so it appears that Josh followed the desired plan.)	• Give praise for any approximation of replacement behaviors • Label Josh's emotions to help him understand what he is feeling • Use a calm voice at all times • Remind Josh what he can do in his beanbag: – Rock, breathe (smell flower, blow out candle)

emotional needs so they can thrive (Mental Health Services Oversight and Accountability Commission, 2020). Calming spaces and the teaching of self-regulation skills are typically part of Tier One Universal Prevention in Multi-Tiered Systems of Support service delivery models. (See appendix for example.) In Josh's case, he was taught to access this station to calm and then communicate his needs/wants through use of his picture cards.

7.2.1.5 Picture Exchange Communication System

The Picture Exchange Communication System (PECS) is a communication system in which cards are printed with either photographs of items or black line pictures to indicate what an individual wants to communicate. PECS was developed by Frost and Bondy in 1985 and has demonstrated effectiveness in helping students with autism and other verbal communication disorders learn to communicate their wants and needs (Koudys et al., 2022).

In Josh's case, all staff and family members were trained using the videos available on the PECS website (https://pecsusa.com/pecs/). All PECS cards were made available across settings: (a) home; (b) school; and (c) daycare. Staff members wore necklaces with the cards on a key ring that were easily detachable, and copies of the cards were available on a wall where Josh could have instant access.

7.2.1.6 Sixty Beats Per Minute Music

In mood regulation research, data found that people intuitively use music to modify their emotional states to calm, soothe, or encourage themselves. Further, brain science studies have found that listening to music set at approximately 60 beats per minute, with no sudden changes in tempo, can have a calming effect on learners (Tervaniemi et al., 2021). Thus, in Josh's plan, such music was played in the amygdala recalibration stations provided at home, school, and daycare.

7.2.1.7 Video Modeling

Video modeling is a valuable tool that supports the acquisition and generalization of skills for students with and without emotional and behavioral disorders. A video typically includes self- or peer-modeling of a skill or behavior applied effectively within a setting (Galligan et al., 2022). These videos can be produced organically using readily available video editing tools. Video models can include adults, peers, and targeted students. Research has demonstrated that video modeling is a sound practice for teaching a wide variety of skills, especially for students with ASD (Zarate & Maggin, 2021). Josh was recorded utilizing the amygdala recalibration station and PECS cards appropriately; the video was shown to him to reinforce procedures.

7.2.1.8 Encourage Communication Through Teaching and Modeling

Because communication was deemed the primary function of Josh's behaviors, a component of his behavior intervention plan included the teaching and reinforcement of communication via PECS cards, as summarized below (Table 7.4).

Table 7.4 Josh's BSP: communication component

Revise	Replace	Reframe
Have PECS cards available in all settings (home, daycare, and school) Have a PECS notebook with pictures for when Josh is in the community	Staff and family model choosing a PECS card to request something Staff and family prompt Josh to choose a PECS card to request something	Whatever Josh requests using PECS cards is granted Positive praise is given for choosing a communication card

7.2.1.9 Encourage Social-Emotional Behaviors for Productive Integration into General Education School

A primary goal for Josh was reintegration to the general education setting with supports, where he would have access to typically developing peer models and the general education curriculum. Evidence indicates that exposure to neurotypical peers with more advanced social skills and language abilities can improve the social and language abilities of children with ASD (Fasano et al., 2021). This component of Josh's plan is summarized in the following Table 7.5.

7.2.1.10 Outcomes

Josh graduated from the day program and his BSP was faded. Gradually, he transitioned to his home high school from his special school, where he was segregated from typically developing peer models. Once he was stable in the new setting, students were reverse integrated into his classroom. At the time of transfer, he had 111 words he was using functionally, and he was completing the same work as the moderate-level students. Josh was successful in daycare and attended respite weekends once a month with zero problematic incidents.

Josh's teacher and paraprofessional remained with him until his graduation. He now works 4–6 hours per day at a grocery store bagging groceries. His boss purposefully schedules employees his age at the same time as Josh so that when he takes his break, he has peers to talk to in the break room. The manager reports that people love to go through Josh's line because he meticulously puts all the frozen items together, all the canned items together, and so on. He is in a Special Olympics bowling league and has friends that come to his home and friends he visits. His mother reports that Josh is happy and that he finally has the dignified life that we promised her he would have.

Table 7.5 Josh's BSP: social-emotional component

Revise	Replace	Reframe
• Provide picture cues of the correct way to exhibit expectations: – Walking in hallway – Seated in chair – Looking at adults for directions	• Take video of Josh engaging in correct behaviors through selective editing and verbally labeling those behaviors as correct on the video	Give positive behavioral praise for all approximations of expectations as they occur • Train the family and all staff to follow the same expectations

7.2.2 *Example 2: Charlie Connors (Pseudonym)*

7.2.2.1 History

Charlie was a 9th-grade student diagnosed with autism and bipolar disorder, and he did not use words to communicate. Charlie also had pseudo-achondroplasia (PSACH). This disease causes extreme pain in the joints and leads to early osteoporosis. Charlie was adopted by parents who also had PSACH disease and were familiar with the pain he felt when asked to walk too far or do repetitive tasks. The staff in Charlie's previous setting had dealt with many problematic behaviors, resulting in use of restraints on him. They had not taken his PSACH and physical limitations into consideration when placing demands on him. Once he entered the new classroom, these factors were considered and the only behavior the team wished to target was his self-injurious behavior. Charlie would bite himself on the forearm with enough force to cause a callous buildup, but not break the skin. His mother reported that Charlie had engaged in self-injurious behavior since he was about 2 years of age (Table 7.6).

Charlie's biting behavior was operationalized to distinguish occurrences from nonoccurrences to promote accurate data collection.

7.2.2.2 Analysis of the Behavior

Data were collected for 2 weeks (10 school days). The first week, Charlie bit himself during three trigger points: (a) being told "no" when requesting to do something other than his work; (b) learning that pizza was a choice for lunch and having to wait for 3 hours until lunchtime; and (c) hearing a loud, sudden noise in the hallway. In the second week while watching for these specific triggers, Charlie only engaged in the biting behavior once, despite many instances of the three identified triggers. It was hypothesized that there was a setting event pairing with the three triggers that needed to be determined. After 3 months of data collection, it was determined that the setting event was a runny nose. Charlie's behavior is summarized in the following Table 7.7.

Although the team was able to identify the setting event and triggers, the impacT, or what the behavior helped Charlie gain or escape, was initially unknown. A behavior support team meeting with his family was held and the findings shared. Charlie's

Table 7.6 Charlie's operationalized behavioral definition

Target	Operational definition	Possible examples	Possible non-examples
Self-injurious behavior (SIB), particularly biting	Charlie would use his teeth to bite his forearm	Biting self on the forearm with enough force to cause a callous, but not enough force to break the skin	Biting objects Sucking on arm with lips Licking arm with tongue

Table 7.7 Charlie's triple T summary statement

Trigger	Target	ImpacT
When Charlie had an infected, runny nose paired with any of the following three triggers: (1) Being told no (2) Having to wait 3 hours for pizza (3) Hearing a loud, sudden noise in the hallway	Charlie would engage in the biting behavior	Initially unknown Communicate or escape distressing triggers and/or pain, determined after conference with mother

mother requested a copy of the data to share with his pediatrician. She said, "The doctor never believes me as to how many sinus infections he has and here we have the data to show her how many he has had in just 3 months." When she said, "sinus infections," it occurred to the team that sinus infections typically result in headache pain. At times, headaches can cause individuals to engage in behaviors to distract from pain, such as digging fingernails into the palm. It was hypothesized that Charlie was most likely biting himself to get relief from the headache, albeit temporary relief. He was escaping pain through attenuation, meaning pain was diminished when he engaged in sensory stimulation, including biting (Karsh et al., 2018). The team's hypothesis was confirmed when Charlie's mother provided the data to his doctor, and she prescribed medication for allergic rhinitis. With treatment, the infection abated, and the self-injurious behavior stopped (Table 7.8).

Charlie's case underscores the importance of identifying setting events, as well as antecedents, or triggers in our model in determining what elicits a behavior.

7.2.2.3 Outcomes

The medication decreased the number of sinus infections Charlie encountered. Once he realized he could communicate his pain, he was very compliant in letting staff know what he needed. Twenty-three years later, Charlie's callous bite mark has almost faded from his forearm. His parents have passed away; however, his sister reports that he still uses his communication cards, has few headaches, and his group home staff reports zero instances of biting himself.

7.2.3 Example 3: Rissa Raine (Pseudonym)

7.2.3.1 History

Rissa was a 5-year-old child diagnosed with ASD and Down syndrome. The target behavior for intervention was noncompliance. The school hired a behavior therapist from a nearby state who instructed school personnel to put Rissa in a basket-hold when she was noncompliant. The definition of a basket-hold by Magee & Ellis (2001) is the confinement of a student by placing him/her face down on the floor

Table 7.8 Charlie's triple R (BSP) amended with new information

Revise	Replace	Reframe
The pediatrician prescribed medication for allergic rhinitis Communication cards were added to Charlie's communication notebook to notify staff of headaches (these were different from his joint pain communication cards) The nurse administered Acetaminophen, as needed for headache pain Charlie was given access to the sensory room with dim lights and a chance to let the medication take effect Charlie was given a cool compress for his forehead	Charlie was taught how to use the communication cards to indicate a headache	Charlie was praised for communicating his physical needs

Table 7.9 Rissa's operationalized behavioral definition

Target	Operational definition	Possible examples	Possible non-examples
Noncompliant behavior	Child is given a task to complete and refuses to complete the task	Verbally saying "no" when given a task Sitting and staring at task and not beginning to work when requested to do so	Asking to be excused to use the restroom Requesting help to understand directions Saying, "this is hard" however still attempting to do the work

Table 7.10 Rissa's triple T summary statement

Trigger	Target	ImpacT
Demand given	Noncompliance	Adult intervention with restraint (escape, attention, sensory?)

while restraining his/her arms or placing the individual in a chair and restraining his/her arms. This form of restraint is used to protect the student from causing bodily harm to self or others. However, the basket-hold can restrict breathing and, thus, is illegal in many school districts. It was deemed an unnecessary response to Rissa's noncompliance behaviors. Because this was considered to be a crisis, an immediate plan was designed and implemented without collecting baseline data (Table 7.9).

Rissa's noncompliant behaviors included work refusal and were characterized by her responding "no" to a task or sitting and staring when prompted to begin work (Table 7.10).

Rissa's trigger was identified as a demand being placed on her. When she exhibited noncompliant behaviors as operationalized above, staff applied the basket-hold. However, Rissa's impact was unknown. Hypotheses included temporary escape from work, adult attention, and sensory input (Table 7.11).

Table 7.11 Rissa's triple R BSP

Revise	Replace	Reframe
Interventionists quickly surveyed and discovered Rissa's reinforcer was a 25-piece puzzle Purchases were made of the following: • A wide variety of 25-piece puzzles • Jelly bracelets to use for a token economy • A floor-level TV tray for home and school • Cheap timers that ticked for a few seconds after the timer elapsed (one for home and school)	Staff, family, and student were trained on the token economy Every time Rissa complied with a demand, she was given a jelly bracelet; five jelly bracelets, resulted in a five-minute break with a puzzle Rissa was taught how to set the timer for 5 minutes When the timer sounded, if Rissa could place the TV tray with the puzzle on a designated shelf, she earned a bracelet (one step closer to her next break)	Staff and family were trained to give positive behavior praise by giving Rissa a bracelet for any approximation of compliance with a demand If Rissa was noncompliant, they were not to restrain her but to remind her to try to earn a break

Token economies, such as the one employed with Rissa, are individual-specific; not all students are motivated by the same reinforcers. The team determined that Rissa was reinforced by access to 25-piece puzzles and implemented a system whereby she could earn bracelets (tokens) for acceptable, appropriate behavior. Five bracelets could be traded for five-minutes working on a puzzle, a preferred activity. It is important to note that tokens must be administered with consistency and fidelity and result in a preferred item and/or activity. Within these systems, tokens are universal, but can be exchanged at a later time for a preferred reinforcer, making token economies easy to implement and effective (Hackenberg, 2009).

7.2.3.2 Outcomes

The interventionists stayed for an entire school day and modeled for the staff how to implement the token economy. The staff was amazed at how much work Rissa completed and how well she worked for the bracelets and the puzzle break. Her mother was also trained that evening and was excited about implementing the system at home. Phone calls to her mother found that Rissa was able to meet demands of the home environment in areas such as staying at the table and eating dinner with the family, getting dressed in the morning, and picking up her toys. Initial phone calls to the school staff also reported success. However, an interventionist visited one month later and found the staff restraining Rissa. When questioned, they said it was easier to restrain her than to implement all of the steps in the token economy. The interventionist then stayed an entire week, modeled for the staff, and helped them see that while it might take more planning, Rissa was learning and complying with commands. The staff finally agreed to follow the token economy, and subsequent first and second-grade visits found that school staff could thin Rissa's reinforcement schedule from five-bracelet tokens to ten bracelets and then, finally, 15 bracelets before she was permitted to access the puzzles.

7.2.4 *Example 4: Ryan Apple (Pseudonym)*

7.2.4.1 History

Ryan was a 31-year-old male with ASD, bipolar disorder, obsessive-compulsive disorder, intellectual disabilities, and mild cerebral palsy. While his behaviors had been aggressive when he was younger, those behaviors had dissipated. The biggest issue at age 31 was his refusal to get up in the morning when staff tried to rouse him. His typical responses included "maybe later," "pretty soon," or "five more minutes." Ryan hit the snooze button repeatedly. The staff was quite upset by this refusal and resorted to (a) yelling; (b) threatening to take away the items most important to him; and (c) bribing him. None of these tactics worked. The main support staff quit over this particular issue (Table 7.12).

Ryan's behavior was defined as remaining in bed when roused, barring illness or a late previous night (Table 7.13).

It was determined that the impacT for Ryan was gaining access to a preferred activity of staying in bed and sleeping longer (Table 7.14).

Rather than duplicate this scenario with new staff starting, it was decided to put a proactive plan in place. Ryan was very motivated by food choices. The new staff

Table 7.12 Ryan's operationalized behavioral definition

Target	Operational definition	Possible examples	Possible non-examples
Refusing to get up in the morning	Ryan is given the command to get up and get ready, but remains in bed	Upon being told it was time to get up, Ryan would verbally respond with one of the following: • Maybe later • Pretty soon • Five more minutes	Ryan was sick and needed to stay in bed due to an illness Ryan had been up late at a function the evening before

Table 7.13 Ryan's triple T summary statement

Trigger	Target	ImpacT
Told to get up	Refuses	Gains access to preferred activity of sleeping longer

Table 7.14 Ryan's triple R BSP

Revise	Replace	Reframe
Make noise at least five minutes before Ryan gets up, so he is semi-awake (e.g., playing music in restroom above his bedroom) Set up a Premack condition of gaining a desired food item if he complies	Model for Ryan what is meant by getting up on first request Explain to Ryan that he will gain his desired meal if he complies with the first request	Refrain from showing anger or disappointment if Ryan refuses to get up after the first request Make the staff choice for breakfast and throw away the desired breakfast if it was premade

on the first night before helping Ryan retire to bed for the evening, told him that if he got up the first time they came into his room in the morning, he could choose whatever he wanted for breakfast. However, if he did not get up at the first request, the staff would choose his breakfast. The staff asked him his preference for breakfast, and he replied, "Pancakes." The staff agreed that if he got right up, he could have pancakes, and if he did not get up, the staff would choose something like bacon and eggs or oatmeal (not his preferred breakfast).

7.2.4.2 Outcomes

The first morning, the staff went into Ryan's room and announced that it was time to get up after making a lot of noise above his bedroom to ensure he was fully awake when they entered his room. Ryan responded with "five more minutes" when requested to get up. The staff just said, "okay," and went to the kitchen and put Ryan's pancake breakfast in the trash. They also poured water over the pancake enough that it still looked like a pancake, but would disintegrate if picked up from the trash. Staff prepared a bowl of cinnamon oatmeal and toast for Ryan and had it on the table in his spot.

Ryan came out and requested a pancake. The staff cheerily said, "It's a bummer, I had to throw the pancake away because you did not get right up, but I made you some oatmeal and toast." Ryan reached for the pancake in the trash and discovered that it could not be picked up. He finally ate his oatmeal and toast. He went to work that day, and the staff received emails that he was slow and appeared sad all day. The staff assured his job coach and other concerned employees that he would be happier and faster the next day.

The next night the staff went through all the nighttime routines and asked Ryan what he wanted for breakfast in the morning—if he got up the first time they requested. Ryan again asked for a pancake. The staff said, "That will be great." The next morning, music was playing in the bathroom above Ryan's bedroom, and lots of noise was made as staff descended the stairs. As staff were about halfway down the stairs, Ryan exclaimed, "I'm up. I'm up." He was standing on the rug beside his bed by the time the staff got to his room. He had his pancakes for breakfast and did not have trouble getting up in the morning again.

7.3 Cultural Considerations in Intervention Design

In the preceding examples, different systems and reinforcers were employed across individuals and settings. The principles of ABA posit that an effective behavioral intervention must be rooted in the function, or purpose a behavior serves. Once the function has been determined, or at least hypothesized, a more desirable behavior can be taught and reinforced that satisfies the same function (Gischlar & Riffel, 2020). However, intervention design is much more complex than simply considering behavioral function. Rather, treatment packages also should focus on procedures that are socially relevant and culturally appropriate. A contextual fit between the intervention components and the values of families, teachers, schools, support personnel, and community agency providers must be considered as paramount, if a plan is to be acceptable and effective (Bal, 2018).

As example, Fong et al. (2016) offer the following case to illustrate the important role culture should play in intervention design. A young female child, Raina, was referred for an assessment due to her "withdrawn" behavior in the classroom. School personnel noted that Raina became especially withdrawn after receiving verbal praise and, eventually, she stopped engaging in behaviors that might warrant praise. In the course of analyzing the behavior, school personnel met with Raina's family and learned that, in her culture, the whole (i.e., community) holds more value than the individual; in other words, Raina's family and larger community did not value individual praise. However, school personnel considered the norm for the school's culture and suggested that praise should be delivered to Raina privately. In this case the school professionals imposed their own values and recommended an intervention component that was incongruent with Raina's and her family's values (Fong et al., 2016). There is potential for an intervention that does not consider the culture and values of the student and family to be ineffective, or worse, harmful. Certainly, practitioners need to be aware of cultural identity—their own and the client's—and should know how to access and implement appropriate culturally-based resources, such as trainings and self-reflection. In our examples, family values and preferences were considered in the design of each intervention to ensure social acceptability.

7.4 Summary

Within this chapter we have provided a new competing pathways model that should aid teachers, service providers, and parents in designing and implementing function-based interventions for children, adolescents, and adults. Our Triple T-Triple R model is grounded in the science of applied behavior analysis, but has been simplified with more accessible language to enable those without behavioral training to develop sound interventions. The model has been applied to real-world cases throughout the chapter, which the reader should find helpful as exemplars when completing a chart for a student or offspring. Throughout our examples, evidence-based intervention components have been detailed to further support the reader. Finally, the appendix offers a blank Triple T-Triple R framework and example treatment components to aid in the design of plans (Figs. 7.1, 7.2, and 7.3; Tables 7.15 and 7.16).

Table 7.15 Blank triple T-triple R framework

Trigger	**Target**	**ImpacT**
Revise	**Replace**	**Reframe**

Table 7.16 Amygdala recalibration station

Revise	Replace	Reframe
Assign an area in the room for the station (This is not a time-out or punishment area) Items to have in station: • Blue vinyl beanbag chair • Green shaggy carpet (not a necessity—but a nice nature approach) • Nature pictures • Calming tools (squeeze balls, glitter water bottles, pompons, or other manipulatives depending on the level of the students • Headphones attached to 60 bpm source • Sachets sprinkled with lavender oil (check for allergies first) • Posters of calming activities • Dim the lights in this area of the room (the custodian can unscrew the bulbs in the panel—so this area is not as bright)	Teach students about the brain and how it works when anger erupts Utilize videos to teach self-calming activities	Behavior specific praise for use of self-regulation skills Calm your voice to 60 bpm using a "singsong" voice Speak toward the student's right ear—but not up close and creepy 😊 If you see the tell-tale signs of an amygdala out of control, turn on the 60-bpm music and dim the lights in the room; keep teaching

Appendix

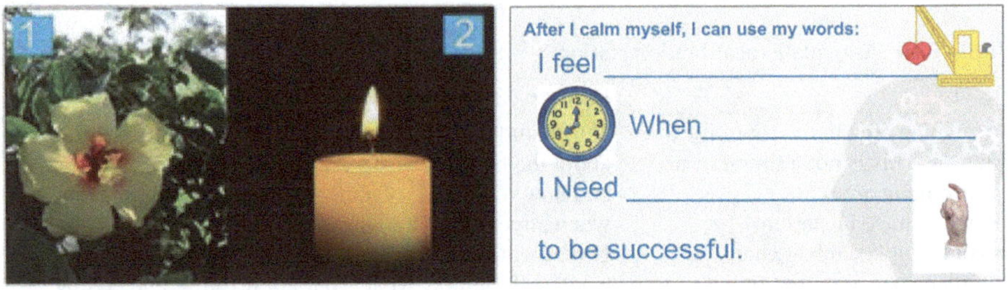

Fig. 7.1 Power card for calming example

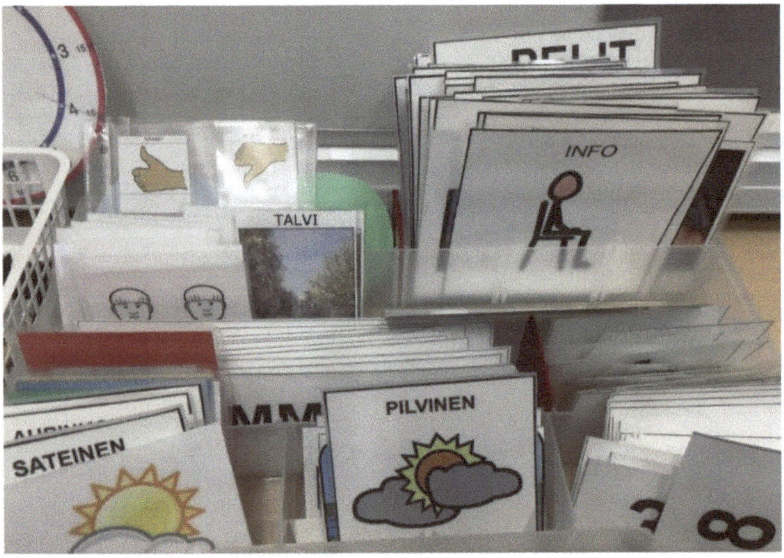

Fig. 7.2 Picture exchange communication system

Co-regulation with a Non-verbal Student

When it appears that Josh is getting mad, the staff should use the communication board to help Josh understand what is happening. The goal is for Josh to be able to say, “I feel ______________ when ___________________. I need _________________ to be successful.” Adults use the words to help Josh identify his feelings with co-regulation.

I feel

When

I need

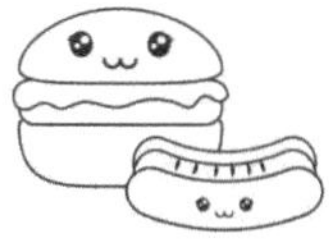

Fig. 7.3 Co-regulation with a nonverbal student. The focus is on four basic emotions: madness, sadness, frustration, and happiness. As the adult co-regulates with Josh, these four emotions are used to identify his feelings. A conversation about what to do when individuals experience these feelings should ensue. Josh should then be encouraged to identify the trigger for his emotions by having a variety of things known from data collection to be triggers for him: (**a**) restroom needs; (**b**) hunger; (**c**) fatigue; and (**d**) boredom. Finally, there should be various items available for him to communicate what he needs to succeed (e.g., a restroom break, food or drink, a work break)

References

Alberto, P. A., Troutman, A. C., & Axe, J. (2022). *Applied behavior analysis for teachers* (10th ed.). Pearson Education.

Bal, A. (2018). Culturally responsive positive behavioral interventions and supports: A process–oriented framework for systemic transformation. *Review of Education, Pedagogy, and Cultural Studies*. https://doi.org/10.1080/10714413.2017.1417579

Donaldson, A. L., & Stahmer, A. C. (2014). Team collaboration: The use of behavior principles for serving students with ASD. *Language, Speech, and Hearing Services in Schools, 45*, 261–276.

Fasano, R. M., Perry, L. K., Zhang, Y., Vitale, L., Wang, J., Song, C., & Messinger, D. S. (2021). A granular perspective on inclusion: Objectively measured interactions of preschoolers with and without autism. *Autism Research, 14*, 1658–1669. https://doi.org/10.1002/aur.2526

Flower, A., McKenna, J. W., & Haring, C. D. (2017). Behavior and classroom management: Are teacher preparation programs really preparing our teachers? *Preventing School Failure, 61*, 163–169. https://doi.org/10.1080/1045988X.2016.1231109

Fomby, P., & Mollborn, S. (2017). Ecological instability and children's classroom behavior in kindergarten. *Demography, 54*, 1627–1651. https://doi.org/10.1007/s13524-017-0602-2

Fong, E. H., Catagnus, R. M., Brodhead, M. T., Quigley, S., & Field, S. (2016). Developing the cultural awareness skills of behavior analysts. *Behavior Analysis in Practice, 9*(1), 84–94.

Galligan, M. R. L., Suhrheinrich, J., & Kraemer, B. R. (2022). Video modeling for high school students with autism spectrum disorder. *Journal of Special Education Technology, 37*, 126–134. https://doi.org/10.1177/0162643420945594

Gischlar, K. L., & Riffel, L. A. (2020). Designing behavioral interventions that work: The Triple T – Triple R competing pathways model. *Educational Considerations, 46*(1). https://doi.org/10.4148/0146-9282.2221

Hackenberg, T. D. (2009). Token reinforcement: A review and analysis. *Journal of the Experimental Analysis of Behavior, 91*, 257–286. https://doi.org/10.1901/jeab.2009.91-257

Hanley, G. P., Iwata, B. A., & McCord, B. E. (2003). Functional analysis of problem behavior: A review. *Journal of Applied Behavior Analysis, 36*, 147–185. https://doi.org/10.1901/jaba.2003.36-147

Hieneman, M. (2015). Positive behavior support for individuals with behavior challenges. *Behavior Analysis in Practice, 8*, 101–108. https://doi.org/10.1007/s40617-015-0051-6

Hojonski, R. L., Gischlar, K. L., & Missall, K. N. (2009). Improving child outcomes with data-based decision-making: Collecting data. *Young Exceptional Children, 12*(3), 32–44. https://doi.org/10.1177/1096250609333025

Iovannone, R., Anderson, C., & Scott, T. (2017). Understanding setting events: What they are and how to identify them. *Hammill Institute on Disabilities, 26*(3), 105–112. https://doi.org/10.1177/1074295617729795

Iwata, B. A., & Dozier, C. L. (2008). Clinical application of functional analysis methodology. *Behavior analysis in practice, 1*(1), 3–9. https://doi.org/10.1007/BF03391714

Johnston, J. M., Foxx, R. M., Jacobson, J. W., Green, G., & Mulick, J. A. (2006). Positive behavior support and applied behavior analysis. *The Behavior Analyst, 29*, 51–74. https://doi.org/10.1007/BF03392117

Karsh, N., Goldstein, O., & Eitam, B. (2018). Evidence for pain attenuation by the motor system-based judgment of agency. *Consciousness and Cognition, 57*, 134–146. https://doi.org/10.1016/j.concog.2017.11.012

Koudys, J., Perry, A., & McFee, K. (2022). Picture exchange communication system® (PECS®) use in a community setting: A preliminary investigation. *Journal of Developmental & Physical Disabilities, 34*, 829–852. https://doi.org/10.1007/s10882-021-09826-5

Lauderdale-Littin, S., & Brennan, M. (2018). Evidence-based practices in the public school: The role of preservice teacher training. *International Electronic Journal of Elementary Education, 10*, 369–375.

Lloyd, B. P., Weaver, E. S., & Staubitz, J. L. (2017). Classroom-based strategies to incorporate hypothesis testing in functional behavior assessments. *Beyond Behavior, 26*(2), 48–56. https://doi.org/10.1177/1074295617711145

Magee, S. K., & Ellis, J. (2001). The detrimental effects of physical restraint as a consequence of inappropriate classroom behavior. *Journal of Applied Behavior Analysis, 34*, 501–504. https://doi.org/10.1901/jaba.2001.34-501

Oakes, W. P., Schellman, L. E., Lane, K. L., Alan, E., Powers, L., Diebold, T., & Gaskill, T. (2018). Improving educators' knowledge, confidence, and usefulness of functional assessment-based interventions: Outcomes of professional learning. *Education and Treatment of Children, 41*. https://doi.org/10.1353/etc.2018.0018

Tervaniemi, M., Makkonen, T., & Nie, P. (2021). Psychological and physiological signatures of music listening in different listening environments—An exploratory study. *Brain Sciences, 11*, 593.

Trump, C. E., Pennington, R. C., Travers, J. C., Ringdahl, J. E., Whiteside, E. E., & Ayres, K. M. (2018). Applied behavior analysis in special education: Misconceptions and guidelines for use. *Teaching Exceptional Children, 50*, 381–393. https://doi.org/10.1177/0040059918775020

von der Embse, N. P., Kilgus, S. P., Eklund, K., Ake, E., & Levi-Nielson, S. (2018). Training teachers to facilitate early identification of mental and behavioral health risks. *School Psychology Review, 47*, 372–384. https://doi.org/10.17105/SPR-2017-0094.V47-4

Zarate, K., & Maggin, D. M. (2021). Using and intensifying video modeling for students with emotional and behavioral disorders. *Beyond Behavior, 30*, 24–31.

Chapter 8
Improving the Vocal Abilities of Children with Autism

Santoshi Halder

Abstract This study explored the effectiveness of echoic and exemplar training in improving the vocal abilities of two children with autism. The first participant was a 5-year-old boy with cat's eye syndrome, and the second was an 8-year-old boy with autism. Both participants attended a special education school and were identified as having a phonological disorder. Using an AB design, the study assessed the impact of the ABA training on articulation. Results showed significant improvements, with gains of up to 57% for the first participant and 71% for the second, indicating the effectiveness of ABA based echoic & exemplar training in enhancing the articulation in both the participants and generalization.

Keywords Behavioral intervention · Phonological disorder · Vocal production · Vocal imitation · Developmental disabilities · Echoic & exemplar training

8.1 Introduction

Over 30% and 50% of individuals with autism may not develop the ability to imitate speech and could remain minimally verbal throughout their lives (Johnson, 2004; Mirenda, 2003). In the 2000–2001 school year, over 700,000 students in U.S. public schools were classified under special education for speech or language disorders (Roy, 2003). Communication difficulties can lead to challenging behaviors, such as tantrums and aggression, negatively impacting academic performance.

Children with autism may struggle with motivation to learn and may engage in behaviors like tantrums, inattention, and a reluctance to participate. Traditional teaching strategies may not be effective to engage them. Applied behavior analysis (ABA) based intervention can leverage natural motivations showing significant

S. Halder (✉)
Department of Education, University of Calcutta, Kolkata, West Bengal, India

S. Halder et al. (eds.), *Applied Behavior Analysis-Based Interventions for Autism Spectrum Disorder*, https://doi.org/10.1007/978-981-95-2889-9_8

progress in treating children with developmental disabilities, including autism (Smith, 1998). Children with phonological disorders often have difficulty matching sounds to words (Eikeseth & Nesset, 2003), necessitating interventions that focuses on enhancing their echoic repertoire through vocal imitation training (Lovaas, 2003). The intervention involves having children repeat sounds and words using techniques like shaping and prompting and reinforcement strategies. Generalized verbal imitation is essential for language training (Horne & Lowe, 1996), and once a child masters articulation, the applied behaviour based intervention ensures the skill generalizes across varied contexts.

8.2 Review of Related Literature

The articulation needs of children with developmental disabilities are significant, and various strategies and therapies have been implemented as interventions. However, the success rates of these approaches can vary widely among individuals and across different strategies. There is a notable lack of published research detailing experimental efforts to train these children in improving their articulation. Partington & Sundberg (1998) provided data indicating increases in verbal production through various methods (Baker & McLeod, 2011; Pace, 2011). However, research on the functional effects of these programs and the generalization of responses remains limited. Koegel et al. (1998) demonstrated that reinforcing strategies can enhance both the rate and accuracy of speech production in children with autism who have severe vocal production deficits (Miliotis et al., 2010).

Phonemes and syllables are the basic building blocks of a person's vocal behavior. Increasing the frequency and variety of these units in young children who do not typically develop them may improve the chances of developing vocal responses. Nevertheless, research indicates that not all interventions produce effective results, as pointed out by Peturstdottir et al. (2011). Esch et al. (2009) demonstrated the benefits of a direct reinforcement procedure using lag schedules, which promote speech variability. Peturstdottir et al. (2011) replicated an enhanced stimulus-stimulus pairing (SSP) strategy utilized by Esch et al. (2009) to increase vocalizations in children with autism, showing significant increases in both target vocalizations and nontarget vocalizations above baseline levels among participants.

Studies involving typically developing children with articulation disorders have shown that training on the correct articulation of speech sounds (phonemes) can often leads to generalization. Interestingly, none of these studies examined whether participants could generalize their training to other contexts where no explicit training was provided. There are very few studies documenting generalized imitation among children with articulation disorders (Ross & Greer, 2003).

Interventions for children with developmental delays, including autism, at the prelinguistic and early language stages have shown significant effect. Thus, it is crucial that these interventions occur as early as possible. The articulation abilities of children with autism are often a significant concern, as their speech can be unintelligible. However, research on interventions using behavior analytic approaches to improve articulation remains limited. Despite evidence suggesting benefits from generalization to similar words, speech, or different settings, very few studies have been conducted to experimentally establish generalization among children with various disabilities.

Limited empirical evidence supporting the specific use of behavior analytic principles as interventions for communication in children with developmental delays in India has been found. Consequently, the present study aimed to explore whether echoic and exemplar training could improve vocal abilities in children with phonological disorders and whether improved articulation might lead to generalization and transfer to similar untrained words among subjects with various disabilities. The articulation needs of children with developmental disabilities are significant, and various strategies have been implemented as interventions. However, the success rates of these approaches can vary widely among individuals and across different strategies. There is a notable lack of published research detailing experimental efforts to train these children in improving their articulation.

Phonemes and syllable units are the building blocks of vocal behavior. Increasing the frequency and variety of these units in young children who do not typically develop them may improve the chances of developing vocal behavior. Nevertheless, research indicates that not all interventions produce effective results. A recent study by Peturstdottir et al. (2011) investigated the factors that might account for the successes and failures of these procedures in clinical practice. Esch et al. (2009) demonstrated some preliminary benefits of a direct reinforcement procedure using lag schedules, which promote speech variability. Peturstdottir et al. (2011) replicated an enhanced stimulus-stimulus pairing (SSP) procedure utilized by Esch et al. (2009) to increase vocalizations in children with autism, showing significant increases in both target vocalizations and nontarget vocalizations above baseline levels among participants.

Studies involving typically developing children with articulation disorders have shown that training on correct articulation of speech sounds (phonemes) can often be generalized. Interestingly, none of these studies examined whether participants could generalize their training to other contexts where no explicit training was provided. There are very few studies documenting generalized imitation among children with articulation disorders (Ross & Greer, 2003). Interventions for children with developmental delays, including autism, at the prelinguistic and early language stages have shown dramatic benefits. Thus, it is crucial that these interventions occur as early as possible. The articulation abilities of children with autism are often a significant concern, as their speech can be unintelligible. However, research on interventions using behavior analytic approaches to improve articulation remains limited. Despite evidence suggesting benefits from generalization to similar words, speech, or different settings, very few studies have been conducted to experimentally establish generalization among children with disabilities.

8.3 Methodology

8.3.1 *Participant Selection*

Two boys with phonological disorder were chosen for this study. The first was a 5-year-old with developmental delays in a special school, while the second was an 8-year-old with autism, also in a special school. Both faced significant articulation and phonological challenges, making their speech difficult to understand.

8.3.2 *Setting*

The intervention was executed in a classroom setting by the researcher. Each participant received one hour-long session per day: Only one session was held each day, and parental consent was obtained to comply with BCBA ethical guidelines (forms are in the appendix).

8.3.3 *Procedure*

8.3.3.1 Experimental Design

An AB design was used to evaluate whether the intervention improved the articulation of target sounds, which are specific word groups. Data were collected before and after the intervention to see if enhanced articulation of target sounds also improved related words. The aim was to determine if this improvement could generalize to similar, untrained words.

8.3.3.2 Target Selection

Initial speech target selection was done on the basis of data taken on single sounds (a-z) pre-training assessments by two well-trained special educators. The first participant was unable to articulate ten single sounds: /f/, /g/, /j/, /l/, /m/, /n/, /r/, /s/, /t/, /v/. The second participant had difficulty in articulating the sounds: /d/, /h/, /j/, /n/, /r/, /x/, /z/.

An AB design was implemented to assess whether the intervention or training resulted in improved articulation of target sounds. Data were collected for pre- and post-intervention to determine if improved articulation of the target sounds was connected to better articulation in related words that share similar sounds. The aim was to assess whether this improvement could generalize and transfer to other similar, untrained words.

Table 8.1 Target words for Participants 1 & 2

		Target sounds	Target words (a set of seven words)
Target words for Participant 1	***Target word Set 1***	/g/	**Gap,** Got, Gas, Gun, Gay, Gup, Gun
	Control group word Set 2	/n/	Net, Nit, Nut, Nap, Nib, Nod, Nob
	Control group word Set 3	/s/	Sun, Sat, Sit, Sip, Sag, Sub, Sad
Target words for Participant 2	***Target word Set 1***	/j/	**Jam**, Job, Jug, Joy, Jar, Jog, Jet
	Control group word Set 2	/r/	Rat, Red, Rub, Rap, Rag, Rug, Rig
	Control group word Set 3	/h/	Hat. Hit, Hip, Hop, His, Ham, Hot

The final selection of the targeted phonemes was made after a thorough analysis of baseline data for both participants. Participant 1 was unable to echo any of the words containing the phonemes (/g/, /n/, /s/). Therefore, a set of words containing these phonemes was developed for Participant 1. Participant 2 faced difficulties with the phonemes (/j/, /r/, /h/), leading to the creation of a set of words for this participant as well. Ultimately, a group of seven distinct target words was selected for each participant, as they exhibited severe difficulties in articulating them. This resulted in three sets of seven target words, each corresponding to the selected phonemes for both participants. Word Set 1, containing the phoneme (/g/), was designated as the first target for Participant 1, while Set 1 with the phoneme (/j/) served as the initial target for Participant 2, and Sets 2 and 3 functioned as a control group (see Table 8.1).

8.4 Response Definition and Data Collection

8.4.1 Assessment of Mastery

The vocal imitation of target words was the dependent variable from a predetermined set (see Table 8.1). This was evaluated through pre-training and post-training test results. A correct response was considered when the participant accurately imitated the target word within 5 seconds, and all other responses were categorized as incorrect.

8.5 Testing and Training Sequence

Data assessment at baseline (pre-training test sessions) was conducted for all the target words in Sets 1, 2, and 3 for both participants. The assessment involved vocal imitation of the target words prior to training. The intervention commenced once a stable data point was identified. Intervention began with one word from Set 1 for each participant. Post-training data were collected for all three sets after every four intervention sessions. If the target word achieve less than 100% accuracy, training continued for that word. Conversely, if the word was mastered, a new word was selected. This testing cycle, every four sessions, continued until both participants achieved 100% accuracy for each set.

8.6 Baseline (Pre-Training) and Post-Training Tests

The baseline & post-training tests assessment was conducted through test sessions, which included both baseline and post-training evaluations. Each test session evaluated all three sets of words in the target list in the same order as they appeared (see Table 8.1). As a result, each test session assessed the newly mastered target word, the remaining six words containing the same sound, and the other 14 target words from the other two-word groups in Sets 2 and 3. The inclusion of the other target word group was necessary to establish experimental control.

8.7 Training

Training Sessions-Echoic Teaching Procedure: Training began for both Participants 1 and 2 with Set 1. Set 1 was with phoneme (/g/) for Participant 1 and phoneme (/j/) with Participant 2. The first target from Set 1 for Participant 1 was the word /Gap/, and for Participant 2, the word /jam/. In an hour training session, 6–8 articulation training sessions were conducted during each session of an hour. Each sitting lasted on average 5–10 minutes, with a 2- to 5-minute break between each session. Approximately 15–25 articulation trials were conducted during each session. The number of trials for each session and also the time of each session varied across the sessions, depending on the motivation of the participants. A preferred edible or toy was given for a correct echoic. In addition, tokens were given for compliance and attending throughout the 5- to 10-minute session and the break, given accordingly.

Articulation training started by ensuring that strong reinforcement was readily available and visible to the learner to enhance motivation to have correct responses. Before introducing any target words, 2–3 easy imitation and echoic tasks were presented in quick succession. Following this, the full target word was introduced, such as "gap."

If the student responded correctly within 5 seconds, then they were given immediate edible or toy as reinforcement. If the learner responded incorrectly, the word was presented two more times. At any point, the learner provided a correct response, he was reinforced. If the learner did not give a better response, the participant was reinforced after eliciting a mastered skill, such as an easy imitation. After three incorrect responses to the target word then the trainer would implement additional articulation training.

If the student tended to leave out or incorrectly pronounce individual sounds, e.g., when the trainer said gap the student said "ap" or replaced the sound, e.g., "jap," then trainer would focus on the single sound which the student had difficulty for a few consecutive trails and provide reinforcement when this was correctly produced on its own. The sound was taught by exaggerating mouth, lip, and tongue movements and differentially reinforcing better attempts at the sound. Once the student was attempting the single sound, the trainer returned to training the target full word up to three times. If the student was able to produce all the sounds but the word was still unclear, e.g., they said it too fast, inconsistently dropped sounds for the word etc. then the parts of the word were presented separately and then closer and closer together, e.g., "g"—"ap" were presented separately and then closer and closer together until the word was presented as a whole.

8.8 Reliability/Interobserver Agreement (IOA)

Interobserver agreement (IOA) was assessed following BCBA guidelines. Two observers, each with over one year of experience in behavioral analysis and working with individuals with developmental disabilities, were selected to record the IOA. They achieved 100% agreement during the baseline phase and 30% agreement during the training sessions, scoring on all probes with each participant. IOA was calculated by dividing the number of agreed observations by the total number of agreed and disagreed observations, then multiplying by 100 $\frac{sum\ \ of\ \ agreements}{sum\ \ of\ \ agreements + sum\ \ of\ \ disagreements} \times 100$. Data recorded on the probe sheets required at least 80% agreement between the two observers for inclusion. The IOA for all assessments ranged from 85% to 100%, indicating strong reliability for all evaluations conducted in the study. An AB design was used to evaluate if the intervention improved the articulation of target sounds, which are specific word groups. Data were collected before and after the intervention to see if enhanced articulation of target sounds also improved related words. The aim was to determine if this improvement could generalize to similar, untrained words. A copy of the IOA data sheet is included in Appendix C.

8.9 Result and Interpretation

Figures 8.1 and 8.2 illustrate the results from the test sessions conducted during the baseline phase, followed by training sessions over a span of one and a half months for the selected articulation intervention in this study. These figures clearly show that both participants had zero correct articulations during the baseline period. However, after the training sessions began, both participants, despite their differences in the nature of developmental disabilities, demonstrated significant improvement in their target words.

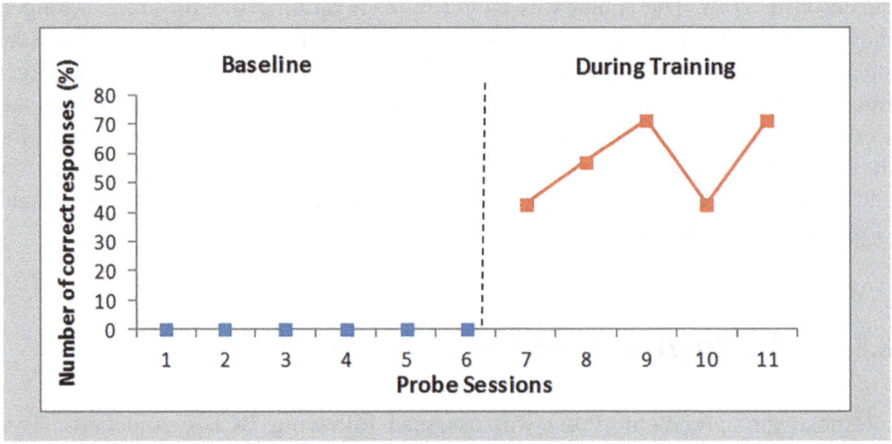

Fig. 8.1 Number of correct responses in the word Set 1 for Participant 1 at baseline and during experimental phases

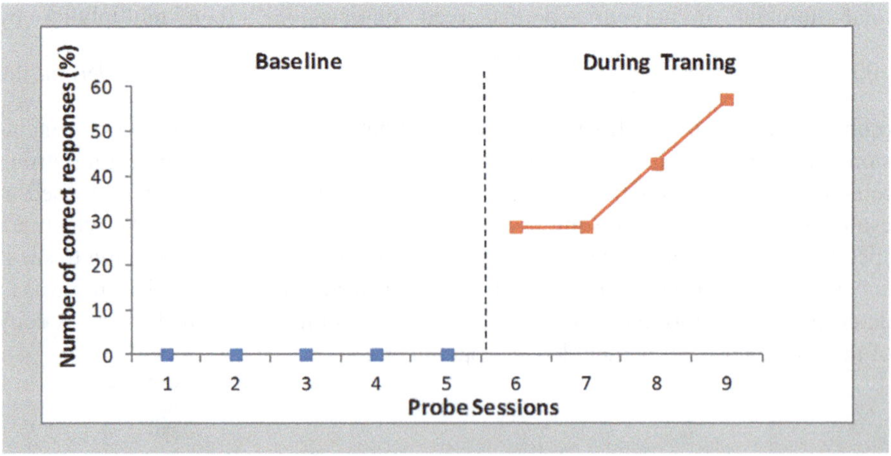

Fig. 8.2 Number of correct responses in the word Set 1 for Participant 2 at baseline and during experimental phases

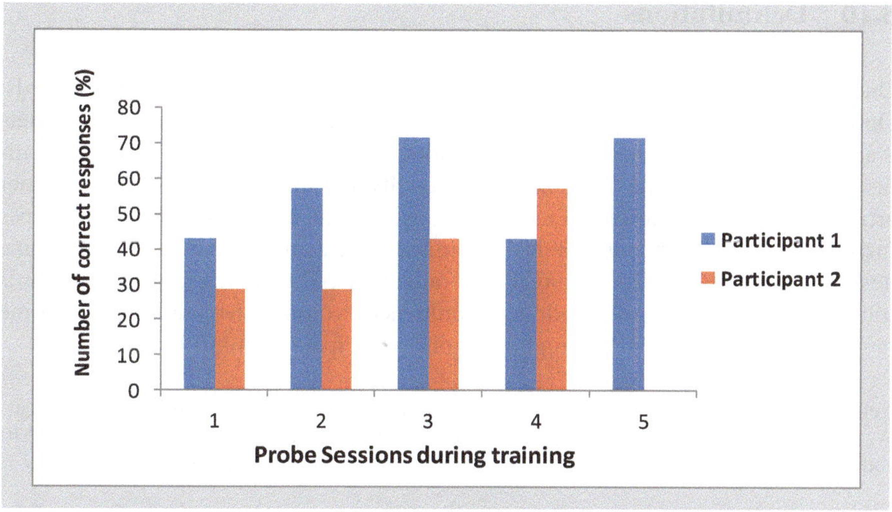

Fig. 8.3 Comparative graphical representation of probe sessions during training sessions of the two participants (1 and 2)

It is important to note that Participant 1 was unavailable for several days due to illness after the fourth probe session. Due to the study's time constraints, the next target sounds were not introduced, which resulted in this phase functioning only as a control condition for both participants. For Participant 1, performance remained at zero for Sets 2 and 3 throughout the study. In contrast, Participant 2's performance remained at zero or near zero, highlighting the effectiveness of the articulation intervention in the study.

The current graphical data (Fig. 8.1) for Participant 1 indicates that they achieved mastery of the target sound (over 70%) with training focused solely on the first word, "Gap." However, Participant 1 underwent additional training sessions to master the target set of words and sounds (Fig. 8.3).

Participant 1 improved the number of correct responses in Set 1 from 42% to 71%. However, Participant 2 improved the number of correct responses in Set 1 from 28% to 57 % only.

This study shows that vocal imitation through echoic and exemplar training improves articulation in children with developmental delays. It highlights the importance of response generalization in articulation interventions in applied behavior analysis, demonstrating that training on one word can lead to mastery of untrained words. The intervention was effective for both participants, despite their developmental delays, emphasizing the value of echoic and exemplar training.

8.10 Delimitations

Due to time constraints, the study could not complete training for all target words. Only the first two words were initiated for the first participant, and training for Sets 2 and 3 could not be started. External factors, such as participant absences and illnesses, also impacted the outcomes. Additionally, the study did not address whether articulation was generalized in natural settings, which could have provided deeper insights. The use of only an AB design limited conclusions, and a multiple baseline design would have yielded stronger generalizations. The varying number of words trained for each participant could have influenced comparative outcomes, as some target sounds were more challenging for one participant than for the other.

Acknowledgment The work was carried on at Amrit Somani Autism Center, ASMC, Kolkata, West Bengal, India. I acknowledge the support and assistance provided by Namita Somani, ASMC and Julianne Bell, BCBA, Former Director, ASMC, Kolkata, West Bengal, India

References

Baker, E., & McLeod, S. (2011). Evidence-based practice for children with speech sound disorders: Part 1 narrative review. *Language, Speech, Hearing Services in Schools, 42*, 102–139.

Eikeseth, S., & Nesset, R. (2003). Behavioral treatment of children with phonological disorder: The efficacy of vocal imitation and sufficient-response-exemplar training. *Journal Applied Behavioural Analysis, 36(3)*, 325–337. https://doi.org/10.1901/jaba.2003.36-325

Esch, B. E., Carr, J. E. & Grow, L. L. (2009). Evaluation of an enhanced stimulus–stimulus pairing procedure to increase early vocalizations of children with autism, *Journal Applied Behavioural Analyses, 42*(2), 225–241. https://doi.org/10.1901/jaba.2009.42-225

Horne, P. J., & Lowe, C. F. (1996). On the origins of naming and other symbolic behaviour. *Journal of Experimental Analyses of Behaviour, 65*(1), 185–241. https://doi.org/10.1901/jeab.1996.65-185

Johnson, C. P. (2004). Early clinical characteristics of children with autism. In V. B. Gupta (Ed.), *Autistic spectrum disorders in children* (pp. 96–134). Marcel Dekker.

Koegel, R. L., O'Dell, M., & Dunlap, G. (1998). Producing speech use in nonverbal autistic children by reinforcing attempts. *Journal of Autism and Developmental Disorders, 18(4)*, 525–538.

Lovaas, O. I. (2003). *Teaching individuals with developmental delays: Basic intervention techniques*. Pro-Ed.

Miliotis, A., Sidener, T., Reeve, K., Carbone, V. J., Radar, L., Sidener, D., & Delmolino. (2010). Stimulus-stimulus pairing of vocalizations: A systematic replication and evaluation of number of target sound per trial. *Journal of Applied Behavior Analysis*. (in press).

Mirenda, P. (2003). Toward functional augmentative and alternative communication for students with autism: Manual signs, graphic symbols, and voice output communication aids. *Language, Speech, and Hearing Services in Schools, 34*, 203–216.

Pace, J. (2011). Critical Review: Is PROMPT an effective treatment method for children with speech production disorders?

Partington, J. W., & Sundberg, M. L. (1998). *The Assessment of Basic Language and Learning Skills (ABLLS)*. Pleasant Hill: Behavior Analysts, ASIN B0006RMKGY, Massachussets, USA

Peturstdottir, A. I., Carp, C. L., Matthies, D. W., & Esch, B. E. (2011). Analyzing stimulus-stimulus pairing effects on preferences for speech sounds. *The Analysis of Verbal Behavior, 27*, 45–60.

Ross, D. E., & Greer, R. D. (2003). Generalized imitation and the mand: Introducing first instances of speech in young children with autism. *Research in Developmental Disabilities, 24*, 58–74.
Roy, A. (2003). *A Comparative Study of Special Education in India and China* M.A Dissertation. University of Honkong, The HKU Scholars hub, http://hdl.handle.net/10722/30306
Smith, T. (1998). Outcome of early intervention for children with autism. *Clinical Psychology: Science & Practice, 6*, 33–49.

Chapter 9
Applied Behavior Analysis-Based Strategies for Transitioning to Inclusive Education Settings

Sarah C. Mead Jasperse, Michelle P. Kelly, Melissa L. Oliver, Elena Couldrey, and Maryam Al Hammadi

Abstract Initial applied behavior analysis services for children diagnosed with autism spectrum disorder often start in a highly structured or familiar environment, such as the home or a clinic, with the ultimate goal of transitioning to a more inclusive setting. As behavior analysts work with clients and their support networks to plan for transitions to inclusive education contexts, they can utilize a variety of behavior analytic strategies to promote successful transitions. This chapter summarizes both pre-transition strategies and post-transition strategies that behavior analysts can implement as students move to inclusive education settings. Then, two case studies of successful transitions into inclusive education settings in the United Arab Emirates are offered as examples of how such strategies have been integrated and utilized in real-world contexts.

Keywords Autism spectrum disorder · Applied behavior analysis · Least restrictive environment · Mainstream schools · United Arab Emirates

S. C. Mead Jasperse (✉) · M. P. Kelly
Emirates College for Advanced Education, Abu Dhabi, United Arab Emirates
e-mail: Sarah.Mead@ecae.ac.ae; mkelly@ecae.ac.ae

M. L. Oliver · M. Al Hammadi
Mohammed bin Rashid Center for Special Education Operated by The New England Center for Children, Abu Dhabi, United Arab Emirates
e-mail: moliver@neccuae.org; malhammadi@neccuae.org

E. Couldrey
The New England Center for Children–GCC Consulting Division, Abu Dhabi, United Arab Emirates

S. Halder et al. (eds.), *Applied Behavior Analysis-Based Interventions for Autism Spectrum Disorder*, https://doi.org/10.1007/978-981-95-2889-9_9

When children diagnosed with autism spectrum disorder (ASD) begin receiving applied behavior analysis (ABA) services, they may start in a highly structured environment, such as their home or an ABA clinic, with a goal of transitioning to more naturalistic environments, such as a school, as soon as they are ready to participate successfully in the less-structured environment (The Council of Autism Service Providers, 2024). In fact, many regulatory bodies and funding entities mandate the development of transition goals from the outset of services. For example, initial authorization forms that must be submitted to insurance companies in order to access funding to begin ABA services often have a section that requires a description of the expected discharge plan (see Virginia's Department of Medical Assistance Services Initial Service Authorization Request form for an example; Department of Medical Assistance Services (2021)). Likewise, special education law in the United States (Individuals with Disabilities Education Act, 2004) requires that students with disabilities are educated in the least restrictive environment possible. Therefore, behavior analysts working with preschool- or school-aged children in intensive treatment contexts often are tasked with developing and implementing plans for successful transitions to inclusive education settings. In the design of those plans, they should look to evidence-based behavior analytic strategies that can be utilized before and after the transition to promote success in the inclusive environment.

The purpose of this chapter is to offer a brief summary of pre-transition and post-transition strategies that behavior analysts and educators can use when supporting children diagnosed with ASD through transitions to inclusive education settings (the post-transition environment) and to share two case studies of successful examples of transitions into inclusive education settings in the United Arab Emirates (UAE).

9.1 Applied Behavior Analytic Strategies to Promote Successful Transitions to Inclusive Education Settings

9.1.1 Pre-Transition Strategies

Preparation for a transition to an inclusive education setting begins long before the transition occurs. All members of the child's support network—including family members, educators, behavior analysts, and allied health professionals—and the child themself should contribute to the development of transition goals and transition planning. Behavior analysts should regularly self-evaluate the support network's adherence to a productive interprofessional collaboration model (Bowman et al., 2021) and a family-centered care approach (Brown et al., 2022). The child's perspectives, preferences, and contributions to the development of transition goals and plans can be incorporated by using assent-based practices throughout service delivery (Breaux & Smith, 2023). Finally, while engaging in transition planning, behavior analysts can advocate for goals that will promote meaningful outcomes in the post-transition environment and beyond (Bahry et al., 2023). After individualized and meaningful goals are developed by an interprofessional team using a family-centered and assent-based approach, a behavior analyst can begin using a variety of ABA-based strategies to best prepare the child for the transition while they still are receiving services in the pre-transition setting.

9.1.1.1 Incorporating Incidental Teaching Strategies

A behavior analyst might want to start by evaluating the teaching strategies being used in the pre-transition environment and determining where and how more incidental teaching strategies can be incorporated. There are plenty of choices of strategies to use when teaching new skills. Based on the needs of the learner and the skill being taught, behavior analysts could choose to use strategies or combinations of strategies, such as chaining, shaping, prompting, and more. When planning for a transition to an inclusive education setting, one may want to place a priority on strategies that utilize an incidental teaching approach. While highly instructor-directed strategies, such as discrete-trial teaching, might result in speedy acquisition, incidental teaching has been shown to lead to greater generalization and spontaneous engagement in skills (Miranda-Linné & Melin, 1992). For example, when teaching the identification of and response to signs and symbols that a student might encounter in an inclusive education environment (e.g., danger, exit), a behavior analyst might want to incorporate incidental teaching of the signs to increase the likelihood that the student will be able to respond correctly when coming across the signs in their post-transition environment.

9.1.1.2 Selecting an Appropriate Communication System for the Post-Transition Environment

When a child with ASD has complex communicative needs, a critical decision that must be made in the pre-transition environment is what type of communication system is the best fit for the child, for their communication goals, and for their communication contexts. If substantial time, effort, and resources are going to be expended to teach an augmentative and alternative communication (AAC) system in the pre-transition environment, then it probably would be wise to ensure that the selected system is an appropriate match for the expected post-transition setting. If, for example, substantial time is spent teaching a high-tech AAC system with a proprietary application that requires expert programming by a clinician familiar with the app but there are not any trained personnel in the post-transition environment who can oversee the system, then time spent teaching the use of that AAC system (and money spent purchasing it!) may have been wasted. While working in close collaboration with a speech-language pathologist, behavior analysts may want to conduct an ecological inventory of both the pre-transition and expected post-transition environment prior to selecting an AAC system (Reichle et al., 2019). Once an AAC system is selected, other variables within the system also can be aligned with the post-transition environment (e.g., vocabulary, language of instruction).

9.1.1.3 Moving from Individualized Instruction to Group Instruction

One major difference that a child may experience when moving from an intensive intervention environment to an inclusive education setting is a shift in teacher-to-student ratios. A typical staffing pattern in early intervention ABA autism services is a 1:1 ratio of behavior technicians to children (The Council of Autism Service Providers, 2024). That is, each learner receives individualized instruction. However, most general education environments have a ratio of one teacher to an entire class of students. Inclusive education environments might have a few more teachers or instructional aides available to support students' additional needs, but a 1:1 ratio would not be typical of an inclusive setting. Even if a student has a dedicated paraprofessional with them, the student still is likely to need to attend to and respond to instruction and feedback from a shared classroom teacher. Therefore, behavior analysts may want to consider moving from individualized instruction to group instruction in the pre-transition environment so the child already has experience with group instruction prior to joining an inclusive education setting. This could be done by fading any number of variables—the number of learners in a group instruction context, the amount of time spent in a group instruction context, the number of skills taught in a group instruction context, and more. While practicing learning in a group instruction context, behavior analysts can incorporate opportunities to teach skills that will be necessary in a classroom setting, such as waiting for teacher attention, recruiting assistance, sharing materials, cooperating with peers, and advocating for one's needs and preferences.

9.1.1.4 Promoting Generalization Across Teaching Staff

Another result of individualized instruction is that learners may become used to working with a specific person or a small group of people in the pre-transition environment. If a child has developed a robust repertoire of functional skills and academic skills in the pre-transition setting but only reliably utilizes that repertoire with a few people, then there is a high probability that those skills will not transfer over to the post-transition environment. One approach to combating this issue would be to promote generalization across teaching staff in the pre-transition environment rather than exclusively focusing on skill building in a single 1:1 teacher–student relationship. In 1977, Stokes and Baer offered nine approaches to programming generalization, and two of them might be particularly useful when promoting generalization of skills across teaching staff. First, behavior analysts might incorporate sequential modification. In this approach, the child would be taught a new skill to a mastery level with their primary instructor in the pre-transition setting. Then, their performance would be assessed with a novel instructor. If the child does not perform the skill to the mastery level with the novel instructor, then teaching would begin with the novel instructor in the same manner. Once mastery is achieved with the novel instructor, performance would be assessed with a third instructor. This pattern of assessing and teaching would be continued until the student is able to complete the skill at a mastery level with a new instructor without having to go through the teaching procedure with that instructor. A more proactive approach would be to utilize sufficient exemplars in the initial teaching. In this case, instead of training a skill to mastery with a single instructor, the child would practice the skill to mastery with a variety of instructors simultaneously. If sufficient instructors are included in the initial training, then the skill should generalize to any novel instructor after mastery. No matter what approach the behavior analyst uses to promote generalization, the case probably can be made for a child having exposure to and learning from multiple instructors in the pre-transition setting.

9.1.1.5 Promoting Generalization Across Environments

When preparing for transitions to an inclusive classroom, similar considerations should be made regarding generalization across environments. Once again, if a child can only utilize their skills in the pre-transition setting, such as their home or an early intervention clinic, then they will not be prepared to succeed in the post-transition setting. To promote generalization across environments, behavior analysts might want to utilize another of the strategies described by Stokes and Baer (1977)—program common stimuli. Here, the approach would be to incorporate as many stimuli as possible from the post-transition environment into the pre-transition environment. For example, if the post-transition environment uses tablets for learning and teaching, then tablets should be used in the pre-transition environment. If the post-transition environment requires school uniforms, then the school uniform should be used in the pre-transition environment. This will require the behavior analyst to collaborate closely with the personnel in the post-transition setting to identify particularly salient and requisite stimuli to bring into the pre-transition environment.

9.1.1.6 Teaching Self-Advocacy Skills, Self-Help Skills, and Other Skills with Practical Implications

As the child and child's support team identify transition goals and prepare for transition planning, they may want to prioritize teaching self-advocacy skills, self-help skills, and other skills that will have practical implications for the student's immediate experience in the inclusive education setting.

Self-advocacy skills are crucial for a number of reasons as children move into their post-transition environment. As discussed previously, staffing ratios often shift during the transition, so the student may not have someone constantly monitoring their needs and advocating on their behalf. Being able to do things such as request a bathroom break, ask to leave an environment they do not want to be in, or seek help to solve a problem can profoundly impact a student's wellbeing in an inclusive setting. Next, as students spend more time in inclusive, less restrictive environments, including post-secondary work or educational contexts, they may need to advocate for themselves in order to access the supports, accommodations, or services they need in order to participate in a full and meaningful way (Schena et al., 2023). Finally, individuals diagnosed with ASD already are at a higher risk of abuse and victimization during their lifetimes (Weiss & Fardella, 2018), and this risk may be compounded when ABA programs place a high value on compliance over self-advocacy and do not teach critical safety skills, such as saying no and withdrawing consent/assent (Mathur et al., 2024). As students move from closely monitored pre-transition environments to less supervised post-transition environments, arriving with a repertoire of self-advocacy skills could be a significant protective factor.

Mastery of self-help skills, or self-care skills, such as toileting, completing hygiene routines, eating, and managing time, may facilitate a smoother transition to an inclusive education setting if they mean that students can access more environments, reinforcers, and learning opportunities. In other words, any self-help skill that could be considered a behavioral cusp (Bosch & Fuqua, 2001) could be an excellent target for practicing in the pre-transition environment in preparation for maximum participation in the post-transition environment. However, behavior analysts also should be vigilant to avoid a hyperfocus on total independence as a blanket goal for all skills. There are many acceptable and effective ways to complete tasks without total independence (e.g., choosing to complete the task of cutting one's hair by booking an appointment at the salon rather than by getting out scissors and chopping it off independently is generally acceptable and effective). When behavior analysts hold neurodiverse clients to a higher degree of expectation of independence compared to the rest of society, this is problematic and not in alignment with the neurodiversity paradigm (Breaux, 2023).

Self-advocacy skills and self-help skills are two categories of skills that could have practical implications on a student's experience in an inclusive setting. Any additional skills that can increase a student's well-being, safety, or ability to participate in the learning environment should be considered for teaching in the pre-transition setting.

The pre-transition strategies summarized in this chapter are only some of the options that behavior analysts have available to them when planning for a child's transition to an inclusive education setting. Different strategies may be more or less useful at different points in time prior to the transition, and the behavior analyst should use their clinical judgment, while working within their scope of practice and scope of competence (Brodhead et al., 2018), to select effective and evidence-based strategies to individualize for their pre-transition students.

9.1.2 Post-Transition Strategies

While the pre-transition strategies primarily are approaches that behavior analysts can use when providing ABA services in the pre-transition environment, the post-transition strategies that follow are ABA-based techniques that educators in inclusive environments can incorporate into their settings to promote successful transitions for students diagnosed with ASD. After a transition to an inclusive education setting, a behavior analyst may or may not continue involvement as part of a student's support team. If a behavior analyst is going to discharge a client as soon as they enroll in the mainstream school, then the behavior analyst should proactively work with the post-transition teaching and clinical team to facilitate a smooth transition. This may involve making suggestions for effective post-transition strategies or incorporating other pre-transition strategies as requested by the post-transition team. If a behavior analyst is going to continue to be part of a student's support team, either on a consultative basis or by providing or overseeing ABA services in the post-transition setting, then an ongoing collaborative relationship with the complete post-transition support team will be critical.

9.1.2.1 Implementing Reinforcement Programs Designed for Inclusive Classrooms

One of the most proactive and thoroughgoing ABA-based strategies that an educator can use in an inclusive classroom is a thoughtful reinforcement program designed for use in that environment. Behavior analysts can support the design of reinforcement systems in the post-transition environment by dispelling any misconceptions and sharing the many options that are available. For example, if personnel in the post-transition environment think that reinforcement programs are synonymous only with prize boxes, sticker charts, and the like, then behavior analysts can clarify that reinforcement programs can be customized to suit any context or population. One type of reinforcement program that might be particularly suited to the inclusive education setting is one based on healthy contingencies (St. Peter & Marsteller, 2017) or healthy behavioral practices (Kamana, 2019; Kanaman, 2022).

In a healthy contingencies model, a teacher would make an effort to deliver common social reinforcers after desired behavior (e.g., offering a break after completing work) and withhold those reinforcers after problematic behavior (e.g., not giving lots of attention after an inappropriate statement). This approach would be taken with all students in the classroom—not just with the student with ASD—and would serve to promote prosocial behaviors and discourage disruptive behaviors. In a healthy behavioral practices model, teachers would incorporate four strategies into their teaching—providing plentiful positive interactions, delivering effective instructions, promoting activity engagement, and responding to disruptive behavior with healthy contingencies as described previously. Neither the healthy contingencies model or the healthy behavioral practices model involves complex schedules of reinforcement, requires extensive training in ABA, uses specialized materials, or takes excessive time to implement. Thus, these approaches may be appealing to and feasible for inclusive classroom teachers.

In some cases, more individualized systems of reinforcement might be indicated, especially if the systems are designed to promote the generalization of skills learned in the pre-transition environment to the post-transition environment. If this approach is selected, then behavior analysts may want to be mindful of creating a system that is not only effective and feasible but also one that minimizes any potential stigmatization of the student (Han et al., 2022) by avoiding reinforcement programs that might result in the student being bullied, targeted, or otherwise excluded in the environment.

9.1.2.2 Differentiating Instruction and Providing Accommodations and Modifications

While differentiating instruction and providing accommodations and modifications in the inclusive education environment have long been within the scope of practice of general and special education teachers, behavior analysts can offer useful contributions as educators figure out how to best differentiate for a student in the post-transition environment. For example, strategies for differentiation in the classroom could include identifying component skills of a complex response, implementing peer tutoring, prompting, incorporating competency-based teaching, using data to monitor student progress, and teaching self-management skills (Pozas & Schneider, 2019) and all have empirical support in the ABA literature. When a behavior analyst's expertise overlaps with strategies used in differentiated instruction, they may be able to provide consultation about how to best implement the strategy with the student in the post-transition environment. The same logic extends to accommodations or modifications made for the student. If the proposed accommodations or modifications are related to behavior analytic strategies, then a behavior analyst's input could be valuable. For example, if the team in the post-transition environment is considering an accommodation that allows the student to take frequent breaks, then a behavior analyst's guidance about how to deploy that accommodation while preventing the emergence of problematic contingencies could be critical to the student's success.

9.1.2.3 Incorporating Active Student Responding Activities

As students transition into the inclusive education environment, one concern might be students' levels of academic engagement. If a student is used to working only in individual or small-group instruction contexts in the pre-transition environment, then they may struggle to stay engaged with the academic content and learning process when they are one of many students in a classroom. This concern is an important one as students' opportunities to respond (OTR) have been linked to academic and behavioral outcomes, with higher OTR being correlated with better outcomes (Stitcher et al., 2009). Teachers in inclusive classrooms can increase OTR for students with and without special educational needs by incorporating active student responding (ASR) activities, such as choral responding, response cards, and guided notes (Twyman & Heward, 2018).

9.1.2.4 Creating and Following Behavior Contracts

Behavior analysts may want to consider partnering with personnel in the post-transition setting to co-develop a behavior contract with the student that will help set them up for success in the inclusive setting. Behavior contracts involve creating clear, written statements of expected behavior, the consequences for engaging in or not engaging in the expected behavior, and other details of how, when, and by whom the consequences will be delivered. They have been shown to be effective – both in decreasing disruptive behavior and increasing academic outcomes—across a number of contexts (Bowman-Perrott et al., 2015). When students are preparing to transition to an inclusive educational setting, behavior contracts could be an effective, assent-based method for delineating and agreeing to shared expectations post-transition.

9.1.2.5 Using Classwide Approaches and Group Contingencies

Finally, educators in inclusive classrooms might want to incorporate group contingencies and classwide approaches to maximize the inclusive experience for students. Similar to reinforcement programs, group contingencies could take a number of effective forms in the inclusive classroom, but any contingencies that promote cooperation in support of whole-class success would be reasonable strategies to consider (for examples of group contingencies in general education classrooms, see Beaver et al., 2023). One extensively researched application of a group contingency in classrooms is the Good Behavior Game (GBG; Flower et al., 2014). While there has been a call for more research about using the GBG in inclusive classrooms specifically (Jornevald et al., 2024), there are instructional guides available for behavior analysts to share with general education teachers about how to use the GBG in general (Joslyn et al., 2020) and in inclusive settings (Lastrapes, 2013). A variation of the GBG that may be particularly useful in an inclusive setting is the Good Inclusion Game (GIG; Dillenburger & Coyle, 2019; Graham et al., 2024). In the GIG, the contingencies are placed on cooperative behavior, such as communication and sharing, to promote behaviors that make the classroom a more inclusive and collaborative place for everyone.

Similar to the pre-transition strategies, the options for post-transition strategies described here represent only a sample of the ABA-based possibilities available for supporting students in inclusive education settings. The selection of strategies for any given student should be individualized based on the needs of the student and the environment.

9.2 Case Examples from the United Arab Emirates

Of course, selected strategies typically are not used in isolation as they are primarily described here. They can be used in combination—either concurrently or consecutively—and should be continuously evaluated for effectiveness and social validity. Next, to demonstrate how multiple strategies can be synthesized during a transition to an inclusive education setting, two case examples of students who made successful transitions in the UAE will be shared.

9.2.1 Special and Inclusive Education in the United Arab Emirates

The UAE is a constitutional federation of seven emirates that is located in the Gulf region of the Middle East (U.ae, 2024). As of 2022, the reported population of the UAE was just over ten million (Ministry of Cabinet Affairs, 2024b). Approximately 11% of the population are UAE Nationals (Emirati), and the remainder of the population is made up of expatriate residents (Ministry of Foreign Affairs, 2024).

While special classrooms have been legally mandated in mainstream UAE government schools since 1981, it was not until 2006 that the UAE government significantly reevaluated its approach to supporting students with special educational needs and disabilities (Gaad, 2019; Gallagher, 2019). Federal Law 29/2006 came in direct response to the UAE's ratification of the United Nations' Convention on the Rights of People with Disabilities (UNRCPD, 2000), which ensures equal educational rights for individuals with special needs (Ministry of Cabinet Affairs, 2024a). Then, the national strategy for people with disabilities was launched by His Highness Sheikh Mohammed bin Rashid Al Maktoum, Vice President and Prime Minister of UAE and Ruler of Dubai, in April 2017, and the term "people of determination" was initiated to highlight these individuals' abilities and not their disabilities (Kelly et al., 2024). Readers are encouraged to consult Gaad (2019) for a comprehensive history of special and inclusive education in the UAE.

In the UAE, free, government-provided schools are generally only available to UAE Nationals and private schools are primarily comprised of expatriate residents, although Emirati students may enroll in private schools and pay for their education (Gallagher, 2019). The UAE has taken many steps to fulfill its commitment to students of determination by implementing policies and mechanisms that promote inclusive education practices and enhance equal access across both public and private school systems (Massouti et al., 2024).

9.2.1.1 Public Schools

In 2008, the MOE established the Special Education Department (since renamed the People of Determination Department) to protect the rights of students of determination and ensure equal opportunities are provided to all students (U.ae, 2024). The 2020 Ministerial Resolution No. 647 on the policy of inclusive education directs government schools to "cater to the needs of students of determination and provide them with the best education services" (U.ae, 2024). Some of the free services and facilities offered by the ministry include accessible buildings, specialized intervention services (e.g., speech and language sessions), devices and assistive technology, and professional development for teachers.

9.2.1.2 Private Schools

The Dubai government has enacted several laws (including Dubai Law No. 2 of 2014 and Executive Council Resolution No. 2 of 2017) to promote the inclusion of students of determination in the private education sector (Massouti et al., 2024). To comply with local laws and regulations, the Knowledge and Human Development Authority (KHDA, 2017) issued the Dubai Inclusive Education Policy Framework (DIEPF), which includes ten standards and corresponding actions that promote inclusivity and equity in schools and provide guidelines for establishing inclusive learning environments that cater to the needs of all learners (Massouti et al., 2024). In Abu Dhabi, the Department of Education and Knowledge (ADEK) published an inclusion policy for schools, which went into effect in October 2023, that mandates that Abu Dhabi schools must accommodate all students with additional learning needs and, if unable to do so for a particular student, must provide documented evidence explaining their limitations.

9.2.2 Applied Behavior Analysis in the United Arab Emirates

Applied behavior analysts in the UAE have faced a range of challenges, such as limited access to resources, professional isolation, ethical dilemmas, and the complexities arising from the diverse cultural backgrounds of both clients and staff (Bhuptani, 2024; Olsen & Kelly, 2020). Despite these obstacles, significant progress has been made in the UAE, including successful interprofessional collaborations, translation efforts, an increase in the dissemination of research outputs, and enhanced access to ASD support and services (see Kelly et al., 2024). Regarding service delivery, Kelly et al. (2024) reported that there are over 35 centers with at least one certified behavior analyst on site in the UAE, and, as of August 2024, there were 1053 Behavior Analyst Certification Board (BACB) certificants in the UAE, comprising 6 Board Certified Behavior Analysts-Doctoral® (BCBA-Ds®), 144 Board Certified Behavior Analysts® (BCBAs®), 44 Board Certified Assistant

Behavior Analysts® (BCaBAs®), and 859 Registered Behavior Technicians® (RBTs®; BACB, 2024). The BACB (2023) expressed hope that the next era of behavior analyst credentialing outside the United States and Canada will involve a commitment to country-specific standards that support the continued growth of the profession in many countries. In line with this, National Occupational Standards (NOS) for Applied Behavior Analysts were developed in the UAE using a five-phase model: (a) preparation, (b) development, (c) review, (d) validation, and (e) endorsement by the National Qualifications Council (Kelly & Trifyllis, 2022).

9.2.3 Special Considerations for Inclusive Education in the United Arab Emirates

With the mandates for inclusive education in both public and private schools in the UAE and behavior analysis growing as a field in the country, behavior analysts are increasingly likely to be part of transition planning for students who are getting ready to shift from ABA centers to mainstream schools. Besides utilizing evidence-based ABA strategies as described previously to support the transition, there are a few other special considerations that must be addressed when students move to inclusive education settings in the UAE.

In contrast to other countries that primarily use a neighborhood-based public school system to education, the heavy reliance on the private school approach in the UAE, especially for expatriate residents, sometimes makes it difficult to identify an inclusive education setting into which students with ASD can transition as some schools have entrance criteria that are difficult for students of determination to meet. Even when these criteria are met, available enrollment for students of determination often is already at capacity. Then, if students are provided with school placements, support staff may have limited training, an important consideration to ensure a genuinely inclusive education system (Massouti et al., 2024) and inclusive education teachers may not be prepared to implement ABA-based strategies in their classrooms. Arabic-speaking special educators were interviewed in Saudi Arabia, a nearby Gulf country, to explore the challenges they faced and their perceptions of ABA-based intervention for students with ASD (Almutlaq, 2021). Findings showed that although teachers viewed ABA-based strategies as effective for students with ASD, they held misconceptions about ABA and felt inadequately prepared to carry out these strategies.

Another special consideration relates to curriculum. Given that over 200 nationalities call the UAE home and approximately 89% of the population identify as expatriates (Ministry of Foreign Affairs, 2024), it is not surprising that a wide array of curricula are offered to students (and sometimes several curricular track options are offered within a school), including American, Australian, British, Canadian, French, German, Indian, International Baccalaureate, Italian, Pakistani, and international hybrids of these (Gallagher, 2019). For behavior analysts working to support students transitioning to inclusive education settings in the UAE, familiarity with a wide variety of curricula and approaches to education is crucial, as Individualized Education Plans are not standardized and vary significantly between schools, requiring adaptability and a thorough understanding of the unique requirements of each setting.

Finally, for behavior analysts working in the UAE, it is important to not only understand Emirati culture but also to gain knowledge of other cultures, as they likely will work with families from diverse educational backgrounds, religions, and cultural backgrounds. Olsen and Kelly (2020) provided valuable guidelines for working with Arab-Muslim families, emphasizing the importance of understanding Islamic principles, cultural formalities, norms, and gender roles. As well as commonly targeted behaviors, such as social skills, communication, and adaptive living skills, behavior analysts in the UAE are often asked to address culturally-specific behaviors. These may include using specific greetings, learning to recite the Quran, performing the five daily prayers and ablution, wearing specific dress, fasting during the month of Ramadan, and using water for cleansing after toileting, among other behaviors. These skills may be of particular importance as behavior analysts help their clients prepare to transition to more inclusive environments.

With these considerations in mind, the following case examples of Rashid and Hazim (pseudonyms), two young students living in the UAE, are offered as examples of how ABA-based strategies can be implemented in the pre-transition and post-transition environments to support transitions from full-time ABA-based programming to inclusive education settings.

9.2.4 Case Example 1: Rashid

9.2.4.1 Case Background

Rashid is a 6-year-old student in the UAE who was diagnosed with ASD at the age of three. His mother noticed that he made limited eye contact, had few attempts to speak or engage with his siblings, experienced prolonged tantrums, and demonstrated a fixation on specific toys. Following his diagnosis, Rashid enrolled in a center for autistic students in Abu Dhabi that utilized ABA-based interventions. The same behaviors were observed in this context. After an initial adjustment period, Rashid began to make progress in communication and social skills, as well as in academic areas, such as counting and reading. His rapid progress across the year and half at the center led the family and his school team to consider whether Rashid was ready to transition to a mainstream school setting where support would be faded over time.

9.2.4.2 Transition Goals and Special Considerations

In the UAE, acceptance of ASD has become more widespread in the recent past and an understanding of how to meaningfully integrate students, both within and outside of schools, has become more apparent through the availability of resources and visible indicators of inclusivity. These indicators include, for example, designated quiet spaces, access to modified resources, and additional staff to support students with individualized needs. Such supports were evident in the school to which Rashid transitioned.

The center coordinated Rashid's transition with a plan to gradually reduce full-time support as Rashid demonstrated readiness for greater independence. His team worked collaboratively to prepare him for the inclusive setting, focusing on the following goals:

1. Build confidence and independence in the school environment: Ensure Rashid becomes comfortable navigating the school by following the classroom teacher and peers.
2. Decrease support: Transition from a center-based program with individualized programming to a mainstream setting with a low teacher-to-student ratio and whole-group instruction.
3. Establish classroom readiness: Teach and practice the skills necessary for school success, including following classroom routines, learning new academic skills, and managing time.
4. Establish social skills readiness: Develop strategies for Rashid to build successful relationships with peers and navigate challenging social interactions.

9.2.4.3 Pre-Transition Strategies

From the time Rashid entered the center-based program, preparations for a less restrictive environment were ongoing. He was taught foundational skills that improved his ability to learn from his natural environment, such as attending, responding to a conversation partner, and engaging in play skills, among others. To prepare for the transition to a mainstream education setting, Rashid experienced smaller transitions first to ease the process and fade support. He started in a 1:1 teacher-to-student ratio, receiving intensive instruction and comprehensive support throughout the school day. As he gained more independence, he moved to a 1:2 instructional ratio but with similar support levels.

When Rashid demonstrated greater independence with task completion and social skills, he transitioned to a classroom within the center-based setting that offered the chance to participate in whole-class group instruction several times a day with a support teacher available as needed. This classroom was designed to replicate an inclusive classroom environment, allowing Rashid to practice independent movement and other skills necessary for success in a mainstream setting.

During his time in the center-based program, Rashid learned through discrete-trial teaching and natural environment teaching with many opportunities for group learning. The level of support he received was tailored to his needs, with an emphasis on fostering independence. By the time he was ready to transition, Rashid had shown that he was prepared for a less restrictive setting.

Before the transition, Rashid visited his new school, and the school staff observed him at the center. Additionally, the center's team met with the school to review Rashid's behavior support program, areas of interest, as well as areas of concern raised by the family. Collaboration with the mainstream school was a crucial element of the successful transition.

9.2.4.4 Post-Transition Strategies

After transitioning to the mainstream setting, the school assumed full responsibility for Rashid's support and education. Various strategies were implemented post-transition to ensure a successful entry into an inclusive education setting for Rashid. The center maintained a collaborative relationship with the mainstream school, offering support as needed. It was agreed that Rashid would begin in the mainstream setting with a support teacher hired and trained by the school and that the behavioral interventions already in place would continue and would be faded as deemed appropriate by the mainstream team.

In addition to general recommendations, the center met with the school's Head of Inclusion to discuss the need for accommodations and modifications for in-class and homework assignments, as well as the implementation of a meaningful reinforcement system. The center's staff later trained the support teacher and classroom teacher on how to use the reinforcement system effectively. Rashid earned points for following classroom rules, completing his work, and displaying other positive behaviors. This system was implemented discreetly, as it was not a classroom-wide program. Rashid used his points to access preferred items or visit preferred locations within the school.

The center also recommended continuing ABA services during the school day to support Rashid's transition, focusing on enhancing his social skills and managing new and challenging tasks. The support teacher working with Rashid had ABA training but was not certified or licensed as a behavior analyst.

9.2.4.5 Successes, Ongoing Challenges, and Future Goals

Throughout Rashid's transition to mainstream education, significant improvements were observed in his social skills, academic achievements, and independence in scheduled activities. His most notable progress was in adapting to significant changes in his daily routine. Rashid engaged in structured play with his peers with minimal support and followed instructions from the classroom teacher. The support teacher was able to gradually reduce assistance in specific classes, allowing Rashid to complete independent and group work with minimal help. These successes were largely due to the thorough preparation before the transition and the ongoing collaboration between the center and the school.

However, Rashid continued to face challenges, particularly in forming friendships with his peers. He struggled to interpret social cues and required ongoing coaching from the support teacher to navigate these difficulties. The focus remained on developing Rashid's social skills and gradually transitioning support responsibilities from the support teacher to the classroom teacher and peers.

9.2.5 *Case Example 2: Hazim*

9.2.5.1 Case Background

Hazim is a 5-year-old boy in the UAE who was diagnosed with ASD when he was 3 years old. He began receiving clinic-based ABA services at that time after being referred for services by his pediatrician. Initially, Hazim presented with challenges surrounding expressive and receptive language and social interactions with others. He also presented with deficits in prosocial behavior; more specifically, he would often shout, throw items, and/or flop to the floor when presented with a nonpreferred task or instruction. During the two years that Hazim received clinic-based ABA services, he made significant progress in various areas, including following directions, transitioning between tasks and activities, functional communication, and self-regulation. In light of Hazim's growth and progress across the years, the family and clinic team all agreed that it was time to support Hazim to transition into an inclusive school setting.

9.2.5.2 Transition Goals and Special Considerations

After meeting with the school to better understand the expectations surrounding student behavior in the classroom, transition goals that specifically targeted inclusion-readiness skills were developed. The transition goals included: following directions in a group setting, following routines, making requests, and developing play skills. One special consideration that the transition team had to plan for was Hazim's transportation. While his parents were able to drive Hazim to the clinic, Hazim's new school was located on the other side of the city, a 30-minute drive from their home. So, a plan had to be made for how to help him learn how to safely ride on a school bus.

9.2.5.3 Pre-Transition Strategies

In order to effectively prepare for the upcoming transition into the inclusive school setting, the teaching style used by the behavior therapists working with Hazim shifted from discrete-trial instruction to more naturalistic teaching strategies. This shift allowed Hazim to access naturally-occurring reinforcement, similar to the type of reinforcement that he would access in the mainstream school setting. The clinic team also began to shift from 1:1, individualized instruction to group instruction during clinic sessions. More specifically, ABA sessions included group activities (e.g., group lessons, circle time, group play) to prepare Hazim to successfully navigate, enjoy, and learn during the collaborative instructional experience that he would encounter in the classroom.

Generalization was also heavily prioritized during the pre-transition phase. During the weeks leading up the transition, Hazim worked with various behavior therapists in the clinic to ensure that he was able to successfully perform learned skills across multiple people. Additionally, Hazim's reinforcement schedule was thinned to match that of what would be typical in the classroom. During the weeks leading up to the transition, reinforcement schedules consisted of intermittent praise with scheduled play times to emulate the type of reinforcement that Hazim likely would experience in the classroom. Lastly, an emphasis was put on helping Hazim to independently manage the daily activities that he would encounter in the classroom. For instance, prior to starting academic work during ABA sessions, the therapist working with Hazim would use least-to-most prompting techniques to guide him in gathering his materials for the lesson (e.g., walking to his workspace, sitting in his seat, getting his pencil).

9.2.5.4 Post-Transition Strategies

Once the transition into the mainstream school setting was complete (i.e., Hazim was attending mainstream school for the entirety of the school day), support from his behavior analyst continued to be provided to ensure that the school team understood how to provide consistent, effective, and individualized support to Hazim. The support from the behavior analyst focused heavily on post-transition strategies that included differentiated instruction and whole-class reinforcement systems.

When working with the school team on how to provide differentiated instruction for Hazim, the behavior analyst worked collaboratively with the classroom teacher to ensure that classroom instruction was tailored to meet Hazim's individual needs. For example, the behavior analyst and classroom teacher worked together to ensure that tasks and assignments were modified and that expectations for assignments and assessments were developed based on Hazim's skill levels. This consisted of utilizing tools such as visuals aids and choice boards in addition to providing Hazim with multiple options of how to complete a task or assignment. While this focus on differentiated instruction was critical in ensuring that Hazim's unique learning needs were met in the classroom, the strategies put in place also benefited many other students in the class who displayed diverse learning needs.

Given that Hazim did not have 1:1 support in the classroom (he instead was supported by the classroom's teaching assistant who worked with several of the children in the class), the behavior analyst worked with the classroom teacher to develop whole-class reinforcement systems that would benefit not only Hazim but all of the other students in the class as well. The reinforcement system created consisted of students earning points for following three predetermined and agreed-upon rules that were explicitly taught and reviewed with the class. Once earned, students could exchange their points to "buy" different rewards from the class reward menu. The classroom teacher praised students intermittently throughout lessons for following the class rules, and points were delivered to individual students at the end of each lesson.

9.2.5.5 Successes, Ongoing Challenges, and Future Goals

In the months after the transition to the mainstream school setting, Hazim's successes were largely due to the collaborative relationship between the school team and the behavior analyst. The school team was willing to learn and was consistently open to new ideas and adopting strategies that ultimately would help Hazim to be successful in the classroom. The behavior analyst worked to ensure that the suggestions made and strategies put in place were sustainable and achievable for both the classroom teacher and the support teacher to implement even while having many other students in the class also needing support support.

Despite the overall success of Hazim's transition, there continued to be ongoing challenges. More specifically, as Hazim continued to progress through his academic career, it became increasingly more challenging to ensure that tasks and assignments were differentiated to meet his needs due to the increase in academic expectations and rigidity of the school curriculum for older students. Being mindful of these challenges from the onset of the transition helped ensure that the team was able to proactively plan for ways to mitigate these challenges while simultaneously working to ensure the continued success of Hazim in the school setting.

9.3 Conclusion

This chapter covered what can be an incredibly important time in the life of a child with ASD—a transition into an inclusive education setting. The role a behavior analyst can take during this time is crucial as ABA-based strategies in the pre-transition and post-transition environment can help set the student up for success. The strategies summarized in this chapter and then demonstrated in the case examples are just highlights of the options available to behavior analysts. Regardless of the strategies used, behavior analysts are encouraged to consult the literature, collaborate with the student's support network, and include the student in the transition planning.

References

Almutlaq, H. (2021). Saudi special educators' perceptions of applied behavior analysis for students with autism. *World Journal of Education, 11*(4), 18–30. https://doi.org/10.5430/wje.v11n4p18

Bahry, S., Gerhardt, P. E., Weiss, M. J., Leaf, J. B., Putnam, R. F., & Bondy, A. (2023). The ethics of actually helping people: Targeting skill acquisition goals that promote meaningful outcomes for individuals with autism spectrum disorder. *Behavior Analysis in Practice, 16*, 672–695. https://doi.org/10.1007/s40617-022-00757-x

Beaver, B. N., Ré, T., Griffith, A. K., Zhang, D., & Schoener, M. A. (2023). A systematic literature review of group contingencies within general education classrooms. *Contemporary School Psychology, 28*, 421–434. https://doi.org/10.1007/s40688-023-00448-6

Behavior Analyst Certification Board. (2023). *Recent changes to the BACB's international focus.* https://www.bacb.com/wp-content/uploads/2022/01/Recent-Changes-to-International-Focus_220711.pdf

Behavior Analyst Certification Board [BACB]. (2024). *Region-specific certificant data.* https://www.bacb.com/services/o.php?page=101134

Bhuptani, N. (2024, May 27). *Pioneering behavior analysis in the United Arab Emirates: Challenges, solutions and the road ahead* [Invited paper session]. 50th Annual Convention of the Association for Behavior Analysis International, Philadelphia, PA, USA.

Bosch, S., & Fuqua, R. W. (2001). Behavioral cusps: A model for selecting target behaviors. *Journal of Applied Behavior Analysis, 34*(1), 123–125. https://doi.org/10.1901/jaba.2001.34-123

Bowman, K. S., Suarez, V. D., & Weiss, M. J. (2021). Standards for interprofessional collaboration in the treatment of individuals with autism. *Behavior Analysis in Practice, 14*, 1191–1208. https://doi.org/10.1007/s40617-021-00560-0

Bowman-Perrott, L., Burke, M. D., deMarin, S., Zhang, N., & Davis, H. (2015). A meta-analysis of single-case research on behavior contracts: Effects on behavioral and academic outcomes among children and youth. *Behavior Modification, 39*(2), 247–269. https://doi.org/10.1177/0145445514551383

Breaux, C. A. (2023, May 28). *Neurodiversity-informed applied behavior analysis (ABA): Ethics through the neurodiversity paradigm* [Invited Paper Session]. 49th Annual Convention of the Association for Behavior Analysis International, Denver, CO, USA.

Breaux, C. A., & Smith, K. (2023). Assent in applied behaviour analysis and positive behaviour support: Ethical considerations and practical recommendations. *International Journal of Developmental Disabilities, 69*(1), 111–121. https://doi.org/10.1080/20473869.2022.2144969

Brodhead, M. T., Quigley, S. P., & Wilczynski, S. M. (2018). A call for discussion about scope of competence in behavior analysis. *Behavior Analysis in Practice, 11*, 424–435. https://doi.org/10.1007/s40617-018-00303-8

Brown, K. R., Hurd, A. M., Randall, K. R., Szabo, T., & Mitteer, D. R. (2022). A family-centered care approach to behavior-analytic assessment and intervention. *Behavior Analysis in Practice*. https://doi.org/10.1007/s40617-022-00756-y

Department of Medical Assistance Services. (2021). *Applied behavior analysis initial service authorization request form.* https://www.dmas.virginia.gov/media/4126/applied-behavior-analysis-initial-authorization-form-december-2021.pdf

Dillenburger, K., & Coyle, C. (2019). Education for all: The Good Inclusion Game. *Behavioral Interventions, 34*(3), 338–351. https://doi.org/10.1002/bin.1671

Flower, A., McKenna, J. W., Bunuan, R. L., Muething, C. S., & Vega, R., Jr. (2014). Effects of the Good Behavior Game on challenging behaviors in school settings. *Review of Educational Research, 84*(4), 546–571. https://doi.org/10.3102/0034654314536781

Gaad, E. (2019). Educating learners with special needs and disabilities in the UAE: Reform and innovation. In K. Gallagher (Ed.), *Education in the United Arab Emirates* (pp. 147–159). Springer. https://doi.org/10.1007/978-981-13-7736-5_9

Gallagher, K. (2019). Introduction: Education in the UAE–Context and themes. In K. Gallagher (Ed.), *Education in the United Arab Emirates* (pp. 1–18). Springer. https://doi.org/10.1007/978-981-13-7736-5_1
Graham, S., Keenan, M., & Dillenburger, K. (2024). All for one and one for all: The good inclusion game. *Behavioral Interventions*. https://doi.org/10.1002/bin.2048
Han, E., Scior, K., Avramides, K., & Crane, L. (2022). A systematic review on autistic people's experiences of stigma and coping strategies. *Autism Research, 15*(1), 12–26. https://doi.org/10.1002/aur.2652
Individuals with Disabilities Education Act of 1997, P.L. 105-17, 20 U.S.C. § 1400 et seq. (Reauthorized 2004).
Jornevald, M., Pettersson-Roll, L., & Hau, H. (2024). The Good Behavior Game for students with special educational needs in mainstream education settings: A scoping review. *Psychology in the Schools, 61*(3), 861–886. https://doi.org/10.1002/pits.23086
Joslyn, P. R., Austin, J. L., Donaldson, J. M., & Vollmer, T. R. (2020). A practitioner's guide to the Good Behavior Game. *Behavior Analysis: Research and Practice, 20*(4), 219–235. https://doi.org/10.1037/bar0000199
Kamana, B. U. (2019). *Increasing staff healthy behavioral practices in programs for adults with intellectual and developmental disabilities* [Doctoral dissertation, University of Kansas]. KU ScholarWorks.
Kanaman, N. A. (2022). *Assessing and enhancing the maintenance and generalization of staff implementation of healthy behavioral practices using the Performance Diagnostic Checklist–Human Services* [Doctoral dissertation, University of Kansas]. KU ScholarWorks.
Kelly, M. P., Alireza, I., Azzaam, S., Baowaidan, L. M., Gabr, A. A., Taqi, R., & Yateem, S. N. (2024). Applied behavior analysis and autism spectrum disorder in the Gulf region in the Middle East. *Journal of Developmental and Physical Disabilities, 36*, 591–614. https://doi.org/10.1007/s10882-023-09931-7
Kelly, M. P., & Trifyllis, I. (2022). Developing national occupational standards for behavior analysis. *European Journal of Behavior Analysis, 23*(2), 196–214. https://doi.org/10.1080/15021149.2022.2137654
Knowledge and Human Development Authority [KHDA]. (2017). *Dubai Inclusive Education Policy Framework*. https://www.khda.gov.ae/cms/webparts/texteditor/documents/Education_Policy_En.pdf
Lastrapes, R. E. (2013). Using the Good Behavior Game in an inclusive classroom. *Intervention in School and Clinic, 49*(4), 225–229. https://doi.org/10.1177/1053451213509491
Massouti, A., Al-Rashaida, M., & Alhosani, M. (2024). A qualitative study on Dubai's Inclusive Education Policy from school leaders' perspectives. *Sustainability, 16*, 1252. https://doi.org/10.3390/su16031252
Mathur, S. K., Renz, E., & Tarbox, J. (2024). Affirming neurodiversity within applied behavior analysis. *Behavior Analysis in Practice, 17*, 471–485. https://doi.org/10.1007/s40617-024-00907-3
Ministry of Cabinet Affairs (2024a). *Federal law concerning rights of persons with special needs*. https://uaelegislation.gov.ae/en/legislations/1172
Ministry of Cabinet Affairs. (2024b). *Statistics by subject*. https://fcsc.gov.ae/en-us/Pages/Statistics/Statistics-by-Subject.aspx
Ministry of Foreign Affairs. (2024). *Facts and figures*. https://www.mofa.gov.ae/en/the-uae/facts-and-figures
Miranda-Linné, F., & Melin, L. (1992). Acquisition, generalization, and spontaneous use of color adjectives: A comparison of incidental teaching and traditional discrete-trial procedures for children with autism. *Research in Developmental Disabilities, 13*(3), 191–210. https://doi.org/10.1016/0891-4222(92)90025-2
Olsen, P. M., & Kelly, M. P. (2020). Applied behavior analysis with Arab-Muslim populations: The importance of cultural awareness. In B. M. Connors & S. T. Capell (Eds.), *Multiculturalism and diversity in applied behavior analysis: Bridging theory and application* (pp. 140–163). Taylor & Francis/Routledge.

Pozas, M., & Schneider, C. (2019). Shedding light on the convoluted terrain of differentiated instruction (DI): Proposal of a DI taxonomy for the heterogeneous classroom. *Open Education Studies, 1*, 73–90. https://doi.org/10.1515/edu-2019-0005

Reichle, J., Simacek, J., Wattanawongwan, S., & Ganz, J. (2019). Implementing aided augmentative communication systems with persons having complex communicative needs. *Behavior Modification, 43*(6), 841–878. https://doi.org/10.1177/0145445519858272

Schena, D., Rosales, R., & Rowe, E. (2023). Teaching self-advocacy skills: A review and call for research. *Journal of Behavioral Education, 32*, 641–689. https://doi.org/10.1007/s10864-022-09472-7

St. Peter, C. C., & Marsteller, T. M. (2017). A "healthy-contingencies" behavioral intervention. *Journal of Behavioral Education, 26*, 250–263. https://doi.org/10.1007/s10864-017-9267-6

Stitcher, J. P., Lewis, T. J., Whittaker, T. A., Richter, M., Johnson, N. W., & Trussel, R. P. (2009). Assessing teacher use of opportunities to respond and effective classroom management strategies: Comparisons among high- and low-risk elementary schools. *Journal of Positive Behavior Interventions, 11*(2), 68–81. https://doi.org/10.1177/1098300708326597

Stokes, T. F., & Baer, D. M. (1977). An implicit technology of generalization. *Journal of Applied Behavior Analysis, 10*(2), 349–367. https://doi.org/10.1901/jaba.1977.10-349

The Council of Autism Service Providers. (2024). *Applied behavior analysis practice guidelines for the treatment of autism spectrum disorder: Guidance for healthcare funders, regulatory bodies, service providers, and consumers* (3rd ed.). https://assets-002.noviams.com/novi-file-uploads/casp/pdfs-and-documents/ASD_Guidelines/ABA_Practice_Guidelines_3_0.pdf

Twyman, J. S., & Heward, W. L. (2018). How to improve student learning in every classroom now. *International Journal of Educational Research, 87*, 78–90. https://doi.org/10.1016/j.ijer.2016.05.007

U.ae. (2024). *Inclusive education for people of determination.* https://u.ae/en/information-and-services/education/education-for-people-with-special-needs/inclusive-education-for-people-of-determination

UNRCPD. (2000). *United Nation convention on the rights of persons with disability.* www.un.org/disability.

Weiss, J. A., & Fardella, M. A. (2018). Victimization and perpetration experiences of adults with autism. *Frontiers in Psychiatry, 9*, 203. https://doi.org/10.3389/fpsyt.2018.00203

Part III
Technology-based ABA Interventions

Chapter 10
Developing Family-Centered Behavior–Analytic Telehealth Services for Under-Resourced Communities

Sheri Kingsdorf

Abstract When working with children and families impacted by autism, respect for individual and cultural differences is imperative. Client-centered practices should be strength-based, focus on building socially important skills, and address behaviors that challenge. There is evidence that interventions grounded in applied behavior analysis (ABA) constitute best practice. Unfortunately, many areas of the world are struggling to access such services. Frequently, limited public resources are spent on low-intensity interventions that are not evidence-based. In these situations, any professional behavior analysts who do exist tend to be overworked, under-supported, and struggling to provide high-quality services. Not surprisingly, misinformation about ABA tends to thrive in such circumstances. Telehealth services can mediate some of these challenges, especially if they focus on developing culturally competent and sustainable support services. Using telehealth, caregivers can be trained to follow protocols and provide behavioral support services to their own children. This chapter outlines the background and practice of behavior-analytic telehealth services in the context of family-centered behavioral applications. Systematic steps are outlined that facilitate caregiver-mediated change efforts in support of a child's behavior as well as the family's quality of life.

Keywords Telehealth · Cultural-competence · Client-centered programming · Behavioral intervention · Rural communities

There is substantial evidence that interventions grounded in applied behavior analysis (ABA) constitute best practice for supporting autistic children and their families (e.g., Granpeesheh et al., 2009; Peters-Scheffer et al., 2011). However, it can be a challenge finding skilled practitioners of behavior analysis. Behavior analysts demonstrate respect for individual and cultural differences, apply client-centered

S. Kingsdorf (✉)
Institute for Research in Inclusive Education, Faculty of Education, Masaryk University, Brno, Czech Republic
e-mail: sherikingsdorf@mail.muni.cz

S. Halder et al. (eds.), *Applied Behavior Analysis-Based Interventions for Autism Spectrum Disorder*, https://doi.org/10.1007/978-981-95-2889-9_10

practices, and individualize strength-based programming that targets building socially important skills. Becoming such a highly specialized practitioner of behavior analysis requires coursework with a certain number of hours of discretionary content, such as ethics, professional conduct, philosophical underpinnings and principles of behavior, measurement, analysis, experimental design, behavior assessment, and behavior change procedures (Association for Applied Behavior Analysis International, 2018). In addition to coursework, ABA practitioners must complete supervised practicums across numerous competency areas, which typically takes over a year to complete (Behavior Analyst Certification Board, 2021). Such rigors likely influence the limited number of practitioners available to provide ABA-based services to families impacted by autism. Notably, in Europe, there are far fewer behavior practitioners than in North America (Keenan et al., 2015). This lack of available professionals is a widespread problem that is also affecting rural communities in the United States (Mello et al., 2016), as well as countries in the Middle East (Eid et al., 2017), Africa (Ruparelia et al., 2016), Asia (Manohar et al., 2019), and Latin America (Montiel-Nava et al., 2020). In response to the limited access to ABA-based services, some providers have begun exploring remote options. However, the development of such telehealth behavioral services is still a work in progress with an ever-present need for guidance, monitoring, and regulation (Kingsdorf & Pancocha, 2023).

10.1 Behavioral Telehealth

Telehealth, also known as telepractice, is now often considered to encompass training, teaching, or coaching services provided using online delivery and two-way audio-visual communication (Rispoli & Machalicek, 2020). These can be synchronous (happen in real time) or asynchronous. Telehealth practices can offer a number of benefits for autistic children and their families. These benefits include increased access to services, reduced travel time, more cost-effective services, and information about how teaching can be extended to the natural environment. As a result, the use of telehealth practices for delivering services to children and their families has increased in recent years. In fact, a recent literature search by the Behavior Change Institute revealed over 80 telehealth studies that were published since 1997 (Behavior Change Institute, 2020). Additionally, a comprehensive review by McLay and colleagues (2020) found that some early empirical support exists for using telehealth services to deliver interventions to children and adolescents with sleep difficulties. Complementary article reviews by Akemoglu et al. (2019) and Unholz-Bowden et al. (2020) found over 30 studies looking at using telehealth practices to train parents. Overall, the research suggests that telehealth practices can be a valuable tool for providing services grounded in the science of behavior analysis, with a growing body of research that supports its usage. As telehealth technology continues to improve, it is likely that this approach to service delivery will become even more common in the future.

10.2 Family-Centered Behavioral Telehealth

Best practices in behavioral services, whether delivered in-person or virtually, are driven by the needs of the client and their community. Therefore, ABA practitioners who go in and provide services in a vacuum are not supporting the needs of the family, taking the necessary steps to promote generalization, or fully demonstrating compassionate care and cultural competence. This mismatch can additionally be intensified when behavioral telehealth services are provided by those outside the targeted cultural community. Including caregivers, and other members of the client's community, in program development and implementation results in the overall best outcomes for autistic children (Burrell & Borrego Jr, 2012). Collaboration in development creates a framework for service provision that is likely to continue without support from outside professionals (Trudell, 2009) and demonstrates a step toward compassionate ABA-based care (Taylor et al., 2019). However, building meaningful caregiver involvement and relationships within ABA programming can be a challenge for practitioners as it is not a typical component of their training (Taylor et al., 2019). Therefore, making procedures for parental inclusion and family-centered practice more systematic (i.e., building them into training program planning and practitioner fidelity scripts) may increase the likelihood of their implementation, increase the overall efficacy of services, and provide the groundwork for best practices in ABA telehealth that comprehensively support familial needs (Fig. 10.1).

10.3 ABA Telehealth Methodological Components

10.3.1 Practitioner Telehealth Preparation

Services grounded in the science of behavior rely on direct observation to measure changes in a client's skills. Optimal services are conducted in-person, with the client seeing the behavior analyst face-to-face at least four times per year, at 3-month intervals, with regular sessions conducted by a supervised trainee practitioner, student, or caregiver. However, there may be cases where in-person services are not available due to geographic or health reasons. In these cases, telehealth may be an option. The first step in moving to telehealth is to determine if the practitioner is able to offer this type of service. A checklist or a set of questions can be used to help a practitioner assess if they have the additional knowledge needed to run behavioral programming with clients from a distance. Questions that might be included in this assessment are (BAYADA Home Health Care, 2019; Schlaak, 2018)

1. Can the behavioral practitioner/staff access email and the Internet to locate the links and online connections for the telehealth session?
2. Can the behavioral practitioner/staff establish the video and audio connection for the telehealth session?

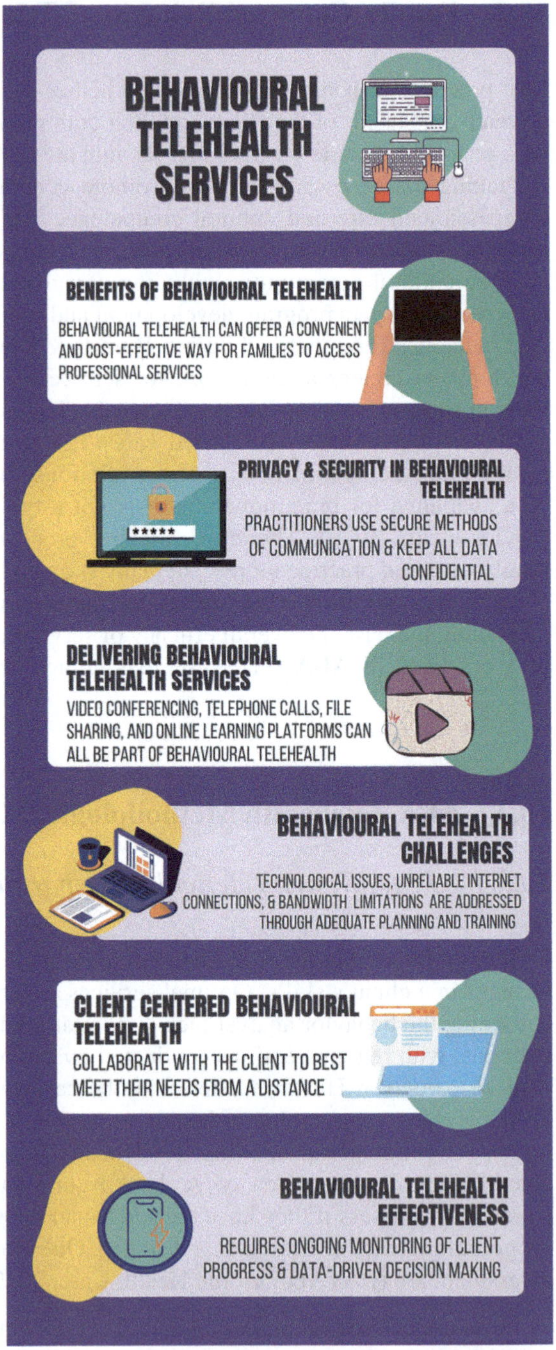

Fig. 10.1 Infographic overview of behavioral telehealth services

3. Can the behavioral practitioner/staff use annotation features of video-conferencing software (e.g., highlighter, arrow, text boxes, chat feature)?
4. Can the behavioral practitioner/staff manage accounts, personal settings, and privacy controls in the online telehealth application?
5. Can the behavioral practitioner/staff solve audio and video problems on their local computer?
6. Can the behavioral practitioner/staff solve problems with software (e.g., loss of mouse, program not responding) on their local computer?
7. Can the behavioral practitioner/staff solve problems with peripheral devices on a local computer (e.g., printer, document camera)?
8. Can the behavioral practitioner/staff use an alternative connection (e.g., telephone, email) with a supervisor to troubleshoot connection problems or to reschedule a session?
9. Can the behavioral practitioner/staff maintain a log of technical difficulties encountered and request assistance with recurring problems?
10. Can the behavioral practitioner/staff independently create needed accounts in new platforms?
11. Can the behavioral practitioner/staff identify the legal issues associated with telehealth practices?
12. Can the behavioral practitioner/staff access a private location where walls are clear of private/inappropriate content, screen out of view of others, and there are no recording devices in the area?
13. Do the behavioral practitioner/staff know to keep any cords, plugs, and peripheral devices clear of walkways?
14. Do the behavioral practitioner/staff know that they should not be using public (shared) Internet connections during sessions?
15. Are the behavioral practitioner/staff knowledgeable of the procedure to contact the office/management for equipment or power failures?

It becomes clear from these sample questions that a relatively high level of technological competence is necessary to successfully implement telehealth services. Additionally, a practitioner looking to offer behavioral-based telehealth services needs to make sure that they are going to be well-received by the local community. Therefore, the practitioner might consider surveying the region, current clients, and stakeholders/funding sources to assess for an interest in telehealth services.

10.4 Considering Telehealth Service Models

After reviewing a practitioner and/or their staffs' ability to provide telehealth behavioral services to clients, it may be necessary to assess which telehealth service delivery model(s) is most feasible. There are two primary approaches to providing telehealth services, each characterized by differences in timing and participation method. The first approach is synchronous, often referred to as real-time support.

This involves interactions such as one-on-one meetings between parents and practitioners or direct service delivery from a behavior practitioner to a child using video-conferencing or telephone communication, as illustrated in the infographic in Fig. 10.2.

The second approach is asynchronous support, where practitioner and client do not need to be present simultaneously. This method encompasses activities like parents sending videos to practitioners, practitioners independently reviewing these videos, parents accessing electronic learning materials, and remotely monitoring various client attributes, such as sleep patterns. The main components in this model are also depicted in Fig. 10.2.

When it comes to providing synchronous didactic instruction or coaching, some studies have demonstrated success using real-time video-conferencing tools like Skype (e.g., Pantermuehl & Lechago, 2015), FaceTime (Boutain et al., 2020), and the Google platform (e.g., Pennefather et al., 2018). In the case of asynchronous telehealth components, some studies have demonstrated success using common file storage applications like Dropbox for video sharing (e.g., Neely et al., 2020), store-and-forward technologies requiring low bandwidth where video recordings from live events and historical data are shared via a secured platform (e.g., Smith et al.,

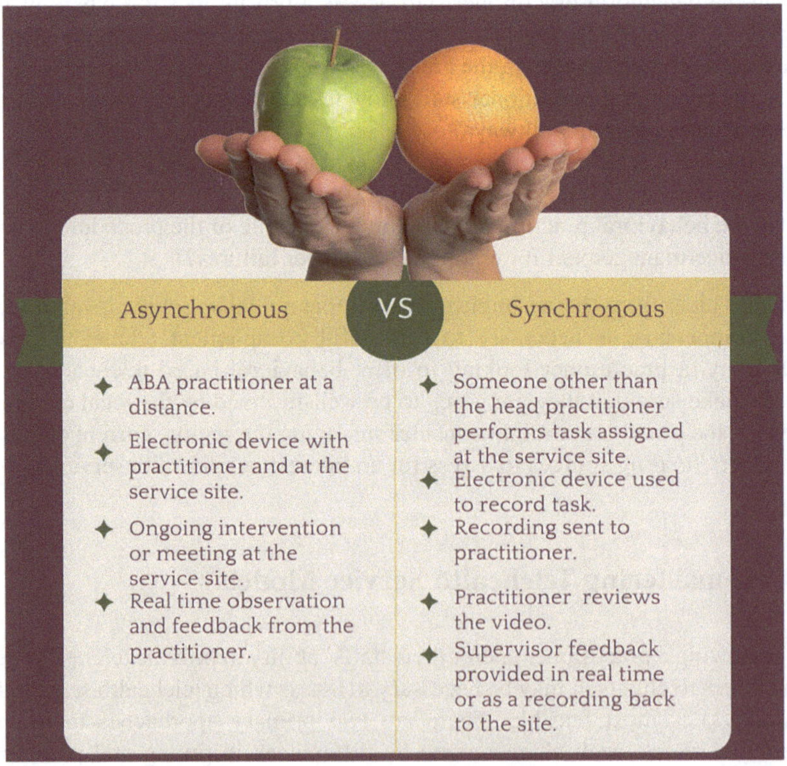

Fig. 10.2 Infographic overview of the two main behavioral telehealth service delivery models

2017), and remote patient monitoring where a person's physiological changes are tracked and shared with a professional (Taj-Eldin et al., 2018). E-learning platforms and Learning Management Systems (LMS) such as Moodle, Blackboard, and Adobe Authorware have been used for independent distance learning to provide information and training to families (Meadan & Daczewitz, 2015). The telehealth service delivery methods that you are most suited to provide as options to your clients will depend on your own time, technological savvy, and service expertise (e.g., demonstrated competency in caregiver training). A further breakdown of what specific services might look like under these models will be reviewed later in this chapter.

10.4.1 Determining Client Telehealth Eligibility

After a behavioral practitioner has determined that telehealth services align with their capabilities and capacity, then it is time to consider specific client needs. First and foremost, it is important to ensure that telehealth services will not do harm to a client in any way. This can be done by conducting a risk assessment specific to the family. A telehealth risk assessment can be conducted over the phone and may use existing risk assessment documents. However, all risk assessments should include questions that assess for the presence of the following inhibiting factors:

- Participation in intense forms of aggression, self-harm, ingestion of nonfood items (pica), running away (elopement), damaging property, or engaging in other dangerous actions.
- Caregivers' resistance or incapability to employ established strategies for managing hazardous behaviors, such as extinction, response interruption, or physical intervention.
- Elevated risk of caregiver injury when implementing essential behavioral protocols.
- Historical difficulties in establishing instructional control between the caregiver and the client during previous in-person service sessions.
- A track record of caregivers struggling to adhere to behavior management plans, which could inadvertently reinforce challenging behaviors.

Additional risk can be assessed by evaluating the overall "functioning level" of the client. See Table 10.1 for recommendations regarding "functioning level" assessment.

Following the risk assessment, the availability of the caregiver should be assessed. Caregivers play a vital role in the provision of telehealth services. Irrespective of the chosen telehealth service delivery model, some level of caregiver participation remains essential for achieving positive outcomes. Hence, it is crucial to evaluate the availability of caregivers' schedules to facilitate these services effectively. The time commitment expected from caregivers varies depending on the chosen telehealth service model, as outlined in Table 10.2, which provides estimated time commitments based on service types. It is important to request caregivers to

Table 10.1 Client-level/prerequisite skill assessments

Low level of prerequisite skills	Medium level of prerequisite skills	High level of prerequisite skills
Lower level of verbal behavior (pre-speaker and pre-listener), missing basic skills, high level of challenging behaviors	Some emerging basic skills, low to moderate level of challenging behaviors, and needs that are manageable by the caregiver. Client can benefit from protocols that are more naturalistic and may involve other household members.	Basic joint attention, motor imitation, echoic, discrimination, ability to follow 1-step directions, ability to sit independently with a device for 10 min, ability to participate in a typical session without caregiver assistance, and low level of safety concerns.

Table 10.2 Caregiver minimum time commitments based on service type

Partial telehealth model	Direct services telehealth model	Caregiver-implemented services	Caregiver consultations	Caregiver asynchronous training
Two hours a week undivided attention, 10 h a week availability, if needed	Two hours a week undivided attention, 10 h a week availability, if needed	12 h a week	4 h a week	No minimum

provide candid assessments of the time they can realistically allocate to participate in telehealth services.

Lastly, although it may not seem as crucial, it is also necessary to assess technology eligibility. Determining the client's Internet connectivity, current software and hardware, technology knowledge, and willingness to learn more technological applications is vital before initiating service planning. A telephone interview can be conducted with the potential client where questions like the following are asked:

1. Do you access the Internet using a wired connection, wireless connection, or through your mobile phone?
2. Does a data limit hinder your Internet access?
3. Do you have a desktop computer, laptop computer, tablet, or phone?
4. Do you have access to a webcam (internal or external)?
5. Do you have access to a headset (headphones with a microphone) for your device?
6. Do you have access to external speakers for your device?
7. What video-conferencing or video chatting applications are you familiar with?
8. What applications do you have accounts with and feel comfortable using?
9. What antivirus software do you currently use?
10. Would you be interested in receiving training on novel technology?

10.4.2 Telehealth Materials

After it is determined that some type of behavioral telehealth services is appropriate and feasible for the client and their family, getting started still requires a lot of preparation. To successfully establish family-centered behavior-analytic telehealth services, a number of specific materials are necessary. Ensure that you have templates created for

- A telehealth-specific confidentiality agreement: the document, in plain language, should cover data access, storage locations, security protocols (for storage, transmission, and disposal), breach response procedures, and the risks tied to data confidentiality lapses.
- A telehealth policy and procedures document: develop clear policies and procedures for conducting telehealth sessions, including appointment scheduling/canceling, billing, emergency protocols, and expectations of caregiver participation and interaction.
- An informed consent form: a plain language document with an overview of the telehealth technologies that will be used, sharing of client data, risks and benefits specific to telehealth participation, and what the client is explicitly agreeing to by participating in services.
- Client telehealth instructions: a brief "how to" guide on how to access technology-specific training, prepare for/entering each telehealth session, and suggestions for maximizing generalization outside of session time.

In terms of technology, you will also need to have purchased and/or created accounts within:

- Secure telehealth platform: choose a HIPAA/GDPR (or other relevant)-compliant telehealth platform or software that ensures the privacy and security of client information.
- Computer or device: a reliable computer, tablet, or smartphone with a stable Internet connection is essential for conducting telehealth sessions.
- Webcam: a good-quality webcam is important for clear video communication.
- Microphone and speakers/headset: ensure clear audio communication with a high-quality microphone and speakers or a headset.
- High-speed Internet connection: a stable, high-speed Internet connection is crucial for uninterrupted video and audio during sessions.
- Cyber privacy and security measures: implement security measures such as encryption, password protection, and two-factor authentication to protect patient data.
- Secure file storage: implement secure cloud storage or data storage solutions to safely store client records and notes.
- Digitized programming resources: create stimuli that will be needed to run skill-acquisition programming and/or the application of behavior change procedures (e.g., token economy materials, behavioral contracts) in an online format that can be viewed and used easily via video-conferencing screen sharing.

- Professional liability insurance: ensure you have appropriate liability insurance coverage for telehealth services, if necessary in your region.
- Technical support: be prepared to access technical support or assistance for any software or hardware issues that may arise during sessions.

Keep in mind that the specific materials and requirements may vary depending on the selected service model and your local regulations. It is important to consult with legal and healthcare/education professionals to ensure compliance with all relevant laws and guidelines when delivering behavioral telehealth services. Additionally, it is imperative to take the individualized needs of the client into consideration by taking steps such as reviewing all documentation provide by the client, planning to conduct skills-based, functional, and preference assessments, and holding numerous meetings with the family to determine their priorities, level of commitment to telehealth services, and application capabilities. These pieces will be discussed in more detail later in this chapter. However, also keep in mind the importance of practicing within the ethical framework of behavioral clinicians. While it is imperative to consult your local regulatory bodies and/or licensing/certification boards for specific guidelines, general best practice tenets should be kept in mind, such as (Behavior Analyst Certification Board, 2020)

- Maximizing telehealth service benefits for the client without doing harm.
- Acting with compassion, dignity, and respect when assessing for eligibility and providing telehealth services.
- Behaving with integrity by being honest with families about the scope and anticipated outcomes of telehealth services, including how outcomes may be more beneficial in a different delivery modality.
- Being guided by the principles of behavior in your telehealth intervention development and applications.
- Ensuring your competence in providing telehealth services to your selected population.

10.4.3 Selecting a Telehealth Model

Finding the model that works best for each family is contingent upon a number of factors. Namely, the feasibility of specific telehealth service delivery models is influenced by both the client's prerequisite skills and the caregiver's capabilities. To review, after establishing general technology eligibility and mitigating risk, further steps are necessary to ascertain the most suitable model, which involves again reviewing (1) client behaviors, (2) caregiver history, (3) schedule availability, and (4) the physical site. The two overarching models of synchronous and asynchronous care were previously introduced (see Fig. 10.2). However, these are further elaborated into four specific options outlined next: (1) the partial telehealth model, (2) direct services telehealth model, (3) caregiver-implemented services model, and (4) caregiver consultations, along with the caregiver asynchronous training (only) model.

Partial Telehealth Model

- Technician delivers services in-person with the client.
- Behavior analyst provides clinical oversight remotely.
- Can allow for continuation of a client's current focused or comprehensive ABA-based treatment program at the recommended dosage (i.e., service hours/intensity) or a partial reduction in dosage.

Direct Services Telehealth Model

- Services are delivered to the client directly via synchronous modalities.
- Can allow for continuation of a client's treatment program at the recommended dosage or a partial reduction in dosage.

Caregiver-Implemented Services Telehealth Model

- Caregivers continue to implement protocols on which they have been trained.
- Behavior analyst coaching caregivers to implement new or modified protocols with the client.
- Can allow the client to receive a reduced level of services, perhaps focused on practicing or developing adaptive behaviors or maintaining daily routines.

Caregiver Consultations Telehealth Model

- Caregivers meet with the behavior analyst remotely to discuss strategies to prevent regression and reduce the likelihood of crisis situations.
- Behavior analyst may provide synchronous training to caregivers on implementing a small subset of protocols.
- Usually focuses on antecedent interventions, crisis prevention, and problem-solving individual concerns with the caregiver.

Caregiver Asynchronous Training Only

- Caregiver participates in asynchronous trainings made accessible via an e-learning platform.
- Trainings can be assigned based on previously assessed family needs.
- Direct and indirect assessments of caregiver and client behavior could be embedded.
- Focuses on providing caregivers with knowledge that they can apply on their own with their child.

Having comprehensive information about a client and his/her caregiver(s) is important to drive the development of family-centered behavior-analytic telehealth services. However, it can be daunting to put all of the information together and select an appropriate service delivery model. Therefore, a decision tree, like the one depicted in Fig. 10.3, can serve as a valuable tool in determining the most suitable telehealth service form for a client, particularly when a fully in-person service delivery model is not feasible. This decision-making process hinges on two primary factors: (1) the availability of caregivers and (2) the client's level of functioning. In a preceding section, we provided a breakdown of the basic time commitments

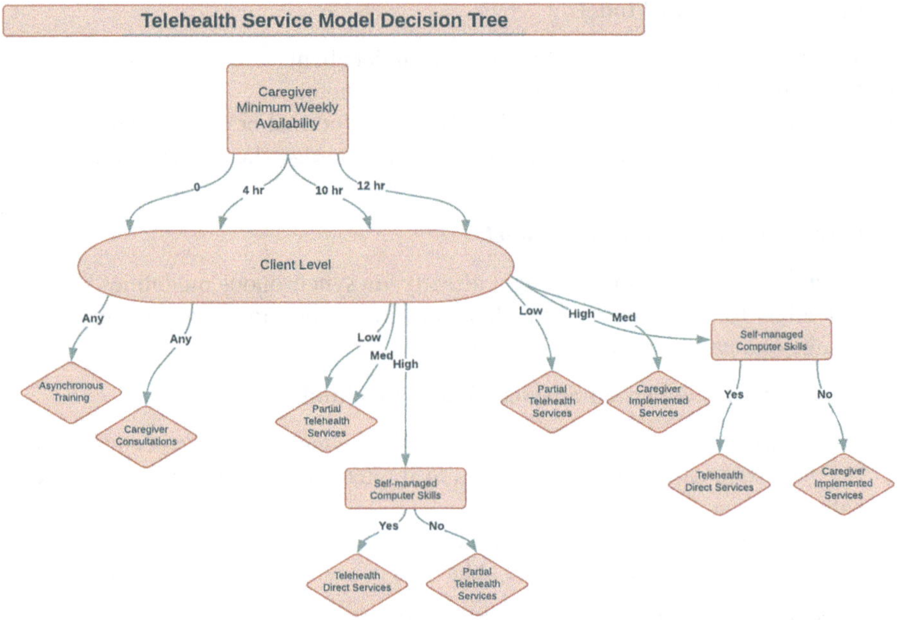

Fig. 10.3 Decision tree for selecting a telehealth service model

expected from caregivers for each model. Additionally, we categorized client functioning into broad levels of "low," "medium," and "high," which are intended as general guidelines. These levels can be correlated with the descriptions found in Table 10.1. The decision tree also accounts for the client's "self-managed computer skills," which encompass a range of abilities related to engaging effectively with digital devices during telehealth sessions. These skills include the capacity to respond to one's name when called on video, relocate to the designated work area as instructed via video, follow previously mastered video instructions (e.g., one-step directions, imitation, or locating materials), identify items on the screen both receptively and expressively (e.g., "touch the tree" or answering questions about on-screen items), pay attention to and respond positively to social praise provided via video, maintain a seated position during video instruction without requiring assistance from others in the room, and focus on the screen without engaging in disruptive behaviors like switching screens, repeatedly pressing buttons, or turning off the device (BHCOE, 2021).

10.4.4 Telehealth Assessment and Data Collection

After an appropriate model of care has been selected, the nuts and bolts of service planning really start. As with all sound behavioral services, assessment is the appropriate place to begin. The process for conducting a client assessment via telehealth to prepare a behavior plan and skill development plan is similar to the in-person services process, but with a few additional steps:

- Have the caregiver mail or email you any needed documents prior to the start of the assessment process by a specified date. This may include an individualized educational program (IEP), past behavior plans, or other relevant documents.
- Schedule indirect assessments via telehealth. This could involve a structured interview over the phone or another video-conferencing platform.
- Provide the caregiver with a checklist for direct assessment site preparation. This checklist should include instructions on how to set up the environment, place the camera, and gather any necessary materials.
- Conduct a comprehensive assessment of the client's strengths and weaknesses. This may involve using a variety of methods, such as interviews, observations, and standardized assessments.
- Establish a contingency plan for termination of the telehealth direct assessment session. This plan should outline what to do if there is a technical issue or other disruption during the session.

10.4.5 Family-Centered Telehealth Intervention Applications

After it has been established that telehealth services are a good match for the family and all of the necessary steps have been taken to prepare for effective session delivery at a distance, including initial assessment, the next step is to start developing services. The actual resources that should be used depend on the specific needs of the family. However, some example scenarios of what telehealth sessions might look like in different formats are provided next.

Naturalistic Family-Run Sessions at a Distance The works of Wacker et al. (2013), Suess et al. (2014), and Hoffman and colleagues (2019) have all found that caregivers can effectively run functional communication training (FCT) with their children as part of telehealth provided services overseen by behavioral professionals. A family-run session when the caregiver is running a protocol, such as FCT, would start by being guided by the individual needs of the family. Prior to the sessions, remote assessment would be done with the child and caregivers to determine the child's preferred items, communication topography, and play setting. The caregivers would then receive training on how to implement the FCT protocol; this can be done without the child present. Following that, the session would start with the computer and camera being set up in a discrete location and connected in real time via a video-conferencing platform to the behavior professional; ideally, the caregiver would have a wireless listening and speaking device in their ear (e.g., "bug in the ear"). The caregiver would set up the natural environment (e.g., playroom) for play with the targeted items in view but unavailable. They would then run the session, playing with the child and following the protocol, using prompts as trained, delivering immediate reinforcement, and providing corrections as specified. The caregiver would simultaneously receive coaching, as prompts and reinforcing or corrective feedback from the behavioral professional through the "bug in their ear." A debriefing session may occur at the end of the play session with the child no longer present. At that time, more performative feedback and training may be provided to the caregiver, as needed.

Direct Therapy-Type Sessions Run with the Child Recently, Ferguson et al. (2020) demonstrated effectively using direct telehealth therapy to teach autistic children comic book characters. Additionally, Nohelty et al. (2021) were successful in using direct discrete trial-type therapy, in conjunction with naturalistic teaching methods, to teach new skills across multiple domains to autistic children at a distance. A direct therapy session where the behavior professional is delivering instruction directly to the client at a distance would also start with individualized assessment procedures. These might be done directly with the child via the telehealth modality. Meaning, the behavior professional would connect with the child and possibly the caregiver (if additional caregiver support was deemed necessary) via a video-conferencing platform. The computer and camera would be directly in front of the child. During an assessment, the practitioner would start by running a preference assessment with the child by sharing images of preferred/potentially reinforcing choices on the screen and having the child select the desired item to work toward. In a direct services telehealth setting, some potential reinforcers that might be easiest for the practitioner to mediate access to are video clips, joint online games, and music. Following preference selection, probe trials might be run to assess the child's knowledge of a certain skill, or teaching trials within an existing program. Regardless, the child would be looking at the computer screen, seeing the practitioner in real time deliver an antecedent and show stimuli, then respond and receive reinforcing or corrective feedback, if appropriate. After a certain number of interlocking contingencies/trials, the practitioner would then mediate access to the reinforcer, ideally engaging in the technology-assisted activity together (e.g., playing a portion of an online game together).

Training Sessions with Only the Caregiver Present The research on training caregivers via telehealth modalities on behavioral procedures is perhaps the most robust of all areas. Enough studies exist that systematic reviews, like that conducted by Unholz-Bowden et al. (2020), have evaluated and shown the effectiveness of caregiver behavior-based training at a distance. However, it has also been shown that this service can take on many different forms. In considering one possible example, a telehealth training session for caregivers might look like the caregiver accessing asynchronous online learning materials on applications of behavior-analytic procedures (e.g., development and application of an in-home behavioral contract). Then, the caregiver might have a live, synchronous, meeting with a behavior practitioner via video-conferencing platform where the information accessed in the asynchronous session is reviewed with specific applications discussed relevant to the family's unique needs. For example, if the asynchronous material covered how to use a behavioral contract, then during the synchronous session between the caregiver and practitioner, a behavioral contract would be created that could be used with the child targeting their specific needs (e.g., daily homework completion).

10.4.6 An Ongoing Family-Centered Telehealth Approach

Regardless of service specifics, keep in mind that active involvement of, and collaboration with, family members is vital to the success of any behavior-analytic-based service. However, when delivered via telehealth it becomes even more crucial. Best practices in behavioral telehealth use a family-centered approach that recognizes that the family plays a crucial role in supporting and promoting positive outcomes for the client and should see benefits of the services themselves. Therefore, family members, including the child when appropriate, should be involved in the goal-setting process, provided with education and training on the basics of behavior analysis, collaborate on decision-making, and participate in sessions to some degree, regardless of the telehealth model. Additionally, it is important for the behavior practitioner to recognize and incorporate the family's cultural values into service planning, offer information on additional support services, bolster empowerment and advocacy, demonstrate flexibility in service development and implementation, and collaborate with other professionals who play an important role in the family's well-being. Taking these family-centric steps in the development and ongoing applications of behavior-analytic telehealth services aligns with the best practices discussed in the work of Antill (2020), where specifics were outlined such as natural environment consideration, education and needs alignment, open-ended qualitative assessments to supplement formal assessments, individualized application of basic training procedures, and ongoing and specific feedback. A number of valuable resources that can promote a collaborative and compassionate care approach in behavior-analytic family-based practices, telehealth delivered or otherwise, have been shared in the work of Brown et al. (2022), such as guiding principles, tools for assessing contextual variables, clinical decision-making models, and visuals for communicating interventions to caregivers.

10.5 Outcomes

10.5.1 Telehealth Benefits

There has been a large increase in the amount of research on behavior-analytic telehealth services. It is no surprise that numerous favorable outcomes have been found. To name only a few examples: e-learning courses have been piloted with families and demonstrated that gains in ABA knowledge could be made when caregivers independently accessed structured learning modules (Kingsdorf et al., 2022), behavioral skills training (BST) was recently used via telehealth modalities to teach caregivers how to implement discrete trial training (DTT) procedures (Gauert et al., 2022), telehealth parent training in naturalistic strategies was used to increase the communication skills of autistic children (Ferguson et al., 2022), and autistic children were successfully directly taught social skills using an intervention with a high level of social validity via a telehealth modality (Cihon et al., 2021). It should be remembered, though, that telehealth is simply a delivery modality. It is not an intervention. Therefore, telehealth services are only as good as the science backing the interventions being delivered. Thus, the behavior-analytic-based interventions that you deliver via any telehealth modality should be systematic, evidence-based, individualized, and focused on improving the family's quality of life by addressing meaningful target behaviors in an ethical manner. Even when provided at a distance, interventions should be a collaborative effort between you, the client, and other family members, and prioritize data collection and analysis to guide decision-making and intervention adjustments.

10.5.2 Avoiding Telehealth Challenges

Telehealth may not be successful for all families. There are a number of reasons why challenges may arise. However, as with any good behavior-analytic practice, being proactive is often the most effective. Therefore, monitoring the outcomes of telehealth sessions by looking at the effectiveness of skill acquisition and behavior programming is essential. If targeted goals fail to improve within a specified decision protocol (e.g., after analyzing five data points; Keohane & Greer, 2005), consider streamlining the protocol or removing the target from the telehealth plan. Conversely, if goals show improvement, gradually increase them, including a slow expansion of remote service hours. Continuously assess service quality to ensure adherence to guidelines by caregivers, on-site therapists, or remote-based therapists. Employ treatment integrity checklists, ideally on a weekly basis, for all programs/targets. If integrity falls below 80%, consider simplifying the protocol or excluding it from the telehealth plan. All of these steps can help avoid telehealth programs that are ineffective or stagnant. Some more specific tips for avoiding and/or assessing telehealth service challenges may include.

Before the session:

- Have automated session reminders sent to those involved in the telehealth session (e.g., client, caregiver, other service providers, therapists).
- Test your equipment and Internet connection. This includes your computer, webcam, microphone, and speakers.
- Find a quiet and private space for your session. This will help you to stay focused and avoid distractions.
- Make sure that you have all of the necessary materials. This may include assessments, stimuli, worksheets, digital token boards, and online games/potential reinforcers.
- Provide your clients with clear instructions on how to connect to the videoconferencing platform, what to prepare, and where to be set up for the session. You may also want to provide them with a backup plan in case of technical difficulties.
- **During the session:**
- Be mindful of your body language and facial expressions. If you are meant to be an observer/coach during the session, then work to minimize yourself as a distraction (i.e., avoid reactivity). However, if you are providing direct services or training, be sure to make eye contact, smile, and remain engaged with your client on the screen (e.g., conditioning yourself as a reinforcer).
- Initial regular check-ins during the session with the clients to make sure that the audio and visual functions of the video-conference platform are working properly.
- Avoid splitting your attention with other browser tabs or technologies that are not relevant to your client and/or the session.
- Have back-up contact information on hand (e.g., phone number of the caregiver) to reach out in case of session and/or technical issues.
- Be prepared to troubleshoot any technical difficulties that may occur (e.g., have a troubleshooting guide prepared and available for you, other included practitioners if relevant, the client, and/or the caregiver).
- **After the session:**
- Review data, create session notes, and follow standardized procedures for analysis/data-based decision-making. Make any necessary changes to programming before the next session.
- Send a follow-up email to all applicable parties with any resources, handouts, assignments, and/or data collection expectations that you discussed during the session.
- Create a feedback loop. If appropriate, consider collecting client feedback data after each session regarding connectivity, content, and the general telehealth experience. Then incorporate the feedback into your next session.
- Check for any technology updates that may be needed before the next session.

10.6 Considerations for Future Research and Practice

Although the delivery of behavior-analytic telehealth services has significantly increased since 2010, there are still considerable strides to be made. For one, reviews of research have found problems with attrition and systematic program adherence (e.g., Kingsdorf & Pancocha, 2023). It may be the case that, especially given the growth of telehealth during the height of a worldwide health crisis, in an effort to meet the needs of families quickly, services were started without the proper preliminary steps. Therefore, future applications of behavior-analytic-based telehealth services should aim to take a more systematic approach to assessing practitioner and client compatibility with remote services, as well as developing intervention plans that are equipped for distance delivery from the onset. Additionally, research in behavioral telehealth has also lacked robust data collection procedures (Kingsdorf & Pancocha, 2023). It is important to remember that behavior-analytic telehealth services should remain grounded in the still-applicable seven dimensions of applied behavior analysis (Baer et al., 1968; Baer et al., 1987). While the field of behavior analysis has considerably evolved over time, even more novel approaches have taken steps to align themselves with the foundations of the science (e.g., Dixon et al., 2020; Vivanti & Stahmer, 2021). The same needs to be done for the telehealth delivery method. Practitioners applying the science in this manner need to be sure to do things like define client-centered meaningful targets behaviorally, safely collect and analyze electronic data, create technological telehealth delivery plans, base family-collaborative interventions on the principles of behavior, program for generalization even at a distance, and evaluate the ongoing effectiveness of remote services.

References

Akemoglu, Y., Muharib, R., & Meadan, H. (2019). A systematic and quality review of parent-implemented language and communication interventions conducted via telepractice. *Journal of Behavioral Education*. https://doi.org/10.1007/s10864-019-09356-3

Antill, K. (2020). Family-centered applied behavior analysis for children with autism spectrum disorder. *Intervention in School and Clinic, 55*(3), 185–191.

Association for Behavior Analysis International. (2018). *Verified course sequence handbook*. Retrieved September 23, 2019, from Abainternational.org website: https://www.abainternational.org/media/155079/abai_vcs_handbook_2018.pdf

Baer, D. M., Wolf, M. M., & Risley, T. R. (1968). Some current dimensions of applied behavior analysis. *Journal of Applied Behavior Analysis, 1*(1), 91.

Baer, D. M., Wolf, M. M., & Risley, T. R. (1987). Some still-current dimensions of applied behavior analysis. *Journal of Applied Behavior Analysis, 20*(4), 313–327.

BAYADA Home Health Care. (2019). *Telehealth employee training and competency checklist*. https://drive.google.com/file/d/16izHB27KIy1UQGQRHNoGTFfxqys6HxZ6/view

Behavior Change Institute. (2020). *Telehealth research summaries*. https://casproviders.org/wp-content/uploads/2020/03/Behavior-Change-Institute-Telehealth-Research-Summaries.pdf

Behavior Analyst Certification Board. (2021). *Board certified behavior analyst handbook*. Littleton, CO.

Behavior Analyst Certification Board. (2020). *Ethics code for behavior analysts*. https://bacb.com/wp-content/ethics-code-for-behavior-analysts/

BHCOE. (2021). *Telehealth: Evidence-based practice in the Time of COVID-19*. https://bhcoe.org/2020/03/telehealth-aba-therapy-ebp-covid-19/

Boutain, A. R., Sheldon, J. B., & Sherman, J. A. (2020). Evaluation of a telehealth parent training program in teaching self-care skills to children with autism. *Journal of Applied Behavior Analysis, 53*(3), 1259–1275.

Brown, K. R., Hurd, A. M., Randall, K. R., Szabo, T., & Mitteer, D. R. (2022). A family- centered care approach to behavior-analytic assessment and intervention. *Behavior Analysis in Practice*, 1–17.

Burrell, T. L., & Borrego, J., Jr. (2012). Parents' involvement in ASD treatment: What is their role? *Cognitive and Behavioral Practice, 19*(3), 423–432.

Cihon, J. H., Ferguson, J. L., Lee, M., Leaf, J. B., Leaf, R., & McEachin, J. (2021). Evaluating the cool versus not cool procedure via telehealth. *Behavior Analysis in Practice*, 1–9.

Dixon, M. R., Hayes, S. C., Stanley, C., Law, S., & al-Nasser, T. (2020). Is acceptance and commitment training or therapy (ACT) a method that applied behavior analysts can and should use? *The Psychological Record, 70*, 559–579.

Eid, A. M., Aljaser, S. M., AlSaud, A. N., Asfahani, S. M., Alhaqbani, O. A., Mohtasib, R. S., Aldhalaan, H. M., & Fryling, M. (2017). Training parents in Saudi Arabia to implement discrete trial teaching with their children with autism spectrum disorder. *Behavior Analysis in Practice, 10*(4), 402–406.

Ferguson, J., Dounavi, K., & Craig, E. A. (2022). The impact of a telehealth platform on ABA-based parent training targeting social communication in children with autism spectrum disorder. *Journal of Developmental and Physical Disabilities, 34*(6), 1089–1120.

Ferguson, J. L., Majeski, M. J., McEachin, J., Leaf, R., Cihon, J. H., & Leaf, J. B. (2020). Evaluating discrete trial teaching with instructive feedback delivered in a dyad arrangement via telehealth. *Journal of Applied Behavior Analysis, 53*(4), 1876–1888. https://doi.org/10.1002/jaba.773

Gauert, S., Rittenhouse-Cea, H., & Rittenhouse-Shaw, K. (2022). Parent implementation of DTT following telehealth instruction. *Journal of Autism and Developmental Disorders*, 1–7. https://doi.org/10.1007/s10803-022-05693-x

Granpeesheh, D., Dixon, D. R., Tarbox, J., Kaplan, A. M., & Wilke, A. E. (2009). The effects of age and treatment intensity on behavioral intervention outcomes for children with autism spectrum disorders. *Research in Autism Spectrum Disorders, 3*(4), 1014–1022.

Hoffmann, A. N., Bogoev, B. K., & Sellers, T. P. (2019). Using telehealth and expert coaching to support early childhood special education parent-implemented assessment and intervention procedures. *Rural Special Education Quarterly, 38*(2), 95–106.

Keenan, M., Dillenburger, K., Röttgers, H. R., Dounavi, K., Jónsdóttir, S. L., Moderato, P., Schenk, J. J. A. M., Virués-Ortega, J., Roll-Pettersson, L., & Martin, N. (2015). Autism and ABA: The gulf between North America and Europe. *Review Journal of Autism and Developmental Disorders, 2*(2), 167–183.

Keohane, D. D., & Greer, R. D. (2005). Teachers' use of a verbally governed algorithm and student learning. *International Journal of Behavioral Consultation and Therapy, 1*(3), 252.

Kingsdorf, S., & Pancocha, K. (2023). Looking at Europe's recent behavioral telehealth practices for children and families impacted by neurodevelopmental disabilities. *International Journal of Developmental Disabilities, 69*(2), 147–162.

Kingsdorf, S., Pancocha, K., Vadurova, H., & Dosedel, T. (2022). Piloting an e-learning applied behavior analysis course for caregivers of children with autism in The Czech Republic. *Journal of Behavioral Education*, 1–32.

Manohar, H., Kandasamy, P., Chandrasekaran, V., & Rajkumar, R. P. (2019). Brief parent-mediated intervention for children with autism spectrum disorder: A feasibility study from South India. *Journal of Autism and Developmental Disorders, 49*(8), 3146. 3158.

McLay, L., Sutherland, D., Machalicek, W., & Sigafoos, J. (2020). Systematic review of telehealth interventions for the treatment of sleep problems in children and adolescents. *Journal of Behavioral Education.* https://doi.org/10.1007/s10864-020-09364-8

Meadan, H., & Daczewitz, M. E. (2015). Internet-based intervention training for parents of young children with disabilities: A promising service-delivery model. *Early Child Development and Care, 185*(1), 155–169.

Mello, M. P., Goldman, S. E., Urbano, R. C., & Hodapp, R. M. (2016). Services for children with autism spectrum disorder: Comparing rural and non-rural communities. *Education and Training in Autism and Developmental Disabilities, 51*, 355–365.

Montiel-Nava, C., Cukier, S., Garrido, G., Valdez, D., Paula, C. S., García, R., Rosoli, A., Irarrázaval, M., & Rattazzi, A. (2020). Service encounters across the lifespan in individuals with autism spectrum disorders: Results from a multisite study in Latin America. *Research in Autism Spectrum Disorders, 79*, 101670.

Neely, L., Hong, E. R., Kawamini, S., Umana, I., & Kurz, I. (2020). Intercontinental telehealth to train Japanese interventionists in incidental teaching for children with autism. *Journal of Behavioral Education*, 1–16.

Nohelty, K., Bradford, C. B., Hirschfeld, L., Miyake, C. J., & Novack, M. N. (2021). Effectiveness of telehealth direct therapy for individuals with autism spectrum disorder. *Behavior Analysis in Practice*, 1–16.

Pantermuehl, R. M., & Lechago, S. A. (2015). A comparison of feedback provided in vivo versus an online platform on the treatment integrity of staff working with children with autism. *Behavior Analysis in Practice, 8*(2), 219–222.

Pennefather, J., Hieneman, M., Raulston, T. J., & Caraway, N. (2018). Evaluation of an online training program to improve family routines, parental Well-being, and the behavior of children with autism. *Research in Autism Spectrum Disorders, 54*, 21–26.

Peters-Scheffer, N., Didden, R., Korzilius, H., & Sturmey, P. (2011). A meta-analytic study on the effectiveness of comprehensive ABA-based early intervention programs for children with autism Spectrum disorders. *Research in Autism Spectrum Disorders, 5*(1), 60–69.

Rispoli, M., & Machalicek, W. (2020). Advances in telehealth and behavioral assessment and intervention in education: Introduction to the special issue. *Journal of Behavioral Education, 29*, 189–194. https://doi.org/10.1007/s10864-020-09383-5

Ruparelia, K., Abubakar, A., Badoe, E., Bakare, M., Visser, K., Chugani, D. C., Chugani, H. T., Donald, K. A., Wilmshurst, J. M., Shih, A., Skuse, D., & Newton, C. R. (2016). Autism spectrum disorders in Africa: Current challenges in identification, assessment, and treatment: A report on the international child neurology association meeting on ASD in Africa, Ghana, April 3-5, 2014. *Journal of Child Neurology, 31*(8), 1018–1026.

Schlaak, H. M. (2018). Professional competencies for E-helpers: A Telepractice resource. *Theses and Dissertations–Communication Sciences and Disorders, 12*. https://uknowledge.uky.edu/commdisorders_etds/12

Smith, C. J., Rozga, A., Matthews, N., Oberleitner, R., Nazneen, N., & Abowd, G. (2017). Investigating the accuracy of a novel telehealth diagnostic approach for autism spectrum disorder. *Psychological Assessment, 29*(3), 245.

Suess, A. N., Romani, P. W., Wacker, D. P., Dyson, S. M., Kuhle, J. L., Lee, J. F., et al. (2014). Evaluating the treatment fidelity of parents who conduct in-home functional communication training with coaching via telehealth. *Journal of Behavioral Education, 23*, 34–59.

Taj-Eldin, M., Ryan, C., O'Flynn, B., & Galvin, P. (2018). A review of wearable solutions for physiological and emotional monitoring for use by people with autism spectrum disorder and their caregivers. *Sensors, 18*(12), 4271.

Taylor, B. A., LeBlanc, L. A., & Nosik, M. R. (2019). Compassionate care in behavior analytic treatment: Can outcomes be enhanced by attending to relationships with caregivers? *Behavior Analysis in Practice, 12*(3), 654–666.

Trudell, B. (2009). Local-language literacy and sustainable development in Africa. *International Journal of Educational Development, 29*(1), 73–79.

Unholz-Bowden, E., McComas, J. J., McMaster, K. L., Girtler, S. N., Kolb, R. L., & Shipchandler, A. (2020). Caregiver training via telehealth on behavioral procedures: A systematic review. *Journal of Behavioral Education.* https://doi.org/10.1007/s10864-020-09381-7

Vivanti, G., & Stahmer, A. C. (2021). Can the early start Denver model be considered ABA practice? *Behavior Analysis in Practice, 14*, 230–239.

Wacker, D. P., Lee, J. F., Padilla Dalmau, Y. C., Kopelman, T. G., Lindgren, S. D., Kuhle, J., et al. (2013). Conducting functional communication training via telehealth to reduce the problem behavior of young children with autism. *Journal of Developmental and Physical Disabilities, 25*, 35–48.

Chapter 11
Enhancing Motor and Verbal Skills in Children with Autism with Video Modeling

Santoshi Halder

Abstract Acquisition of verbal and motor play skills can be a challenging task for the children with autism. The present study examines the effectiveness of video modeling in teaching verbal and motor play skills to children with autism using a video modeling intervention, using a single-subject design with three participants with autism. Participants 1 and 2 achieved 100% mastery in both motor and verbal responses, while participant 3 attained over 73% mastery in motor responses but only 17% in verbal responses. The intervention was personalized to each participant's needs and showed that video modeling intervention resulted in the rapid acquisition of motor & verbal play skills. The study highlights the effectiveness of video modeling in teaching play skills to children with autism.

Keywords Video Modeling · Children with autism · Verbal and motor responses · Multiple baseline design

11.1 Introduction

Designing effective intervention programs for individuals with autism is challenging for professionals. Research demonstrates that visual learning methods, particularly video modeling, are effective for teaching skills to individuals with autism spectrum disorder (ASD) (Bellini et al., 2007; Ganz et al., 2011). These interventions improve attention shifting (Quill, 1995, 1997, 1998), clarify concepts (Peeters, 1997), and aid in maintaining new skills (Krantz & McGlannahan, 1993, 1998). Video modeling uses videos to showcase specific skills, allowing individuals to imitate socially approved behaviors. This evidence based method has successfully

S. Halder (✉)
Department of Education, University of Calcutta, Kolkata, West Bengal, India

S. Halder et al. (eds.), *Applied Behavior Analysis-Based Interventions for Autism Spectrum Disorder*, https://doi.org/10.1007/978-981-95-2889-9_11

taught motor, verbal, and communication skills to children with autism, promoting independent functioning and addressing diverse objectives, including behavioral, self-help, communication, and social skills.

Video modeling is consistently effective for enhancing various skills in students with ASD (Ganz et al., 2007, 2008) enhancing social interactions (Apple et al., 2005; Ganz et al., 2006; Nikopoulos & Keenan, 2003a, 2003b, 2003c), conversation skills (e.g., Sherer et al., 2001), daily living skills (Keen et al., 2007), play skills (MacDonald et al., 2005; Maione & Mirenda, 2006), reduces problem behaviors (Luscre & Genter, 1996), and improves academic tasks (Delano, 2007). A meta-analysis confirms the effectiveness of video modeling for a range of skills (Bellini et al., 2007; Ganz et al., 2011). The current study aims to assess the effects of video modeling on teaching extended motor and verbal play responses to children with autism.

11.1.1 Research Questions

(a) Is video modeling effective for enhancing play skills in children with autism?
(b) Does video modeling enhance motor responses in children with autism?

11.1.2 Methodology

11.1.2.1 Participant Screening

Three participants diagnosed with autism were selected for the study: participant 1 (9 years old), participant 2 (8 years old), and participant 3 (9 years old). The criteria included no severe behavioral issues and no ADHD or inattention challenges. All participants attended the same special school, although participant 3 also went to a mainstream school.

11.1.3 Inclusion and Exclusion Criteria

All participants were verbal and could communicate in simple sentences. They showed an interest in playing with items like play farms. After nearly a year at the special school, they were attentive during video watching. However, none demonstrated modeled play skills when prompted with play items.

11.1.4 Dependent Variable

The dependent variable consisted of the responses described next. Participants were asked to provide both verbal and motor responses within a 2-min time limit when prompted with the statement, "Well, this is a farmhouse, and you may play with it." This 2-minute limit was established based on sample trials conducted by the experimenter, who measured the time required for participants to complete the modeled responses. It was concluded that all responses could be completed within this timeframe, considering the variability in children's pacing.

11.1.5 Experimental Design

The intervention was implemented separately for each of the three participants. All participants began the baseline phase on the same day and at the same time; however, the training phase was personalized to progress individually based on each participant's criteria and mastery before introducing the next stages of the intervention.

11.1.6 Experimental Procedures

The study began with all participants starting on the same day. Each participant was seated in a designated room with a farmhouse toy and given instructions. Baseline data were collected until a stable trend was noted. Intervention phases then began, featuring individualized videos tailored to each participant. Data were recorded, and trends were plotted until mastery was achieved.

11.1.7 Baseline (Condition A): First Stage of the Research Project

During the baseline phase of the study, no consequences were provided for either correct or incorrect responses. The aim was to collect data on whether the participant demonstrated both motor and verbal responses correctly and independently. Gathering baseline data was essential to identify the skills the learner already possessed and assess how much of the target behavior the participants could perform without assistance. The baseline phase was conducted in the same setting as the training phase, with only one probe trial taking place each day. No feedback or instructions were provided during this stage. Probe trials were conducted daily on weekdays, from Monday to Friday, until the criterion was met. Each baseline session lasted a maximum of 2 min, and if participants left their seats or the room for more than 15 sec, the session was terminated before the 2-min mark was reached.

11.1.8 Setting

A separate room within a special school or center was chosen for the study. This room provided a natural environment and contained relevant items as it typically would. A separate table and chair were set up for the child to sit and perform tasks. The door was kept closed throughout the session to minimize distractions, with only the researcher and the primary trainer present.

11.1.9 Assessment Procedure

Baseline data were collected for 2 min during each session. Only one or two sessions were conducted daily to prevent boredom, which could arise from the repetition of the same play item. Data were recorded based on the duration of engagement with the farmhouse play items, focusing on either verbal or motor responses. Each participant was given a single instruction upon entering the room: "Please sit on the chair. This is a farmhouse, and you may play with it."

11.1.10 Planning, Preparing, and Making the Video for the Intervention

The researcher identified the device to be used for displaying the video: a laptop with Windows Media Player. This choice was made because the researcher is comfortable using this technology, and all participants are familiar with the device, ensuring smooth execution of the intervention.

To prepare for video recording, the researcher created a detailed script that included both verbal instructions and motor actions, based on the skills identified during the baseline probes. Developing this script, or task analysis, for the target skill or behavior is essential for effective video modeling. A task analysis breaks down a complex skill into a series of steps, listing all actions necessary to complete the target behavior (Sigafoos et al., 2007).

Following the outlined steps (both verbal and motor responses), the researcher models the behavior herself to record the video according to the script. The goal is to produce a video of satisfactory quality, free of errors, and accurately reflecting the planned content. The detailed list of the script (both verbal and motor responses) is provided in Table 11.1.

11.1.11 Intervention Stage 1 or B1

In the baseline phase, participants watched a video of a play sequence in a separate room away from the classroom. Each intervention phase included two segments: 2 min of video viewing followed by 2 min of performing the targeted behavior

Table 11.1 Modeled motor and verbal responses

S. no.	Motor responses	S. no.	Verbal responses
1	The sheep indicating the **farmhouse**	1.	Sheep says: Wow! Beautiful farmhouse
2.	Sheep on the **farm**	2.	Sheep says: Wow, nice flowers!
3.	Sheep eat the **grass.**	3.	Sheep says: I am hungry
		4.	Sheep says: Yummy grass!
4.	A cow near the farm.	5.	Cow says: Hey sheep… this is my grass, go away
5.	The cow pushes the sheep to go away on the farm.		
6.	Dog near the farm	6.	Dog says: Bhow bhow…hey you both stop fighting bhow bhow
7.	**McDonald the farmer** comes out near the farm.	7.	Farmer says: Hey, you both stop fighting. Time to go home.
8	The farmer on the farm to chase the animals.		
9.	McDonald goes near **wife-merry** to call.	8.	Farmer says: Hey merry, let's go to the market.
10.	The farmer in the car	9.	Drives: Wooooooooooooooooh
11.	Wife in the car		
12.	Both (farmer and his wife drive towards the **market**.		
13.	Wife **gets out of** the car	10.	Merry says to the seller: Give me some vegetables
14.	**Put** the vegetables in the car	11.	Merry says: Thank you
15.	Wife in the car		
16.	Both **drives back** home	12.	Drives: Wooooooh

through motor and verbal responses. The researcher arranged the environment to facilitate this process.

11.1.11.1 Section 1: Modeling Exposure

The researcher showed each participant a video that demonstrated the target behavior in a way similar to the baseline phase, making it more functional. Each learner watched a video featuring the target behavior in the context of classroom routines and activities. The researcher and the child then entered a designated room for instruction. During the video modeling session, the researcher said, "You are going to watch the video," and then played a prerecorded 2-min video (developed by the researcher) that demonstrated the task once.

11.1.11.2 Section 2: Performance Assessment

The researcher provided the materials and instructions for the task: "You can play with the farmhouse." No prompts or reinforcement were given for correct or incorrect responses. The criteria for moving on to the next phase required four consecutive trials with an accuracy rate of 80–100%, based on either motor or verbal responses as modeled. After a minimum delay of 2 min, participants were given access to the same blocks that corresponded to the play sequence shown in the video. Each session lasted 2 min or until participants left their seats for more than 15 sec. No reinforcement, prompting, or correction procedures were implemented by the researcher.

The researcher recorded and analyzed the performance of each learner separately, focusing on the target behavior and noting the specific responses that participants were able to perform independently. If the data indicated that a learner was making progress, instruction continued until mastery was achieved or until the learner reached maximum proficiency. However, if, after collecting and recording data on 3–5 occasions a learner showed no progress, the researcher would begin the next level of intervention. The researcher provided the materials and instructions for the task: "You can play with the farmhouse." No prompts or reinforcement were given for correct or incorrect responses. The criteria for moving on to the next phase required four consecutive trials with an accuracy rate of 80–100%, based on either motor or verbal responses as modeled (Graph 11.1, 11.2, 11.3, 11.4, and 11.5).

11.1.12 Intervention Stage 2 or B2

As participants 2 and 3 were unable to perform the target response as per the expected criteria, so intervention stage 2 was introduced. Participant 2 achieved 100% mastery in motor responses but showed 0% in verbal responses.

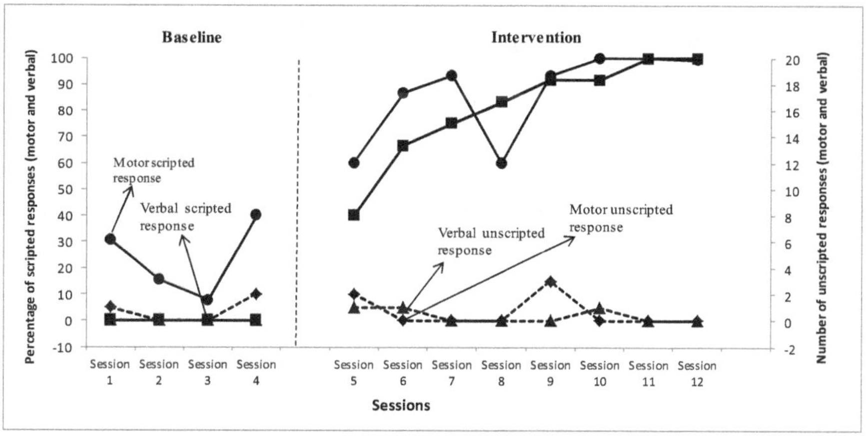

Graph 11.1 Graphical representation of the motor and verbal scripted responses of participant 1

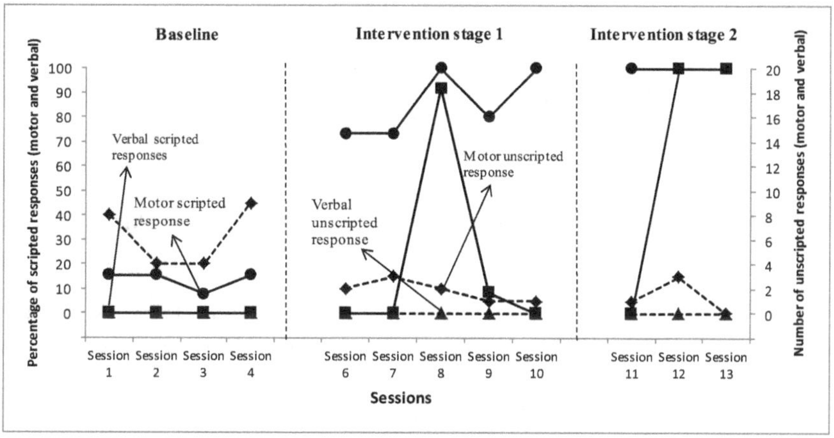

Graph 11.2 Graphical representation of the motor and verbal scripted responses of participant 2

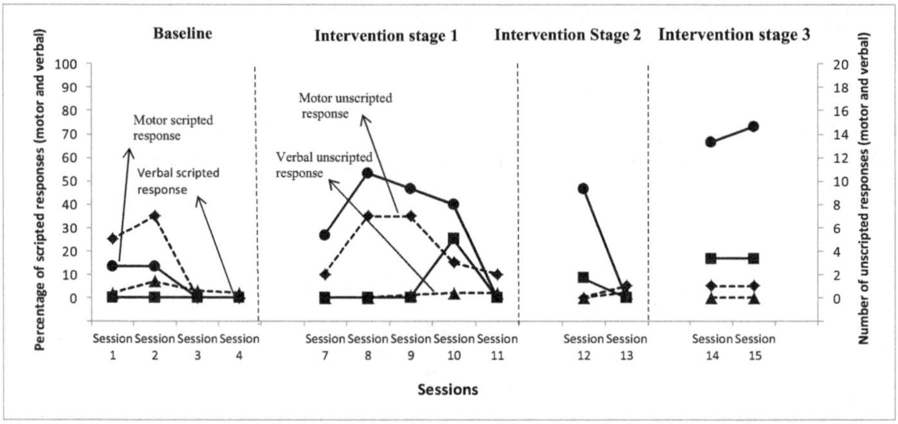

Graph 11.3 Graphical representation of the motor and verbal scripted responses of participant 3

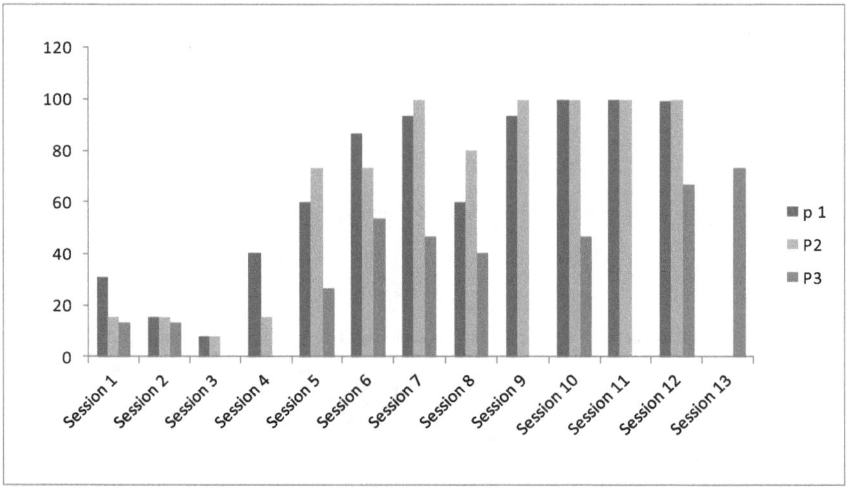

Graph 11.4 Graphical representation of the motor scripted responses (MS) of the three participants

Section 2—Showing the Video: Instruction was introduced before showing the video for participant 2, *"You are going to see the video. You have to see carefully and also listen to what they are saying."*

Section 2—Performance Assessment: Participant was instructed before the performance, *"Sit on the chair. You have to perform the actions and also say."* The participant was demonstrated verbal and motor responses beforehand.

Mastery was achieved by both participants 1 and 2 in both verbal and motor responses, with very little instruction. However, participant 3 was noncompliant in

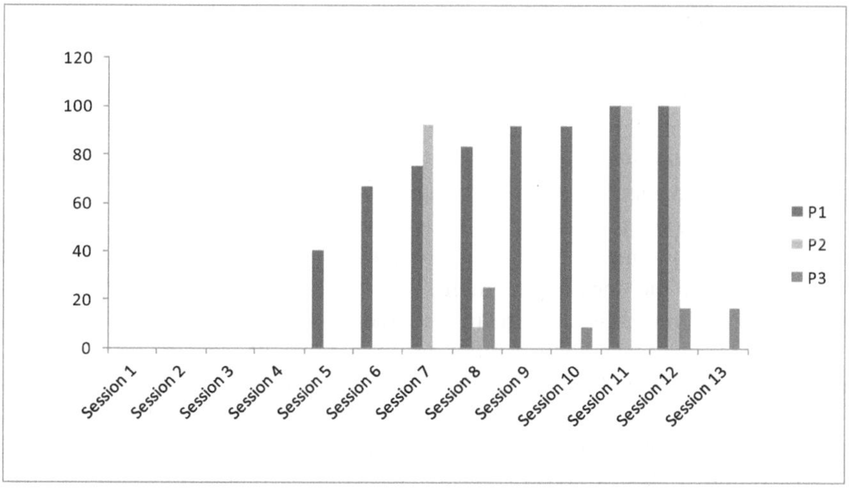

Graph 11.5 Graphical representation of the verbal scripted responses (VS) of the three participants

sitting in one place and playing with the toy, hence interfering with achieving the target. Hence, the next stage of intervention was introduced for the third participant.

11.1.13 Intervention Stage 3 or B3

In this stage, before implementing instruction, reinforcement was introduced. Use of a token was found to be a significant reinforcement based on preference assessment for the participant.

Section 1 of Showing the Video: The child was provided the instruction: *"You are going to see the video. You have to see carefully and also listen to what they are saying. You can attain one token for sitting on the chair and watching the video continuously for 2 min."*

Section 2: Performance Assessment: Additional instruction was introduced before playing with the farmhouse, *"Sit on the chair. You have to perform the actions and also say. If you can perform 5 correct responses (total motor and verbal responses), then you can attain a token."* Also, an example with one motor and one verbal response was demonstrated to the participant beforehand. The participant was provided a token if they performed four responses as per the video shown. The researcher reinforced with a social praise, *"Good job/excellent."* The token was provided at four motor and/verbal scripted responses by the child, and the same was set as a criterion.

11.1.14 Interobserver Agreement (IOA)

Interobserver agreement measures were calculated for 50% of baseline and intervention sessions for all play sequences separately for scripted and unscripted motor and verbal responses by dividing the number of agreements by the number of agreements plus disagreements and multiplying by 100.

For scripted motor responses, the mean agreement was 100%, and for scripted verbal responses, the mean agreement was 99.7% for participant 1. For unscripted motor responses, the mean agreement was 95% (range = 75–100%), and for unscripted verbal responses, the mean agreement was 99% (range = 60–100%).

For scripted motor responses, the mean agreement was found to be 99% (range = 90–100%), and for scripted verbal responses, the mean agreement was 80% for participant 2. For unscripted motor responses, the mean agreement was 90% (range = 70–100%), and for unscripted verbal responses, the mean agreement was 80% (range = 70–100%).

For scripted motor responses, the mean agreement was 100%, and for scripted verbal responses, the mean agreement was 99% for participant 3. For unscripted motor responses, the mean agreement was 95% (range = 75–100%), and for unscripted verbal responses, the mean agreement was 99% (range = 80–100%).

11.2 Results & Interpretation

Participant 1 achieved 100% mastery of the target responses, both motor and verbal, at the first stage of the intervention without any other additional strategies or prompts. The range of numbers of unscripted motor and verbal responses also decreased.

Participant 2 achieved 80–100% mastery in the target responses in the first stage of intervention, but with little instruction and demonstration in the second stage of intervention, achieved 100% mastery in both. The number of unscripted motor responses also decreased from the baseline.

Participant 3 showed an increase in the scripted responses from 13.33% in the baseline to 53.33% in the first stage of intervention. With the introduction of the third stage of intervention, there was a further increase in the performance. However, with the token strategy, further increase was projected in the performance of the child.

Video modeling is an effective intervention strategy to enhance the motor and verbal play skills or responses in these children with autism, as also established in earlier studies (Ganz et al., 2008; Marcus & Wilder, 2009; Nikopoulos & Keenan, 2004, 2006, 2007). The findings also depicted the acquisition of relatively long sequences of verbal and motor responses through VM intervention. The present findings indicate that video modeling can be an effective and efficient teaching medium among individuals with developmental delays such as autism.

11.2.1 Delimitation

Due to time constraints, multiple baseline design was not implemented, which could have depicted the experimental control. The study could not be extended further to establish generalization across settings. The next phase of the desired intervention required for participant 3 was not implemented due to time constraints.

Acknowledgments The work was carried out at the Amrit Somani Autism Center, ASMC, Kolkata, West Bengal, India. I acknowledge the support and assistance provided by Namita Somani, ASMC, and Julianne Bell, BCBA, former director, ASMC, Kolkata, West Bengal, India.

References

Apple, A. L., Billingsley, F., & Schwartz, I. S. (2005). Effects of video modeling alone and with self-management on complimenting-giving behaviors of children with high-functioning ASD. *Journal of Positive Behavior Interventions, 7*(1), 33–46.

Bellini, S., Akullian, J., & Hopf, A. (2007). Increasing social engagement in young children with autism spectrum disorders using video self-modeling. *School Psychology Review, 36*, 80–90.

Delano, M. E. (2007). Improving written language performance of adolescents with Asperger syndrome. *Journal of Applied Behavior Analysis, 40*, 345–351. https://doi.org/10.1901/jaba.2007.50-06

Ganz, J. B., Cook, K. E., & Earles-Vollrath, T. L. (2007). A grab-bag of strategies for children with mild communication deficits. *Intervention in School and Clinic, 42*(3), 179–187.

Ganz, J. B., Kaylor, M., Bourgeois, B., & Hadden, K. (2008). The impact of social scripts and visual cues on verbal communication in three children with autism spectrum disorders. *Focus on Autism and Other Developmental Disabilities, 23*, 79–94. https://doi.org/10.1177/1088357607311447

Ganz, J. B., Earles-Vollrath, T. L. & Cook, K. E. (2011). Video modeling *a visually based intervention for children with autism Spectrum disorder,* Teaghing Exceptional Ghildren July/Aug issue, 8–19.

Ganz, J. B., Gook, K. E., & Earles-Vollrath, T. L. (2006). How to write and implement sociai scripts.: PRO-ED.

Krantz, P., & McGlannahan, L. (1993). Teaching children with autism to initiate to peers: Effects of a script-fading procedure. *Journal of Applied Behavior Analysis., 26*, 121–132. https://doi.org/10.1901/jaba.1993.26-121

Krantz, P. J., & McGlannahan, L. E. (1998). Social interaction skills for children with autism: A script-fading procedure for beginning readers. *Journal of Applied Behavior Analysis., 31*, 191–202. https://doi.org/10.1901/jaba.l998.31-191

Keen, D., Brannigan, K. L., & Guskelly, M. (2007). Toilet training for children with autism: The effects of video modeling. *Journal of Developmental and Physical Disabilities., 19*, 291–303. https://doi.org/10.1007/S10882-007-9044-X

Luscre, D. M., & Genter, D. B. (1996). Procedures for reducing dental fear in children with autism. *Journal of Autism and Developmental Disorders., 26*, 547–556. https://doi.org/10.1007/BF02172275

Maione, L., & Mirenda, P. (2006). Effects of video modeling and video feedback on peer-directed social language skills of a child with autism. *Journal of Positive Behavior Interventions, 8*, 106–118. https://doi.org/10.1177/10983007060080020201

MacDonald, R., Glark, M., Garrigan, E., & Vangala, M. (2005). Using video modeling to teach pretend play to children with autism. *Behavioral Interventions., 20*, 225–238. https://doi.org/10.1002/bin.197

Marcus, A., & Wilder, S. (2009). A comparison of peer video modeling and self-video modeling to teach textual responses in children with autism. *Journal of Applied Behavior Analysis, 42*(2), 334–341. Retrieved from ERIC database.

Nikopoulos, C. K., & Keenan, M. (2003a). Promoting social initiation in children with autism. *Behavioral Interventions, 18*(2), 87–108.

Nikopoulos, C. K., & Keenan, M. (2003b). Promoting social initiations in children with autism using video modeling. *Behavioral Interventions., 18*, 87–108.

Nikopoulos, C. K., & Keenan, M. (2003c). Promoting social initiation in children with autism using video modeling. *Behavioral Interventions, 18*, 87–108.

Nikopoulos, C. K., & Keenan, M. (2004). Effects of video modeling on social initiations by children with autism. *Journal of Applied Behavior Analysis, 37*(1), 93–96.

Nikopoulos, C. K., & Keenan, M. (2006). *Video modelling and behaviour analysis: A guide for teaching social skills to children with autism*. Jessica Kingsley Publishers.

Nikopoulos, C. K., & Keenan, M. (2007). Using video modeling to teach complex social sequences to children with autism. *Journal of Autism and Developmental Disorders, 36*(4), 678–693.

Peeters, T. (1997). *Autism: From theoretical understanding to educational intervention*. Singular.

Quill, K. A. (1995). *Teaching children with autism: Strategies to enhance communication and socialization*. Delmar.

Quill, K. A. (1997). Instructional considerations for young children with autism: The rationale for visually cued instruction. *Journal of Autism and Developmental Disorders, 27*, 697–714. https://doi.org/10.1023/A:1025806900162

Quill, K. (1998). Environmental supports to enhance social-communication. *Seminars in Speech and Language, 19*, 407–422. https://doi.org/10.1055/s-2008-1064057

Sigafoos, J., O'Reilly, M., & de la Cruz, B. (2007). *How to use video modeling and video prompting*. Pro-Ed.

Sherer, M., Pierce, K. L., Paredes, S., Kisacky, K. L., Ingersoll, B., & Schreibman, L. (2001). Enhancing conversational skills in children with autism via video technology. Which is better, "self" or "other" as a model? *Behavior Modification, 25*(1), 140–158.

Part IV
Multidisciplinary ABA-based support

Chapter 12
Acknowledging the Expertise of School-Based Professionals: An Evaluation of Their Collaboration Competencies

Miriam C. Boesch, M. Alexandra Da Fonte, Sarah C. Hammonds, Brittney L. Goscicki, Alexandra Candelaria, and Kimberly N. Bowers

Abstract Effective collaboration among professionals is a critical aspect of supporting students with autism in school settings. Typically, this involves a range of practitioners, including special education teachers, speech-language pathologists, and behavior analysts. This chapter evaluated whether professional preparation and ethical standards set by these professionals' governing organizations—Council for Exceptional Children (CEC), American Speech-Language-Hearing Association (ASHA), and the Behavior Analyst Certification Board (BACB)—address collaborative practices. This chapter reviewed and analyzed the standards from these organizations, focusing on the extent and nature of content related to collaboration. Results revealed that less than 11% of standards across the three organizations addressed collaboration. Additionally, key themes were identified and analyzed within these collaboration-related standards to better understand the core elements of collaboration emphasized. Findings highlight a need for more comprehensive standards across organizations. Ensuring that these standards are adequately addressed in the training and preparation of these professionals could improve collaborative efforts and enhance outcomes for students with autism in schools. As such, the call-outs are highlighted for professional preparation programs, professional development training, and school settings to increase professionals' knowledge and skills on collaborative practices.

Keywords Collaboration · Competencies · Educational teams · Professional skills · School teams · Teamwork

---

M. C. Boesch (✉) · A. Candelaria
University of North Texas, Denton, TX, USA
e-mail: Miriam.boesch@unt.edu; Alexandra.candelaria@unt.edu

M. A. Da Fonte · S. C. Hammonds · B. L. Goscicki · K. N. Bowers
Vanderbilt University, Nashville, TN, USA
e-mail: Alexandra.dafonte@vanderbilt.edu; Sarah.hammonds@vanderbilt.edu; Brittney.l.goscicki@vanderbilt.edu; Kimberly.n.bowers@vanderbilt.edu

S. Halder et al. (eds.), *Applied Behavior Analysis-Based Interventions for Autism Spectrum Disorder*, https://doi.org/10.1007/978-981-95-2889-9_12

12.1 Introduction

With an estimated 1 in 100 children worldwide with a diagnosis of autism spectrum disorder (ASD), it continues to be one of the most prevalent childhood diagnoses (World Health Organization, 2023; Zeidan et al., 2021). Various countries are seeing an increase in autism diagnoses over the past 10 years, specifically in Australia, France, South Korea, Taiwan, and the United States (Zeidan et al., 2021). In the United States, 13%, or approximately 975,000, of students are served under the eligibility category of autism of the Individuals with Disabilities Education Act (National Center for Education Statistics, 2024). Autism is characterized by deficits in social interactions and communication, along with repetitive or restrictive behaviors. Students with autism can range from requiring minimal support to requiring a substantial amount of support (American Psychiatric Association, 2013). Students with autism can vary greatly in the severity of their characteristics and may present with intellectual disability, language deficits, or significant behavioral challenges (Xu et al., 2019).

Given that individuals with autism have a broad range of characteristics and areas of need (e.g., communication, social, cognitive, behavior, and other adaptive skills), it is typically expected that professionals from various disciplines are involved in providing intervention services (Donaldson & Stahmer, 2014) such as academic instruction, functional life skills, applied behavior analysis, augmentative and alternative communication practices, and other services. For those receiving services in public schools, special education teachers are their primary service provider. Other common service providers include speech-language pathologists, behavior analysts, occupational therapists, and physical therapists (Cox, 2012; Donaldson & Stahmer, 2014). The *ASHA 2020 School Survey Report* found that 91.7% of the school-based speech-language pathologists worked with students with autism. While 57% of board-certified behavior analysts work with students with autism and 7–12.5% work in schools with this population (Association of Professional Behavior Analysts, 2015; Layden, 2023).

12.1.1 Collaboration

A key element of supporting students with autism is the need for all stakeholders to engage in effective collaborative practices. Montiel-Overall (2008) defined collaboration as a "trusting working relationship between two or more equal participants involved in shared thinking, shared planning, and shared creation of integrated instruction" (p. 150). Collaboration is important because it can contribute to student success by sharing each other's expertise, improving efficiency between professionals, and compiling resources (Kelleher et al., 2008). Additionally, collaboration allows professionals to understand their respective roles, form relationships with one another, work toward common goals that are in the best interest of the student

(Alant et al., 2012), and increase problem solving and planning (Chung & Stoner, 2016). When members of the school team collaborate, there is an increase in positive intervention outcomes while having a greater impact on the student's development (Borg & Drange, 2019). Alternatively, the absence of effective collaboration has the potential to limit student growth and cause frustration between family members and professionals (Emmons & Zager, 2018; Strunk et al., 2017).

To mitigate potential challenges and achieve effective collaboration, some possible strategies for professionals include (a) obtain adequate resources by providing additional time and potential additional funding for team members; (b) be committed to the student; (c) respect fellow team members' backgrounds; (d) have an open and frequent line of communication through regularly scheduled meetings, phone calls, and emails; and (e) provide staff members with a positive view of collaboration so that all stakeholders are aware of the potential positive outcomes (Johnson et al., 2003). Professionals need to be willing to compromise and accept new ideas from others, be open to accepting feedback, and use others' expertise in a nonjudgmental manner. Each team member needs to feel respected and recognize each stakeholder has a unique skill set and knowledge to contribute to the group (LaFrance et al., 2019).

12.1.2 Governing Professional Organizations of Professional Standards

In many parts of the world, professional and ethical standards for school-based professionals (including collaboration standards, if any) are often determined by governing professional organizations within their respective countries. The expectation is that professional preparation programs that prepare special education teachers, behavior analysts, speech-language pathologists, require that their graduates adhere to these ethical and professional standards. For instance, in India, the National Professional Standards for Teachers (NCTE, 2023) serves as the governing body for special education teachers. Similarly, the Republic of Korea Ministry of Education (n.d.) is the cabinet-level division of the government in South Korea. They set the professional standards for their special education teachers. While in Canada, professional standards for special education teachers are developed by provinces such as the British Columbia Ministry of Education (2016).

In the United States, the professional standards for school-based professionals are developed across two entities. The State Department for each state is the regulatory agency for the professionals' licensures, and they set standards of practice for professionals working in their state. The second entity that sets professional standards is the professional organization of the professionals' respective area. Specifically, the Council for Exceptional Children (2025) is an organization focused on improving the outcomes of individuals with disabilities through the development of professional and ethical standards for special education teachers, professional training, and government advocacy. While the American Speech-Language-Hearing Association (2023a) is a professional and accreditation organization that supports speech-language pathologist and audiologists through the creation of professional standards, advancement of research, and establishment of professional practice. Similarly, Behavior Analyst Certification Board (BACB, 2023) is a nonprofit corporation that establishes and promotes professional practices of standards for behavior analysts.

12.1.3 Statement of Purpose

Given the need for school-based professionals to adopt a team approach in providing applied behavior analysis, communication, functional, and academic services to students with autism, it would seem logical for all governing professional organizations to include standards addressing collaborative practices. Collaboration is a critical aspect of working with students with complex communication needs, including those with autism. Yet, there is little information about the applicability of collaborative practices (Alant et al., 2012). Based on the importance of teamwork to effectively support students with autism, the purpose of this chapter is to highlight the collaboration competencies expected of three primary school-based professionals (i.e., special education teachers, speech-language pathologists, and behavior analysts). Specifically, the following research questions (RQs) are addressed:

1. Based on the analysis of preparation and ethical standards from their respective governing professional organizations to what extent are school-based professionals expected to be trained on collaborative practices?
2. What target concepts or competencies specific to collaborative practices are addressed in the professional and ethical standards within each governing professional organizations for school-based professionals?

12.2 Method

To determine the training of special education teachers, board-certified behavior analysts, and speech-language pathologists, the respective professional preparation and ethical standards from each affiliated or governing organization were reviewed and analyzed.

12.2.1 Procedures

The professional preparation and ethical standards for each affiliated or governing organization were extracted from the organization's website and added to a Microsoft Excel spreadsheet. Specifically, the standards were from the (a) Council of Exceptional Children (CEC, 2020) Initial Practice-Based Professional Preparation Standards, and Code of Ethics, special education teachers; (b) American Speech-Language-Hearing Association Standards for the Certificate of Clinical Competence in Speech-Language Pathology (Council for Clinical Certification in Audiology and Speech-Language Pathology of the American Speech-Language-Hearing Association, 2018) and Code of Ethics (ASHA, 2023b), speech-language pathologist; and the (c) Behavior Analyst Certification Board (BACB, 2017) fifth Edition Task List and Ethics Code, board-certified behavior analyst. Each set of professional and ethical standards was coded based on the extent to which it targeted professional competencies in "collaboration" or "collaborative practices."

A two-phase coding process was implemented. In phase 1, each preparation and ethical standard was reviewed to determine if it focused on collaboration as a competency. For the purpose of chapter, *collaboration* was referred to a standard that outlines the complex process of teamwork. That is, a process that includes two or more people who plan for positive outcomes. This may include but is not limited to components of theories or principles, practices, strategies, professional communication or dispositions, the importance of shared values, or professional communication strategies (Green et al., 2015; Griffiths et al., 2021; Montiel-Overall, 2008; see Fig. 12.1 for an example of collaboration for students with autism).

In phase 1, each standard was coded by assigning a "1" if it addressed collaboration, and a "0" if it was not addressed. If any part of the standard addressed any aspect of collaboration, that standard was assigned a "1." For example, standard ICSI.7. S2 from CEC states, "Collaborate with families and others in assessment of individuals with exceptionalities" explicitly addresses collaboration and was therefore coded as a "1." Conversely, BACB ethics standard, 3.13 addresses,

> Behavior analysts make referrals based on the needs of the client and/or relevant stakeholders and include multiple providers when available. Behavior analysts disclose to the client and relevant stakeholders any relationships they have with potential providers and any fees or incentives they may receive for the referrals. They document any referrals made, including relevant relationships and fees or incentives received, and make appropriate efforts to follow up with the client and/or relevant stakeholders.

In this example, this item was coded "0" because the focus of the standard was referring clients and other services rather than directly on how to collaborate with the individuals mentioned within the standard.

In phase 2, only standards that were determined to address collaboration were coded to create themes that identified the key concepts. The themes were determined by interpreting the intent of the standard (Creswell & Creswell, 2022). Each standard was coded by assigning a "1" to the specific theme being addressed within the standard, and a "0" if it was not addressed a specific theme. In this phase, a

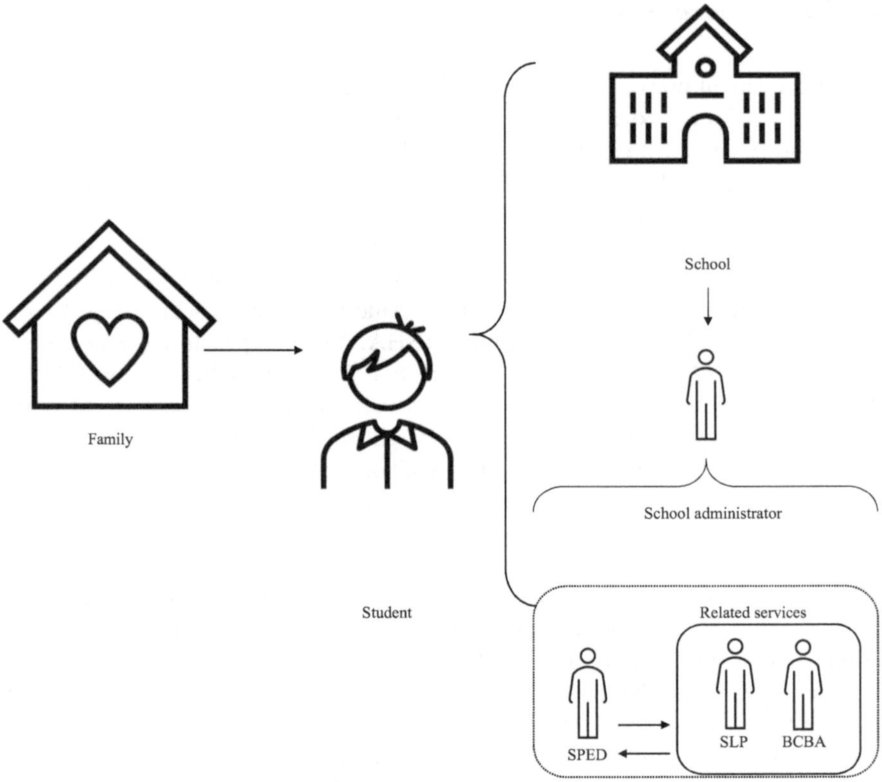

Fig. 12.1 Collaborative teams for students with autism. Note. *BCBA* board-certified behavior analyst; *SLP* speech-language pathologist; *SPED* special education teacher

standard could be coded within a specific concept (theme) or across multiple concepts (themes).

12.2.1.1 Data Analysis Codebook

After completing the extraction of the standards (phase 1), the research team met to develop a codebook. The team represented a range of professions and experience levels. Three team members had special education doctorate degrees and were university faculty in teacher preparation programs. These three team members had between 10 and 30 years of experience in the field and were certified special education teachers. One of the three members was also a board-certified behavior analyst who provided applied behavior analysis supervision and taught bachelor's- and master's-level courses on applied behavioral analysis principles. The fourth member was a project coordinator who held a master's degree and special education teaching licensure and had close to 10 years of experience in the field. The fifth member held master's degree in special education, was currently pursuing a doctoral degree in the same area, and was a board-certified behavior analyst with 7 years of experience. In addition, the project also included a research assistant with a non-educational bachelor's degree, who was currently pursuing a master's degree in special education and applied behavior analysis. The research assistant had 2 years of experience as a Registered Behavior Technician (RBT).

12.2.1.2 Operational Definitions

Operational definitions, examples, and nonexamples were included in the codebook for each of the identified collaboration-related concepts, or competencies. The five themes were (a) *purpose of collaboration*, which was comprised of concepts that focused on the rationale for teamwork, the highlights and challenges of teaming, and theoretical principles of collaboration; (b) *collaboration strategies*, which related to the specific procedures used to implement or increase the effectiveness of teamwork, including when working with other professionals and families; (c) *collaboration roles and responsibilities*, included concepts related to specific knowledge and skills that each team member should possess to effectively distribute tasks among team members, and determine and implement the various types of team models; (d) *professional disposition*, was referred to as the characteristics and level of professionalism expectations that may influence the team structure. This may include, but not limited to, timely completion of tasks, openness to feedback and other's perspectives, and engaging in ethical practices; and (e) *professional communication*, included elements of professionalism related to the ability to "code-switch" by differentiating how to speak in a relatable manner across team members, and willingness to seek or receive input from others.

12.2.1.3 Reliability

Coding reliability was conducted by two coders of the research team. For phase 1, a total of 389 standards were analyzed. The first 30% of the professional standards ($n = 117$) were coded together by the team. The purpose of this coding phase was to refine the codebook as needed and ensure there was consensus among the team prior to coding individually. The remaining professional standards ($n = 272$) were coded by the first coder. A random selection of 30% ($n = 82$) of the professional standards was selected for reliability purpose and was coded by the second coder. Interrater reliability was calculated by dividing the number of agreements by the number of agreements plus disagreements and multiplying by 100%. Reliability ranged from 79.68% to 100% ($M = 90.28\%$). Cohen's kappa (1960) was also calculated, indicating "substantial agreement for all themes and standards across the three organizations" ($k = 0.75$). Similar procedures were used in phase 2. The standards that met the "collaboration" per the operational definition ($n = 46$) were further coded to identify the themes emerging from each standard. The first 30% of the professional standards (n = 14) were coded together by the team. The first coder coded the remaining 32 professional standards, while the second coder coded a random selection of 30% (n = 10) of the professional standards for reliability purposes. Reliability was 95.65% with "almost perfect agreement" (k = 0.91).

12.2.1.4 Data Analysis

Descriptive statistics were used to calculate frequencies and percentages. Frequencies were calculated based on the occurrence of "collaboration" (phase 1) and "competencies and concepts in collaboration" (phase 2) addressed within each standard. Data were also used to make comparisons across (a) collaboration competencies and concepts and (b) professional organizations.

12.3 Results and Discussion

Thematic analyses were conducted on the professional preparation and ethical standards across three professional organizations that govern the training of special education teachers (CEC), speech-language pathologist (ASHA), and board-certified behavior analyst (BACB). Coding of the standards was conducted in two phases. In phase 1 (RQ1), a total of 411 professional preparation (n = 258) and ethical standards (n = 153) were coded, and in phase 2 a total of 42 professional preparation (n = 30) and ethical standards (n = 12) were coded. Results and practical implications are discussed based on the extent to which school-based professionals are prepared to engage in collaborative practices (RQ1) and the specific collaboration concepts and competencies targeted within each organization (RQ2).

12.3.1 Preparation of School-Based Professionals on Collaborative Practices (RQ1)

As shown in Table 12.1, from the total of professional standards (preparation and ethical), only 10.21% of these addressed "collaboration" practices. Interestingly, 62.78% of the professional standards were preparation standards, and the remaining 37.23% were from the ethical standards. These findings are concerning as collaboration in education is considered a beneficial best practice, for supporting teachers and other professionals to effectively serve students with disabilities (Reeves et al., 2017). Furthermore, it has been suggested that interdisciplinary teams that leverage various professionals' expertise are more likely to enhance students' outcomes and reach their targeted goals, more than professionals who work in isolation (Dillon et al., 2021). Unfortunately, despite the importance of collaboration among

Table 12.1 Number and percentages of standards across governing professional organizations

		Standards				Collaboration standards			
		Preparation		Ethics		Preparation		Ethics	
Organizations	*N*	#	%	#	%	#	%	#	%
CEC	140	128	91.40%	12	8.60%	26	86.66%	4	13.33%
ASHA	80	24	30.00%	56	70.00%	3	50.00%	3	50.00%
BACB	169	74	49.70%	85	50.30%	1	16.55%	5	83.33%

Note. *ASHA* American Speech-Language-Hearing Association; *BACB* Behavior Analyst Certification Board; *CEC* Council for Exceptional Children

school-based professionals, often they are ill-prepared on how to effectively collaborate as part of an interdisciplinary team (LaFrance et al., 2019).

A noteworthy finding was the disparity between governing professional organizations in the number of professional standards focused on collaboration skills. Specifically, CEC had significantly more standards that addressed collaboration practices (21.43%), than ASHA (5.88%) and the BACB (3.55%). Interestingly, these findings support the literature as it has been suggested that preparation programs across disciplines tend to focus on content-specific experiences, with little to no time spent teaching interdisciplinary collaborative practices (Bricker et al., 2020). These current findings are concerning given that board-certified behavior analysts are key professionals with expertise in applied behavior analysis and who will need to work with various stakeholders to effectively support students with autism (Monz et al., 2019).

When further analyzing the CEC standards, there were a total of 140 standards, including 128 preparation standards and 12 ethical practices standards, of which 21.43% addressed collaboration practices. A noteworthy finding was that the majority of these were within the preparation standards (86.66%). This is not surprising as special education teachers' roles and responsibilities are to lead the student's instructional or service provision team (Bagley & Tang, 2018). Despite these responsibilities, it has been suggested that special education teachers lack the collaborative skills and competencies needed (Liu & Benoliel, 2022).

Beyond special education teachers' roles and responsibilities, collaborating with other related service providers, such as speech-language pathologist and board-certified behavior analyst, is paramount. Speech-language pathologists are increasingly involved in instructional teams; yet ASHA addressed collaboration practices in only 5.88% of their 102 standards ($n = 46$, preparation standards; $n = 56$, ethical practices standards). These results are interesting as previous findings show that 43% of speech-language pathologists felt ill-prepared to engage in interdisciplinary collaborative practices (ASHA, 2020). These findings are concerning as the amount of training that speech-language pathologist receive on collaborative practices is a factor that predicts their engagement in interdisciplinary collaboration (Pfeiffer et al., 2019). Additionally, most preparation programs that train speech-language pathologist reported having little contact with other disciplines of study as part of their training (Bricker et al., 2020). As such, it is not surprising to learn of reports suggesting that speech-language pathology generally prefers isolated service provision (Ritzman et al., 2006).

Similarly, when analyzing the BACB standards, out of the 169 standards, only 3.55% addressed collaboration practices, and most of these were addressed with the ethical standards (83.33%) rather than the preparation standards (16.66%). It is evident that BACB has a strong emphasis for BCBAs to have an ethical obligation to collaborate with the other service providers (Behavior Analyst Certification Board, 2020). However, a lack of understanding of the roles, responsibilities, and scope of practice of service providers can impede effective collaboration (LaFrance et al., 2019). The lack of collaborative competencies required by the BACB may be a contributing factor to collaboration barriers among stakeholders.

12.3.2 Key Concepts and Competencies in Collaborative Practices (RQ2)

Evidence exists on the need for school-based professionals, such as special education teachers, speech-language pathologists, and board-certified behavior analysts to be strong collaborators (Donaldson & Stahmer, 2014). Thus, it is important for professional preparation programs to provide these school-based professionals with the knowledge and skills needed (Ergül et al., 2013; Price et al., 2023). Unfortunately, based on the current literature and professional preparation standards, some of these professionals may not be gaining the knowledge and skills needed to effectively participate in teams, and understand the importance of collaborative practices. To compensate for the lack of pre-service preparation, professional development training may be needed to enhance these school-based professionals' skills (Ergül et al., 2013; Van der Steen et al., 2020) and enrich their abilities to be effective and collaborative team members (Kennedy, 2016).

To better understand what concepts and competencies were evident in the preparation and ethical standards for collaboration, further analysis was conducted. During the coding, standards could be coded under a single theme (76.19%) or multiple themes (23.80%). When looking at the data by governing professional organizations, most of the CEC's professional standards on "collaboration" were coded under one theme (76.67%; multiple themes = 23.33%), ASHA's "collaboration" standards were coded equally across one theme (50%; multiple themes = 50%), and interestingly, all the BACB's professional standards were coded under one theme.

Additionally, as represented in Table 12.2, the five themes were (a) "purpose and theories" of collaboration (theme 1); (b) "collaboration strategies" (theme 2); (c) "collaboration roles and responsibilities" (theme 3); (d) "professional disposition" (theme 4); and (e) "professional communication" (theme 5). The key concepts and competencies that were mostly addressed across these standards were "collaboration roles and responsibilities" (31.48%) and "collaboration strategies" (29.63%),

Table 12.2 Number of collaboration standards and collaboration key concepts and competencies

Organization	Standards	Collaboration standards	Identified key concepts and competencies				
			CRR	CS	PC	PD	PT
CEC	140	30	14	13	4	7	1
ASHA	102	6	2	3	1	2	1
BACB	169	6	1	0	1	2	2

Note. ASHA American Speech-Language-Hearing Association; *BACB* Behavior Analyst Certification Board; *CEC* Council for Exceptional Children; *CRR* collaboration roles and responsibilities; *CS* collaboration strategies; *PC* professional communication; *PD* professional disposition; *PT* purpose and theories of collaboration

followed by "professional disposition" (20.37%). The two that were least addressed were "professional communication" (11.11%) and "purpose and theories" of collaboration (7.41%). An interesting finding across the three governing professional organizations was that four of the key concepts and competencies were addressed by at least one standard. Although "collaboration strategies" was one of the most addressed, none of the standards in the BABC met the operational definition for this theme. Yet, based on the ethical standards, board-certified behavior analysts are expected to have the skills to communicate their roles in different contexts with other professionals (Kelly & Tincani, 2013; Kelly et al., 2020). In other words, it seems that the BACB preparation standards contradict their ethical standards.

Although there were some similarities across the concepts and competencies addressed across the themes and governing professional organizations, there were some differences. For example, out of the 30 "collaboration" standards from CEC, 14 standards (46.66%) emphasized "collaboration roles and responsibilities" and 13 standards (43.30%) targeted "collaboration strategies." Whereas three out of the six ASHA "collaboration" standards stressed "collaboration strategies" (50%), and two out of the six (33.30%) BABC "collaboration" standards addressed equally "purpose and theories" of collaboration and "professional dispositions." Interestingly, contrary to the BACB, the concept and competencies least addressed by both CEC and ASHA were "purpose and theories" of collaboration (CEC 1 out of 30; ASHA 1 out of 6) and "professional communication" (CEC 4 out of 30; ASHA 1 out 6). It is possible that the differences among these governing professional organizations may be due to the long-standing history on the standards of collaboration in the field of special education (Hernandez, 2013). Unfortunately, despite the longevity of collaboration standards, there is still a lack of pre- and in-service training for this essential skill (Ergül et al., 2013). The lack of training will likely create barriers among professionals and families (Chung & Stoner, 2016).

Despite the concepts and competencies identified from the thematic analysis on collaboration standards, there was a discrepancy between the focus and distribution among governing professional organizations and their preparation and ethical standards. For example, 86.66% of CEC's collaboration standards stemmed from the preparation standards rather than the ethical standards (13.33%). Whereas ASHA's collaboration standards were equally distributed (50% each); and interestingly, the BACB's collaboration standards were 83.33% from the ethical standards, rather than the preparation standards (16.66%). Despite "collaboration" being addressed across the preparation standards of the governing professional organizations, gaps in key concepts and competencies still exist. Consequently, this increases the likelihood of the professionals' having skill deficits in collaboration and may interfere in successfully working with students with autism and their families (Brodhead, 2015; Ergül et al., 2013; Kelly & Tincani, 2013). For board-certified behavior analysts, there is a higher likelihood of having skill deficits given that only a few of the BACB's overall standards (3.55%) addressed "collaboration." In fact, it has been suggested that a lack of pre-service training in collaboration makes it difficult for board-certified behavior analyst to communicate effectively with stakeholders and other professionals (Kelly & Tincani, 2013; Kelly et al., 2020; Rohrer et al., 2021). Yet, the expectation from the BACB is that behavior analysts demonstrate competencies in collaborative practices for their certification (Kelly & Tincani, 2013).

Overall, there were five key concepts and competencies of collaboration that were identified from the professional standards (see Fig. 12.2). These findings support the assertions by Griffiths et al. (2021), who suggested that there were four building blocks to collaboration. As such, preparation programs and professional development training opportunities should focus on increasing these competencies (Griffiths et al., 2021; Hoaglund et al., 2014) and, when possible, providing training opportunities to practices these skills (Hoaglund et al., 2014). By emphasizing

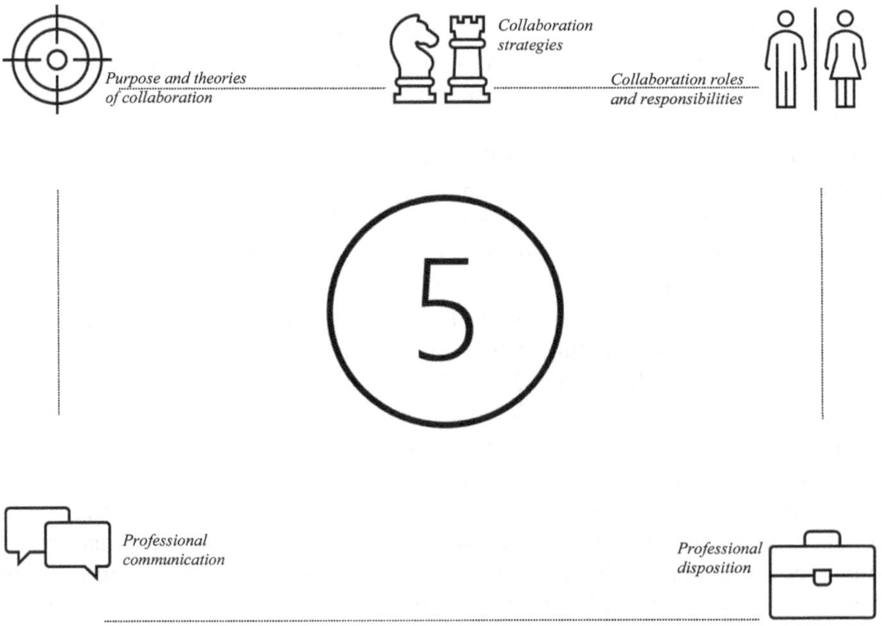

Fig. 12.2 Concepts and competencies addressed in governing professional organizations' standards

training in these areas, it is reasonable to assume that effective and collaborative practices will increase, and therefore, students with autism may receive services that support the maintenance and generalization of their skills (Kelly & Tincani, 2013).

12.3.3 Practical Implications: A Call-out for Future Practices

It is important to highlight that evidence indicates a need for further collaboration training among school-based professionals (Borg & Drange, 2019). As such, to enhance school-based professionals' knowledge and skills in collaborative practices, a call-out goes out to *professional preparation programs* to strengthen the curricula and increase practical training opportunities for these future professionals to practice teamwork skills. More specifically, it is preparation programs are encouraged to emphasize content and experiences related to the "purpose and theories" of collaboration, "collaboration strategies," "collaboration roles and responsibilities," and on the importance of having strong "professional disposition" and "professional communication."

Similarly, a call goes out to school administrators and state departments on the need for further *professional development training*. These training opportunities should address the benefits and challenges in collaboration, strategies on how to decrease the potential challenges, and provide opportunities where participants can practice these skills and learn about the pros and cons of the various types of team models (Henderson et al., 2023). A call-out also to school administrators and school-based professionals to ensure that within the *school setting* roles and responsibilities are clearly established, described, and outlined so that each team member can better understand their respective roles and responsibilities within the team (see Fig. 12.3).

To further help identify which specific competencies are fundamental for school-based professionals in supporting students with autism and their families, further research is needed.

Only through the identification of key concepts can school-based practitioners gain the knowledge and skills needed to implement effective practices. This, in turn, will allow the possibility to increase a holistic team-based approach in the assessment and instruction of students with autism.

12.4 Conclusion

Overall findings suggest that the three governing professional organizations all addressed "collaboration," to some extent. Findings confirm there are differences among these three governing professional organizations as it relates to the preparation and ethical standards. Although one can assume that these disparities may be due to differences across professional licensures, these school-based professionals will need to have strong collaboration skills to effectively work in teams, and in

PROFESSIONAL PREPARATION PROGRAMS
Strengthen the curricula and increase practical training opportunities.

Purpose and theories of collaboration:
- Providing training on the scope of each team member.
- Delivering instruction on collaboration models.
- Presenting information on how others can offer valuable input.

Professional disposition:
- Providing opportunities on differing perspectives.
- Creating evaluation systems to assess professional dispositions.

Professional communication:
- Giving explicit opportunities to practice professional communication.

PROFESSIONAL DEVELOPMENT TRAINING
Provide training that emphasizes the benefits, challenges, and practices of various types of team approaches.

Collaboration roles and responsibilities:
- Attending training on the roles and responsibilities of other professions.

Collaboration strategies:
- Creating opportunities on decreasing interpersonal conflicts.
- Training on conducting holistic assessment and intervention strategies.
- Providing examples on teamwork to support student outcomes.

SCHOOL SETTINGS
Establish clear description and structures of professional roles and responsibilities.

Collaboration roles and responsibilities:
- Assigning roles and responsibilities at the start of service provision.
- Intentionally meeting with professionals to collaborate.

Collaboration strategies:
- Modeling how interventions should be done to supplement the written report.
- Ensuring all goals across domains are addressed with input from others.

Professional disposition:
- Confirming that interventions fit classroom needs.

Professional communication:
- Verifying that everyone understands key terminology.
- Actively listening to others' perspectives.
- Effectively writing instructional plans.

Fig. 12.3 Call-out to increase the knowledge and skills of professionals on collaborative practices

turn, provide high-quality services to students with autism. While currently "collaboration" standards are being considered across professions, it is noteworthy to acknowledge there are differences and may impact how school teams function. As a result, governing professional organizations and professional preparation programs should determine if they are adequately preparing school-based professionals given the existing collaboration standards. In particular, they should assess the extent to which each concept and competency needs to be addressed or prioritized to ensure that all school-based professionals can work successfully in teams.

References

Alant, E., Champion, A., & Colone, E. (2012). Exploring interagency collaboration in AAC intervention. *Communication Disorders Quarterly, 34*(3), 172–183. https://doi.org/10.1177/1525740112455

American Psychiatric Association (APA). (2013). *Diagnostic and statistical manual of mental disorders* (5th ed.). American Psychiatric Publishing.

American Speech-Language-Hearing Association (ASHA). (2023a). *About the American speech-language-hearing association.* https://www.asha.org/about/

American Speech-Language-Hearing Association. (2023b). *Code of ethics.* www.asha.org/policy/

American Speech-Language-Hearing Association (ASHA). (2020). *2020 Schools survey report: SLP caseload and workload characteristics.* http://www.asha.org/Research/memberdata/Schools-Survey/

Association of Professional Behavior Analysts. (2015). 2014 U.S. professional employment survey: A preliminary report. https://www.csun.edu/~bcba/2014-APBA-Employment-Survey-Prelim-Rept.pdf

Bagley, S., & Tang, K. (2018). Teacher leadership in special education: Exploring skills, roles, and perceptions. *Journal of Interdisciplinary Teacher Leadership, 1*(3), 44–63. https://doi.org/10.46767/kfp.2016-0023

British Columbia Ministry of Education. (2016). *Special education services: A manual of policies, procedures, and guidelines.* https://www2.gov.bc.ca/assets/gov/education/administration/kindergarten-to-grade-12/inclusive/special_ed_policy_manual.pdf

Behavior Analyst Certification Board (BACB). (2023). *About the BACB.* https://www.bacb.com/about/

Behavior Analyst Certification Board (BACB). (2017). *BCBA task list* (5th ed.). https://www.bacb.com/wp-content/uploads/2020/08/BCBA-task-list-5th-ed-230130-a.pdf

Behavior Analyst Certification Board (BACB). (2020). *Ethics code for behavior analysts.* https://bacb.com/wp-content/ethics-code-for-behavior-analysts/

Borg, E., & Drange, I. (2019). Interprofessional collaboration in school: Effects on teaching and learning. *Improving Schools, 22*(3), 251–266. https://doi.org/10.1177/1365480219864812

Bricker, D. D., Felimban, H. S., Lin, F. Y., Stegenga, S. M., & Storie, S. O. (2020). A proposed framework for enhancing collaboration in early intervention/early childhood special education. *Topics in Early Childhood Special Education, 41*(4), 240–252. https://doi.org/10.1177/0271121419890683

Brodhead, M. T. (2015). Maintaining professional relationships in an interdisciplinary setting: Strategies for navigating nonbehavioral treatment recommendations for individuals with autism. *Behavior Analysis in Practice, 8*(1), 70–78. https://doi.org/10.1007/2Fs40617-015-0042-7

Chung, Y. C., & Stoner, J. B. (2016). A meta-analysis of team members' voices: What we need and what we do to support students who use AAC. *Augmentative and Alternative Communication, 32*(3), 175–186. https://doi.org/10.1080/07434618.2016.1213766

Council for Clinical Certification in Audiology and Speech-Language Pathology of the American Speech-Language-Hearing Association. (2018). *2020 Standards and implementation procedures for the certificate of clinic competence in speech-language pathology.* www.asha.org/certification/2020-SLP-Certification-Standards

Council for Exceptional Children. (2020). *CEC professional standards.* https://exceptionalchildren.org/standards/initial-special-education-preparation-standards

Council for Exceptional Children. (2025). About us. https://exceptionalchildren.org/about-us

Cox, D. J. (2012). From interdisciplinary to integrated care of the child with autism: The essential role for a code of ethics. *Journal of Autism and Developmental Disorders, 42*(12), 2729–2738. https://doi.org/10.1007/s10803-012-1530-z

Creswell, J. W., & Creswell, J. D. (2022). *Research design: Qualitative, quantitative, and mixed methods approaches* (6th ed.). SAGE Publications.

Dillon, S., Armstrong, E., Goudy, L., Reynolds, H., & Scurry, S. (2021). Improving special education service delivery through interdisciplinary collaboration. *Teaching Exceptional Children, 54*(1), 36–43. https://doi.org/10.1177/00400599211029671

Donaldson, A. L., & Stahmer, A. C. (2014). Team collaboration: The use of behavior principles for serving students with ASD. *Language, Speech, and Hearing Services in Schools, 45*(4), 261–276. https://doi.org/10.1044/2014_LSHSS-14-0038

Emmons, C. L., & Zager, D. (2018). Increasing collaboration self-efficacy to improve educational programming for students with autism. *Focus on Autism and Other Developmental Disabilities, 33*(2), 120–128. https://doi.org/10.1177/1088357616686

Ergül, C., Baydik, B., & Demir, S. (2013). Opinions of in-service and pre-service special education teachers on the competencies of the undergraduate special education programs. *Education Sciences: Theory and Practice, 13*(1), 518–522.

Green, B. N., & Johnson, C. D. (2015). Interprofessional collaboration in research, education, and clinical practice: Working together for a better future. *The Journal of Chiropractic Education, 29*(1), 1–10. https://doi.org/10.7899/JCE-14-36

Griffiths, A., Alsip, J., Hart, S. R., Round, R. L., & Brady, J. (2021). Together we can do so much: A systematic review and conceptual framework of collaboration in schools. *Canadian Journal of Psychology, 36*(1), 59–85. https://doi.org/10.1177/0829573520915368

Henderson, T. B., Ludden, B. J., & Romero, R. A. (2023). The ethical obligations, barriers, and solutions for interprofessional collaboration in the treatment of autistic individuals. *Behavior Analysis in Practice, 16*(4), 963–976. https://doi.org/10.1007/s40617-023-00787-z

Hernandez, S. J. (2013). Collaboration in special education: Its history, evolution, and critical factors necessary for successful implementation. *US-China Education Review Board, 3*(6), 480–496.

Hoaglund, A. E., Brikenfeld, K., & Box, J. A. (2014). Professional learning communities: Creating a foundation for collaboration skills in pre-service teachers. *Education, 134*(4), 521–528.

Johnson, L. J., Zorn, D., Yung Tam, B. K., Lamontagne, M., & Johnson, S. A. (2003). Stakeholder's views of factors that impact successful interagency collaboration. *Exceptional Children, 69*(2), 195–209. https://doi.org/10.1177/001440290306900205

Kelleher, C., Riley-Tillman, T. C., & Power, T. J. (2008). An initial comparison of collaborative and expert-driven consultation on treatment integrity. *Journal of Educational and Psychological Consultation, 18*(4), 294–324. https://doi.org/10.1080/10474410802491040

Kelly, A., & Tincani, M. (2013). Collaborative training and practice among applied behavior analysts who support individuals with autism spectrum disorder. *Education and Training in Autism and Developmental Disabilities, 48*(1), 120–131.

Kelly, E. M., Greeny, K., Rosenberg, N., & Schwartz, I. (2020). When rules are not enough: Developing principles to guide ethical conduct. *Behavior Analysis in Practice, 14*(2), 491–498. https://doi.org/10.1007/s40617-020-00515-x

Kennedy, M. M. (2016). How does professional development improve teaching? *Review of Educational Research, 86*(4), 945–980. https://doi.org/10.3102/0034654315626800

LaFrance, D. L., Weiss, M. J., Kazemi, E., Gerenser, J., & Dobres, J. (2019). Multidisciplinary teaming: Enhancing collaboration through increased understanding. *Behavior Analysis in Practice, 12*(3), 709–726. https://doi.org/10.1007/s40617-019-00331-y

Layden, S. J., Lorio-Barsten, D. K., Gansle, K. A., Austin, K., & Rizvi, S. (2023). Role and responsibilities of school-based behavior analysts: A survey. *Journal of Positive Behavior Interventions, 26*(1), 1–13. https://doi.org/10.1177/10983007231200528

Liu, Y., & Benoliel, P. (2022). National context, school factors, and individual teacher characteristics: Which matters most for teacher collaboration? *Teaching and Teacher Education, 120*, 1–16. https://doi.org/10.3102/2016276

Montiel-Overall, P. (2008). Teacher and librarian collaboration: A qualitative study. *Library and Information Science Research, 30*(2), 145–155. https://doi.org/10.1016/j.lisr.2007.06.008

Monz, B. U., Houghton, R., Law, K., & Loss, G. (2019). Treatment patterns in children with autism in the United States. *Autism Research, 12*(3), 517–526. https://doi.org/10.1002/aur.2070

National Center for Education Statistics. (2024, May). *Students with disabilities.* U.S. Department of Education, Institute of Education Sciences. https://nces.ed.gov/programs/coe/indicator/cgg/students-with-disabilities#suggested-citation

National Council for Teacher Education. (2023). *National professional standards for teachers.* https://ncte.gov.in/website/IntroductionNPST.aspx

Pfeiffer, D. L., Pavelko, S. L., Hahs-Vaughn, D. L., & Dudding, C. C. (2019). A national survey of speech-language pathologists' engagement in interprofessional collaborative practice in schools: Identifying predictive factors and barriers to implementation. *Language, Speech & Hearing Services in Schools, 50*(4), 639–655. https://doi.org/10.1044/2019_LSHSS-18-0100

Price, J. R., Cooper-Duffy, K., Ogletree, B. T., Campbell, J. M., Rose, A. J., Cathey, M., & Chen, K. (2023). Interprofessional education on autism and intellectual disabilities: Program description and initial evaluation. *School Psychology, 39*(4), 419–432. https://doi.org/10.1037/spq0000570

Reeves, P. M., Pun, W. H., & Chung, K. S. (2017). Influence of teacher collaboration on job satisfaction and student achievement. *Teaching and Teacher Education, 67*, 227–236. https://doi.org/10.1016/j.tate.2017.06.016

Republic of Korea Ministry of Education. (n.d.). Organization. https://english.moe.go.kr/sub/infoRenewal.do?m=0105&page=0105&s=english

Ritzman, M. J., Dixie, S., & Coufal, K. L. (2006). A case study of a collaborative speech-language pathologist. *Common Disorders Quarterly, 27*(4), 221–231. https://doi.org/10.1177/15257401060270040501

Rohrer, J., Marshall, K., Suzio, C., & Weiss, M. J. (2021). Soft skills: The case for compassionate approaches or how behavior analysis keeps finding its heart. *Behavior Analysis in Practice, 14*(4), 1135–1143. https://doi.org/10.1007/s40617-021-00563-x

Strunk, J., Leisen, M., & Schubert, C. (2017). Using a multidisciplinary approach with children diagnosed with autism spectrum disorder. *Journal of Interprofessional Education and Practice, 8*, 60–68. https://doi.org/10.1016/j.xjep.2017.03.009

Van der Steen, S., Geveke, C. H., Steenbakkers, A. T., & Steenbeek, H. W. (2020). Teaching students with autism spectrum disorders: What are the needs of educational professionals? *Teacher and Teacher Education, 90*, 1–9. https://doi.org/10.1016/j.tate.2020.103036

World Health Organization. (2023, March). *Autism* https://www.who.int/news-room/fact-sheets/detail/autism-spectrum-disorders

Xu, G., Strathearn, L., Liu, B., O'Brien, M., Kopelman, T. G., Zhu, J., Snetselaar, L. G., & Bao, W. (2019). Prevalence and treatment patterns of autism spectrum disorder in the United States, 2016. *The Journal of the American Medical Association (JAMA) Pediatrics, 173*(2), 153–159. https://doi.org/10.1001/jamapediatrics.2018.4208

Zeidan, J., Fombonne, E., Scorah, J., Ibrahim, A., Durkin, M., Saxena, S., Yusuf, A., Shih, A., & Elsabbagh, M. (2021). Global prevalence of autism: A systematic review update. *Autism Research : Official Journal of the International Society for Autism Research, 15*(5), 778–790. https://doi.org/10.1002/aur.2696

Chapter 13
Considerations for Enhancing Speech-Language Pathology (SLP) and Applied Behaviour Analysis (ABA)-Based Practices

Lina Slim and Dag Strömberg

Abstract This chapter is written from the perspective of two dually certified speech-language pathologists (SLPs) and behaviour analysts (BAs) with extensive international experience. It explores how interprofessional collaboration between SLPs and BAs enhances client outcomes by blending the strengths of each field. By embracing mutual learning opportunities, professionals can create more effective, evidence-based, culturally responsive interventions and partnerships.

Keywords Autism · Applied behaviour analysis · Speech-language pathology/speech-language therapy · Interprofessional collaboration · Evidence-based practice · Cultural responsiveness

Autism spectrum disorder (ASD) is on the rise, with a global prevalence of approximately 1% (Zeidan et al., 2022) and in some areas as high as 2.8% (Maenner et al., 2023). ASD is a neurodevelopmental disorder that may be associated with several coexisting conditions (i.e. medical, genetic, biomarkers, behavioural, cognitive, linguistic; Muskens et al., 2017). Diagnosis requires observation of an individual's behaviour across various domains. Individuals with autism encounter challenges in social communication and social interaction and display restricted, repetitive behaviours, interests, or activities (American Psychiatric Association, 2022). These characteristics are highly individualised, necessitating tailored interventions rather than a one-size-fits-all approach.

Individualisation of intervention does not imply a single-provider approach. On the contrary, to better understand the complex needs a person with autism may experience, a well-informed practitioner should tap into the expertise of

L. Slim
Lina Slim Consulting, Miami, FL, USA

D. Strömberg (✉)
Department of Special Education, Stockholm University, Stockholm, Sweden
e-mail: dag.stromberg@specped.su.se

S. Halder et al. (eds.), *Applied Behavior Analysis-Based Interventions for Autism Spectrum Disorder*, https://doi.org/10.1007/978-981-95-2889-9_13

professionals from different disciplines who can help address the various challenges that a person with autism is facing. Specifically, professionals from different backgrounds, such as speech-language pathology and behaviour analysis may sometimes work on similar goals. Within this shared space, the boundaries may be blurred, potentially leading to misunderstandings and perceived encroachment across scopes of practices (Spencer et al., 2020). To foster clear and respectful communication that promotes comprehensive and evidence-based intervention, speech-language pathologists[1] and behaviour analysts must understand and respect each other's practice, competence, and theoretical backgrounds. This chapter aims to inform regarding each profession's theoretical background, identify areas of strength and opportunities, and how each professional discipline can improve their practice by collaborating to deliver evidence-based, integrated and responsive interventions and supports.

Please note that for purposes of this chapter the authors acknowledge and honour the individual's choice and preferences in terminology. While some prefer the person-first format (person with autism), others prefer identity-first language (e.g. autistic person). Additionally, some advocate using 'autism' instead of 'autism spectrum disorder'. For this chapter, the authors primarily use person-first terminology, with a focus on the primary descriptor being 'autism'. Additionally, for professional disciplines, this chapter will utilise the complete nomenclature (e.g. speech-language pathology and behaviour analysis). Conversely, the abbreviated designations for practitioners in each discipline will be employed, namely speech-language pathologist(s) as SLP(s) and behaviour analyst(s) as BA(s).

13.1 Professional Foundations of Speech-Language Pathology and Behaviour Analysis

The partial overlap in the scope of practice among the professions of speech-language pathology and behaviour analysis highlights the necessity for collaboration, collective understanding, and respect (LaFrance et al., 2019). It is critical to understand that each discipline has complex and comprehensive educational preparation requirements. These requirements include mastery of essential content areas, including foundational concepts and principles, theoretical frameworks, screening, assessments, evaluation, development and implementation of intervention plans, service delivery contexts, and a commitment to professional ethics (LaFrance et al., 2019; & Gerenser & Koenig, 2019). We will review some pertinent areas that are essential to building and establishing collaborative practices between SLPs and BAs.

[1] May also be referred to as speech-language therapists, or speech therapists.

13.1.1 Scope of Practice and Scope of Competence

SLPs and BAs are guided by their scope of practice, scope of competence, and different approaches to interventions. A definition of scope of practice and scope of competence is needed to establish a shared language (Brodhead et al., 2018; Spencer et al., 2020). Scope of practice refers to 'the set of activities that a licensed/certified behaviour analyst [or speech-language pathologist] is authorised to engage in. That authorization is conditioned upon the professional also being competent' (Spencer et al., 2020, p. 3). On the other hand, the scope of competence refers to 'the extent to which a professional can engage in specific clinical activities at a [proficient] level of performance consistent with a specified standard of excellence' (Spencer et al., 2020, p. 3).

Speech-language pathology is a professional field that falls under the discipline of communication sciences and disorders. The scope of practice includes assessment and treatment of a wide range of human communication, speech, language, voice, pragmatics, and swallowing disorders across all ages, and the use of augmentative and alternative communication (AAC) (American Speech-Language-Hearing Association, 2016). Applied behaviour analysis (ABA) is both a science and an applied profession with wide application across various areas of practice. The scope of practice includes assessment and treatment across many socially significant behaviour domains (Heward et al., 2022).

13.1.2 Educational Background

An understanding of education and training requirements will inform practitioners of the rigorous preparation and scope of practice for each professional discipline. Acknowledging this can foster a renewed and reinforced appreciation and respect for the thorough educational background, training, and expertise that each professional discipline brings to a collaborative intervention.

13.1.2.1 Speech-Language Pathology

The educational and training requirements for SLPs are rigorous and extensive and vary internationally, featuring distinct criteria in different regions. While current requirements are stated per country/region/continent, it is important to remain updated on these criteria as degree and licensing regulations may change over time. In the USA, the comprehensive education and training of SLPs are credentialed by the American Speech-Language-Hearing Association (ASHA). ASHA mandates a master's, doctoral, or other recognised post-baccalaureate degree, along with a minimum of 400 h of supervised clinical experience and a Praxis Exam. Recognising the shortage of SLPs and its impact on addressing communication disorders, ASHA

has approved the use of speech-language pathology assistants (SLPAs) as vital support personnel with specific licensing or certification requirements in some states (American Speech-Language-Hearing Association, 2022).
Other countries' educational requirements and mandates are country-specific. These include rigorous coursework with supervised fieldwork clinical hours and a competency exam. The following are some examples: the UK mandates a bachelor's degree in speech and language therapy accredited by the Health and Care Professions Council; France requires a 5-year master's degree in speech therapy, followed by a national exam; Sweden requires a 4-year (magister) degree in speech and language pathology and licensing from the National Board of Health and Welfare; South Africa, a 4-year bachelor's degree in speech-language pathology, and registration with the Health Professions Council; Brazil, a 4-year bachelor's degree in speech therapy and registration with the Regional Council of Speech Therapy; India typically a bachelor's degree in audiology and speech-language pathology, and registration with the Rehabilitation Council of India or state authorities.

13.1.2.2 Behaviour Analysis

BAs follow a rigorous and extensive education and training that varies across the world. For professionals who reside in the USA or Canada, certification is regulated by the Behavior Analyst Certification Board, Inc.® (BACB®, 2023), which was established in 1998. Three levels of certification are available that are accredited by the National Commission for Certifying Agencies (NCCA), the accreditation body of the Institute for Credentialing Excellence (ICE): the Board Certified Behavior Analyst (BCBA®), the Board Certified assistant Behavior Analyst (BCaBA®), and the Registered Behavior Technician (RBT®). In addition, a doctoral designation (BCBA-D) is available for BCBAs who hold a relevant doctoral degree.

The pathway to eligibility for the BCBA® certification includes an Association for Behavior Analysis International (ABAI)-verified course sequence of 315 h of behaviour-analytic coursework and a master's degree from accredited, qualifying and/or recognised higher educational institutions, 2000 h of practical supervised behaviour-analytic fieldwork experience, and passing a competency exam.

The BCaBA® is an undergraduate-level certification in behaviour analysis for practitioners who provide behaviour-analytic services under the supervision of a BCBA. To address shortage of behaviour analysts and the impact that this may have in meeting the needs of individuals with behavioural and communication needs, the BACB® approved a professional designation for frontline practitioners; the Registered Behavior Technician (RBT®). Frontline professionals who are RBT® deliver behaviour-analytic services and practice under the direction and close supervision of a BCBA® and/or an RBT supervisor (BACB, 2023). Additionally, in 37 US states, behaviour analysts are required to not only be certified but also gain a licence to practice (BACB, 2024a, 2024b). In the USA and Canada, there are over a quarter of a million certified behaviour analysts across the various qualification levels.

Outside the USA and Canada, however, there is considerable variation. For regulatory reasons, since January 2023 it is no longer possible for behaviour analysts who reside outside of the USA and Canada to sit for the BACB® exam and become BCBAs. However, there are about 8000 BACB-certified behaviour analysts who gained their qualifications before 2023 and who can retain their certification if they meet biannual re-certification requirements (BACB®, 2023).

In most countries outside of the USA and Canada, behaviour analysis as a profession is neither recognised nor regulated (Keenan et al., 2022), although ABAI-verified master's-level coursework in behaviour analysis still is offered at around 50 universities in 16 European countries. To meet the need for professional regulation, national behaviour analysis organisations are taking the initiative to create certification and licensing bodies for the practice of professional behaviour analysts in their countries. For example, the UK Society for Behaviour Analysis' register of behaviour analysts was accredited by the Professional Standards Authority of the UK, thus formally recognising the profession. In the Czech Republic, the Czech Association for Behaviour Analysis led the development of a law regulating the profession (Zákon, 2017). The qualification levels were modelled on those of the BACB. In France, the Organisation Nationale des Professions de l'Analyse du Comportement is advancing towards professional recognition for French-speaking behaviour analysts. Other countries are progressing with similar developments (Keenan et al., 2022).

Professional groups are developing standards and competency requirements and training for individuals practising as behaviour analysts. The Erasmus+ financed project *Supporting European Behaviour Analysts by Developing Professional Qualifications and Training* (EuroBA) developed Intellectual Outputs to facilitate recognition and mobility of European behaviour analysts. In this project (2020–2023), researchers from universities in six European countries, together with a professional advisory group representing another 16 European countries, created competence profiles that can be used as templates to build educational programmes for behaviour analysts at master-level and pre-bachelor entry level. This project included the creation of an entry-level multilingual online training programme for behaviour technicians using Programmed Instruction and the multimedia program Simple Steps Autism (Keenan et al., 2022).

The European Association for Behaviour Analysis (EABA; https://europeanaba.org) offers a platform for behaviour analysts to work together and support each other across Europe and further afield. EABA's biannual conference and summer schools, located in various countries across Europe, provide a forum for European behaviour analysts to share their experiences, research, and networks.
Representatives of the national behaviour analysis associations of the Nordic countries (Denmark, Finland, Iceland, Norway, Sweden) have formed a collaborative network to address quality assurance and ethical aspects of the field (Keenan et al., 2022). In addition, it is important to note that in several countries where BA is not recognised as a standalone profession, higher education in behaviour analysis may be available for students with diverse professional backgrounds like psychologists, special educators, or SLPs (Dillenburger et al., 2014). In Sweden, for example,

higher education in ABA has been offered as a specialisation for professionals who already possess at least a bachelor's degree in another related domain, such as psychology, special education, occupational therapy, or speech-language pathology. In fact, all current BCBAs educated within the Swedish higher education system had another profession first. The majority of this group of behaviour analysts are dually certified psychologists or speech-language pathologists (Keenan et al., 2022).

13.1.3 Theoretical Background

Different professional disciplines draw from different theoretical backgrounds to inform clinical practice. This applies also to speech-language pathology and applied behaviour analysis (LaFrance et al., 2019). Speech-language pathology draws from multiple theoretical perspectives (LaFrance et al., 2019; Paul et al., 2018), including behaviourism, social constructivism, cognitivism, phonological theory, motor learning theories, and developmental and linguistic theories (Sutton, 2008; Paul et al., 2018).

Behaviour analysis is a natural science that aims to discover 'basic scientific laws that delineate how behaviour-environment relations work' (Cooper et al., 2020, p. 39). The philosophical foundation of behaviour analysis is radical behaviourism where behaviour is considered the subject matter. Behaviour is defined holistically as the interaction of an organism with their environment. In other words, behaviour analysis encompasses the analysis of everything an organism does (anything that can be expressed as a verb), including moving, acting, speaking (i.e. public behaviour), as well as feeling and thinking (i.e. private behaviour or Inners). Mentalistic reifications are exposed as circular reasoning. Pseudo-explanatory nouns that reify observed behaviour are reverted into the relevant descriptive verbs, for example, the noun 'cognition' is returned to the verb 'thinking' or the noun 'emotion' to the verb 'feeling' (Johnston, 2014). While behaviour analysis primarily addresses issues related to the function of social and physical environmental contingencies, genetic, neurophysiological, and developmental factors are acknowledged and included in the analysis (McLaughlin, 2010).

While it is crucial to recognise the different theoretical perspectives of SLPs and BAs, it can be beneficial to recognise that, in certain instances, significant similarities do exist; such as when comparing behaviourist and social constructivist views on language acquisition. In fact, these perspectives have a lot in common, both emphasising the importance of context and social interaction for the development of language and other behaviours (Burkholder & Peláez, 2000).

In sum, several distinctions establish speech-language pathology and behaviour analysis as distinct professions. This distinction is further reinforced by a robust system of behaviour analysis certification in the USA, Canada, the UK, and the Czech Republic. However, this is not the case in other countries where behaviour analysis is not yet fully established as a regulated profession (Keenan et al., 2022).

By contrast, speech-language pathology is fully recognised and established as a regulated profession in most global regions.

13.2 Current State of the Professional Relationship Between Speech-Language Pathologists and Behaviour Analysts

SLPs and BAs who work with individuals with autism can find themselves working on similar goals. While this goal alignment can create opportunities for collaboration, it may also lead to conflict among professionals, particularly related to perceived overlap in the scope of practice (Spencer et al., 2020). In the USA, resolving these conflicts has been an ongoing challenge, given the complex underlying economic (i.e. insurance funding sources) and political forces that maintain them. To address these issues, the governing bodies of both professions have worked with States and regions to develop laws to license practitioners, to increase recognition of the professional fields, and ensure guidelines for lawful, ethical regulations and policies that benefit both practitioners and consumers. These efforts can enhance collaboration between the two professions, fostering increased awareness of the benefits that each discipline offers in assessing and developing interventions for individuals with autism.

Although the profession of behaviour analysis is not yet regulated in many countries outside the USA, SLPs are likely to collaborate with colleagues that are trained in behaviour analysis at least to some extent. These professionals may be competent in behaviour-analytic principles and procedures and may have degrees in other professions. Moreover, SLPs might hold dual certifications (i.e. in 2023 there were 522 dually qualified SLP/BCBAs worldwide, 460 of whom resided in the USA) (Speech Pathology Applied Behavior Analysis Special Interest Group of Association of Behavior Analysis International, December, 2023).

Outside the USA, the situation for the field of behaviour analysis differs significantly from speech-language pathology. Regulation, certification, and funding vary between regional and national health and education ministries. Interdisciplinary models typically claim to incorporate behaviour analysis as an adjunct rather than a primary field. While this approach may diminish disciplinary barriers, lack of adequate training, professional recognition, and familiarity with the science of behaviour analysis has led to scepticism, erroneous assumptions, and misinformation (Keenan et al., 2022).

In sum, professionals seek certification in applied behaviour analysis through credentialing and certifying organisations. Certified behaviour analysts, along with other professionals who may have completed coursework and training in behaviour analysis without certification, collaborate with SLPs across various models, settings, and functions. Despite the persistence of misconceptions and misinformation, their shared goal is to establish effective and meaningful interventions promoting improved educational and health outcomes for those they serve.

13.3 Interprofessional Collaborative Practices

SLPs and BAs engage in various interprofessional collaborative practices, which exist on a continuum based on the level of interaction, integration, and blending of disciplines. In a *multidisciplinary* practice, SLPs and BAs work alongside each other, typically maintaining their distinct roles and responsibilities. Each expert contributes their specialised knowledge to address different aspects of a client's needs. In an *interdisciplinary* practice, SLPs and BAs work together closely, in an integrated manner, fostering a shared understanding and continuous communication between team members toward coordinated care plans, engaging in some joint decision-making and responsibilities. Lastly, in a *transdisciplinary* practice SLPs and BAs come together to engage in mutual learning and shared decision-making. This practice differs from multidisciplinary or interdisciplinary approaches by emphasising the blending and integration of roles rather than simply working alongside each other. This collaborative approach reduces potential concerns about encroachment on areas of practice.

A transdisciplinary practice is particularly effective when ethical principles and learning strategies are shared among team members (Slim & Reuter-Yuill, 2021). An example is illustrated at the Autism Centre for Young Children (Autismcenter små barn) in Stockholm, Sweden. At this publicly funded habilitation centre, all professionals (mainly psychologists, SLPs, and special educators) who are involved in focused or comprehensive intervention programmes operate as generalists. Here, behaviour analysis serves as the foundational science, underpinning all practices and unifying team members with diverse professional backgrounds (Dillenburger et al., 2014). Competence is developed and maintained through a system of staff training, team meetings and supervision, provided by clinical supervisors who have completed the master's-level training in behaviour analysis and autism at Stockholm University. This transdisciplinary approach contributes to providing equality of interventions, with all professionals sharing a common ground, and a culture of continuous learning and support between colleagues (Strömberg, 2019; Tonér, 2023).

13.4 Intersection of Speech-Language Pathology and Behaviour Analysis

The rising prevalence of autism has increased the need for efficient educational and therapeutic services, and families are seeking the most effective approaches for their child with autism. This is a daunting task given the proliferation of information disseminated on social media and reports, which include a mix of science-based and pseudoscientific approaches that may be harmful (Daly & Celiberti, 2021). SLPs and BAs are ethically bound to advocate for the right to effective science-based autism interventions and protect consumers from harmful pseudoscientific treatments (American Speech-Language-Hearing Association, 2005; Behavior Analyst Certification Board®, 2020).

SLPs and BAs are likely to 'share space' and encounter overlapping scopes of practice when working with individuals with autism, especially in areas such as speech, language, communication, swallowing, feeding, and augmentative and alternative communication (AAC). Navigating interprofessional collaboration is likely to prompt discussions about different as well as shared evidence-based practice, including assessment methods and interventions.

13.4.1 Evidence-Based Practice

Evidence-based practice (EBP) has been defined in a variety of ways across organisations and professions. In 2008, ASHA defined EBP as the integration of clinical expertise, evidence (both external and internal), and client/patient/caregiver perspectives (ASHA, 2005; Greenwell & Walsh, 2021; Hall-Mills et al., 2023; Slocum et al., 2014). Similarly, Contreras et al. (2021) describe EBP for behaviour analysts as a decision-making process that combines the best available evidence, clinical expertise, and client values and context. As part of the decision-making process about EBP, Higginbotham and Satchidanand (2019) recognised the need for performance-based data collected by practitioners about the effectiveness of the intervention they select, the client progress, and the potential modifications needed. As such, they proposed an expansion of the triangle to the diamond-shaped EBP model, which includes evaluation after an EBP has been selected. In other words, to inform practice, a practitioner should engage in an ongoing decision-making process that integrates practice-based evidence (Lemoncello & Ness, 2013). It is important to note that EBP should be based on collaborative dynamic interactions between those involved to ensure it leads to individualised, meaningful, and effective interventions.

Establishing consensus on a universal definition of EBP has been challenging. In this chapter, an extension of the Higginbotham and Satchidanand (2019) diamond construct is proposed (see Fig. 13.1). EBP is defined as a decision-making process that integrates

1. Clinical expertise/expert opinion, which refers to the *knowledge, judgement, and critical reasoning* acquired through training and professional experiences.
2. External evidence (empirically supported treatment) (Drisko & Friedman, 2019), which leverages the *best available information* gathered from the scientific literature.
3. Unique set of *personal and cultural circumstances, values, priorities, and expectations* identified by the client and their caregivers.
4. Internal evidence, or practice-based evidence, that refers to the *clinical evidence* derived from high-quality design, implementation, and evaluation of clinical practices using observational data collected during treatment intervention ses-

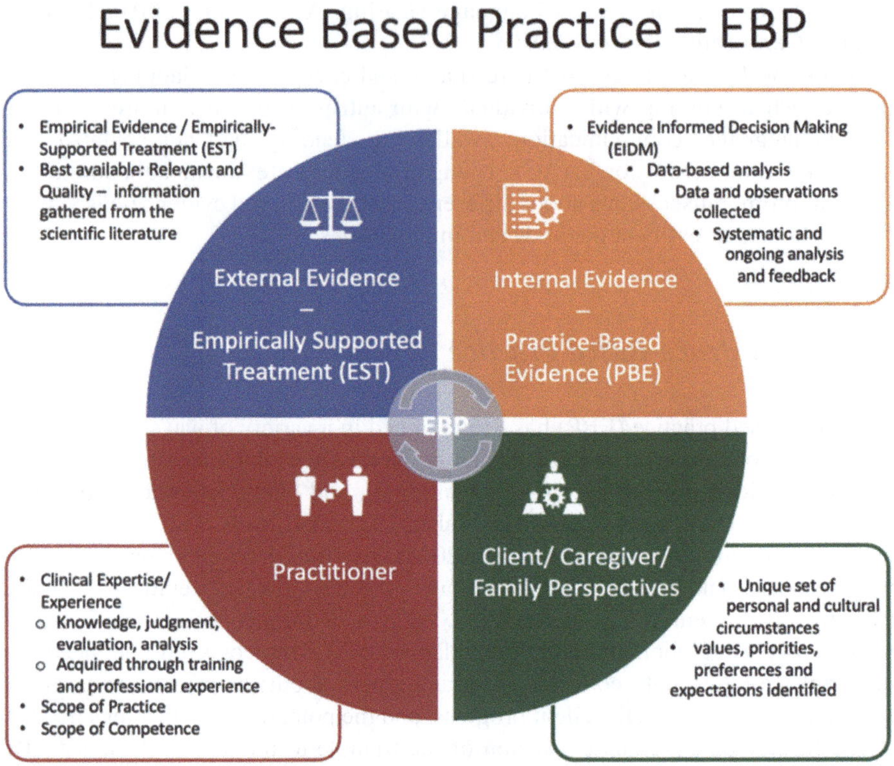

Fig. 13.1 Four components to evidence-based practice (EBP). (*Note.* Adapted by Slim (2021) from Higginbotham and Satchidanand (2019) with the addition of practice-based evidence)

sions (Higginbotham & Satchidanand, 2019; Lemoncello & Ness, 2013; Olswang & Bain, 1994).

It is beneficial for the fields of speech-language pathology and behaviour analysis to adopt and embrace a universal and agreed-upon definition of EBP. This approach will greatly facilitate collaboration in the selection, design, and implementation of effective intervention practices, ultimately leading to more meaningful, socially significant, and sustainable outcomes.

13.4.2 *Assessment*

Prior to conducting assessments, practitioners should have an understanding and respect for the family's and person's cultural norms, values, and preferences. This information will guide the assessment and ensure that it is conducted in a sensitive and responsive manner. When evaluating assessment tools, it is crucial to acknowledge the diversity of tests and modalities available to practitioners. While some are specific to a discipline, others may be utilised by professionals with various disciplinary backgrounds. Speech-language pathology assessment tools may be employed across a variety of modalities and methods, including

- Direct assessments that involve interacting with or observing the individual.
- Indirect assessments that require the assessor to engage with caregivers, parents, teachers, or direct care staff.
- Criterion-referenced assessments that evaluate the individual's acquisition of specific skills, and compare them against a predetermined standard, learning goal, performance level, or other criterion (i.e. Communication Matrix; The Rossetti Infant-Toddler Scale; Autism Diagnostic Interview-Revised; Functional Communication Profile-Revised).
- Norm-referenced assessments that compare the individual's performance to same-age peers of the norm group, using a normal distribution or bell curve (e.g. Preschool Language Scale; Peabody Picture Vocabulary Test; Clinical Evaluation of Language Fundamentals I Fifth Edition; Goldman-Fristoe Test of Articulation™ 3; Kaufman Speech Praxis Test).

Speech-language pathology test batteries offer valuable insights by assessing a range of skills across developmental domains, including articulation, language, auditory discrimination, swallowing, and speech sound concerns. Although not autism-specific, these tools provide valuable information on the structural, physiological, and developmental state of individuals with autism. Therefore, SLPs contribute to the collaborative approach by providing valuable information about a learner's skills, obtained from these diverse tests. Assessment tools commonly used in the field of speech-language pathology highlight strengths, deficits, or concerns, specifically, *what* the learner is demonstrating. However, these tests do not generally offer guidance on the next steps or actions to address these challenges, specifically, *how to* support the learner.

Assessment tools that are utilised by BAs enhance the planning and design of the intervention process by providing practical, operationalised, and individualised guidelines for addressing areas of challenges. While SLPs have access to a wide range of structured, norm-referenced assessments, this is an area where BAs can significantly enhance the collaboration process. Assessment tools that are utilised by BAs usually provide practical, operationalised, and individualised guidelines. For example, behaviourally based tools to assess skills related to communication (e.g. Verbal Behavior Milestones Assessment and Placement Program; Essential for Living; PEAK Relational Training System) often include suggestions of which learning targets to choose and operationalised guidelines on *how* to support the learner. These assessments generally draw from B.F. Skinner's (1957) analysis of verbal behaviour, which provides a useful framework for understanding the functions of various communicative behaviours (i.e. behaviour environment interactions, environmental and motivating conditions that function as discriminative stimuli for the behavioural response).

The general approach to assessment used by BAs is to take a close look at the function of the behaviour of concern (i.e. communication) by using a *functional behaviour assessment* (FBA). A thorough FBA offers a systematic way of understanding the function of behaviours and thus provides a useful basis for decisions regarding evidence-based supports (Hume et al., 2021). FBA can be conducted *indirectly* by using questionnaires or interviews, such as the Functional Analysis Screening Tool (Iwata et al., 2013), Questions About Behavior Function (Matson & Vollmer, 1995), Functional Analysis Interview (O'Neill et al., 1997), or Open-ended Functional Assessment Interview (Hanley, 2012). It can also be conducted *directly*, through behavioural observations or various types of experimental functional analysis, that is, a systematic testing method regarded as the gold standard for comprehending the function of challenging behaviour (Saini et al., 2020). Often, a combination of indirect and direct methods is used.

Challenging behaviours may serve one or multiple functions. The assessment of the functions usually is divided into at least three categories (Melanson & Fahmie, 2023). FBA procedures are arranged to explore whether the challenging behaviours is maintained by

(a) Social-positive reinforcers in the form of attention, tangible items, or activities.
(b) Social-negative reinforcers that function as avoid/escape from a potentially aversive stimulus.
(c) Automatic reinforcers that function to obtain access to sensory stimulation.

Based on the assessment outcome, the practitioner(s), family, and other stakeholders can identify and agree on whether there is a need for an intervention. When an FBA shows that a challenging behaviour serves one of the first two functions (a or b), it can be interpreted 'as if' the behaviour is communicative. In such cases, one of the ways to effectively address the challenging behaviour is by reinforcing a more meaningful functionally equivalent communicative behaviour (for more information on FBA, refer to the Tennyson chapter in this book).

13.4.3 Intervention

Practitioners who provide support services for individuals with autism, including SLPs and BAs, need to advocate for effective science-based intervention to protect consumers from harmful and pseudoscientific treatments and ensure safe and quality health outcomes. To support this advocacy, the National Clearinghouse on Autism and Evidence and Practice (NCAEP) (Hume et al., 2021; Steinbrenner et al., 2020) has identified a number of evidence-based practices (i.e. EST, as referenced in Fig. 13.1), demonstrating evidence of efficacy in promoting positive outcomes, increasing independence, and success for individuals with autism. They have classified evidence-based interventions in three broad categories and conceptualised evidence-based interventions, including

- Focused intervention practices (FIPs).
- Multicomponent interventions, including multiple elements of empirically supported FIP (i.e. Early Intensive Behaviour Intervention, Early Start Denver model, TEACCH program, LEAP model, UCLA Young Autism Program).
- Manualized Interventions Meeting Criteria of Evidence (MIMC), consisting of manualised procedures and package interventions.

Twenty-eight FIPs that are recognised as evidence-based are based on applications of behaviour analysis, such as antecedent-based intervention; differential reinforcement of alternative, incompatible, or other behaviour; discrete trial training; FBA; modelling; prompting; reinforcement; task analysis; time delay; video modelling; and visual supports (Steinbrenner et al., 2020, Table 4.1, p. 42).

Ten MIMCs that have been identified as empirically supported are based on applications of behaviour analysis. They are classified into six categories, including Naturalistic Intervention (i.e. Pivotal Response Training, JASPER, Milieu Teaching), Augmentative and Alternative Communication (Picture Exchange Communication Systems©), Parent-Implemented Intervention (i.e. Project ImPACT & Stepping Stones Triple P), Milieu Teaching, social narrative (i.e. Social Stories™), social skills training (PEERS®), and technology-aided instruction and interventions (i.e. FaceSay®, Mindreading) (Steinbrenner et al., 2020, Table 4.1, p. 42).

13.4.4 How SLP and BA Inform One Another's Practices

Interprofessional collaborative practice includes a range of professionals working together to support service users. In the context of this chapter, the focus is to highlight areas in which BAs and SLPs can work together collaboratively. Table 13.1 highlights the scope of practice for the two professions, and areas where they intersect. The scope of practice of BAs is guided and informed by knowledge of natural laws of behaviour focusing on improving socially significant behaviours without restriction to any specific aspect of human behaviour. Their *scope of competence* refers to the competence of a specific BA who works with a particular service user group (e.g. autistic children) or with a specific behaviour of concern (e.g. food selectivity), while maintaining a performance level that meets a defined standard of excellence (Spencer et al., 2020). As such, BAs who work with children who experience speech and language and/or feeding issues need to be competent in designing systematic, conceptually sound, behaviour-analytic procedures to address these children's behaviours of concern.

The scope of practice of SLPs is to provide sets of activities (i.e. assessment tools and intervention strategies) in support of individuals facing difficulties and challenges with communication, eating, drinking, and swallowing. These include considerations of structural and physiological aspects of speech production and swallowing. As with BAs, an SLP's scope of competence depends on their specialisation with consideration to maintaining a performance level that meets a defined

Table 13.1 Scope of practice for SLPs and BAs

Scope of practice	Speech-language pathologists	Behaviour analysts
Diagnostics of language	✓	
Receptive language	✓	✓
Expressive language	✓	✓
Written language	✓	✓
Functional analysis of speech		✓
Language sampling	✓	
Child development	✓	
Articulation/phonology	✓	
Swallowing	✓	
Feeding	✓	✓
Augmentative and alternative communication (AAC)	✓	✓
Speech	✓	
Fluency	✓	✓
Voice	✓	
Data collection strategies		✓
Behaviour interventions		✓
Functional behaviour assessments (FBA)		✓
Reinforcement		✓
Motivation	✓	✓
Single-case design methodology		✓
Functional communication training (FCT)	✓	✓
Preference assessments		✓
Principles and tactics of effective teaching		✓
Communication/verbal behaviour	✓	✓

standard of excellence (Spencer et al., 2020). SLPs working with children with autism can benefit from collaborating with BAs in their selection and design of individualised intervention practices. A behaviour-analytic approach ensures interventions are socially significant and meaningful, observable and measurable, effective, and data-driven. SLPs must be able to demonstrate that the intervention is responsible for the behaviour change rather than some other variable, operationalise targets and procedures, and systematically implement the intervention, leading to generality and long-lasting behaviour change (Baer et al., 1968). To better understand how both disciplines can inform one another, the following considerations may be helpful:

- BAs adopt a systematic and analytic approach to changing environmental contingencies (independent variables) based on the function of the behaviour of concern (dependent variable).

- SLPs follow a structural organisational scheme that is based on developmental trajectories and physiologic conditions. They also account for health, personal, environmental factors, and the influence that these have on assessment and intervention planning (American Speech-Language-Hearing Association, 2016).
- SLPs typically learn about some specific behavioural strategies, rather than the broader science of applied behaviour analysis (Gerenser & Koenig, 2019). This means that they may use particular manualised procedures, which may not always be consistently and systematically implemented.
- BAs base verbal (communication) and vocal (speech) assessments and interventions on Skinner's functional verbal behaviour analysis. The specialised knowledge and techniques that SLPs have, for example, for encouraging pronunciation, managing swallowing, and regulating respiratory function, complement behavioural procedures by addressing the physiological, structural, developmental and linguistic components of speech and language that are outside most BA's training, thereby enhancing overall communication outcomes.

BAs may not be familiar with the field of speech-language pathology and vice versa. While BAs may focus on verbal and vocal behaviour and eating and feeding problems, the developmental and physiological processes generally are not part of their basic training. This is an area where SLPs can offer expertise to augment intervention programmes. In addition, SLPs use linguistic concepts to understand the processes by which speech and language are acquired and this can contribute in the selection of target behaviour that require interventions. The relevant supports include an understanding of culturally-based developmental and linguistic norms, as well as physiological abilities. Specifically, SLPs can assess the *what* the learner is demonstrating or needs to learn [form/topography], structural and skill deficits, and *why* [pragmatics, function] the learner is communicating.

13.4.4.1 How SLP Informs BA Practice

SLPs draw from multiple toolkits to assess, engage, and develop a learner's communication skills across social, developmental, and language domains. They also take into account environmental, social, and personal factors when designing person-centred and responsive interventions. Their expertise in these areas, combined with knowledge of phonological and linguistic concepts, aids in understanding how speech and language are acquired. This understanding contributes to selecting target behaviours that require intervention and determining the appropriate intervention sequence.

SLPs engage the learner in social play, providing verbal models, and comment (talking) on shared items or activities, using pictures, books, objects, or ongoing events to stimulate language development and social skills. Some specific approaches include incidental teaching, Enhanced Milieu Teaching, More Than Words (Hanen Program adapted to autism), Pre-Linguistic Milieu Teaching, and Milieu Communication Training (Prelock & McCauley, 2021).

Speech interventions focusing on motor production of speech sounds are categorised as *articulation approaches*, while those emphasising the linguistic aspects of speech production are termed *phonological/language-based approaches*. It is common to use both, articulation and phonological/language-based approaches, with the same individual at different times, contexts, or for different reasons. The intervention for speech sound disorders typically follows the following steps: establishment, generalisation, and maintenance.

Target selection is guided by developmental, theoretical, and/or client-specific approaches and the extent of deviation of speech from the norm and its impact on intelligibility. Some examples of intervention methods include Naturalistic Speech Intelligibility intervention, Nonspeech Oral–Motor Therapy, speech-sound perception training, the Nuffield Dyspraxia Programme, the Kauffman Method, Dynamic Temporal and Tactile Cueing, Rapid Syllable Transition Treatment, Integrated Phonological Awareness Intervention, Phonemic Hand Cues, and Prompts for Restructuring Oral Muscular Phonetic Targets.

Further, within their scope of practice, SLPs assess and address speech-language and communication challenges and disorders by implementing augmentative and alternative communication (AAC) (ASHA, n.d.-a). ASHA refers to AAC as a system that 'describes multiple ways to communicate that can supplement or compensate (either temporarily or permanently) for the impairment and disability patterns of individuals with severe expressive communication disorders' (ASHA, n.d.-b). AAC is augmentative when used to complement or supplement speech and alternative when employed as a substitute or to compensate for speech (ASHA, n.d.-c; Beukelman & Light, 2020).

SLP intervention employs a multimodal approach also known as total communication, whereby all means of communication are used based on the context and individual characteristics (Beukelman & Mirenda., 2013). SLPs use AAC to address the individual's full communication abilities; this may include any existing speech or vocalisations, gestures, manual signs, and aided communication, low-tech to high-tech modality. When assessing for and selecting an individualised AAC system, SLPs engage in a dynamic assessment process that includes the broader environmental context consisting of the ecological, cultural, and social and communicative contexts, the communication partners, and the individual's skills, needs, and strengths (Light et al., 2021; Reuter-Yuill et al., 2024). They do so by engaging in an interprofessional, collaborative decision-making process to determine the most effective and culturally meaningful AAC modality needed (Beukelman & Mirenda, 2013; Kasper et al., 2024).

In other words, speech-language pathology can significantly enhance BA practice by offering a deeper understanding of the physiological, mechanical, and linguistic aspects of speech and language. This added context not only expands skillsets and content knowledge but also improves target selection and progression, resulting in interventions that are more comprehensive, cohesive, and effective.

13.4.4.2 How BA Informs SLP Practice

SLPs engage in a practice-based inquiry approach relying on observation of learner behaviour to inform on progress of the intervention, which may require different data collection and analysis approaches and measures (Olswang & Bain, 1994). This approach is enhanced by the integration of behaviour-analytic principles. BAs develop precise interventions by operationalising targets and instructional practices, employing a conceptually systematic and analytic approach to instruction. Their training allows them to identify data collection and selection procedures tailored to the context and goals, establishing metrics for data-based decision-making, and developing performance feedback measurement systems that ensure intervention fidelity. Most importantly, behaviour-analytic programmes are individualised to meet the learner's needs, preferences, and leveraging their strengths, while ensuring meaningful, socially significant, sustainable long-term learner outcomes (Behavior Analyst Certification Board, 2020).

BAs provide function-based interventions that teach skills or establish alternative behaviours by arranging carefully designed contingencies. When the functions of challenging behaviour are related to communication (Melanson & Fahmie, 2023), BAs may recommend Functional Communication Training (FCT; Hume et al., 2021; Tiger et al., 2008). Behaviour of concern that has a communicative function is replaced by socially important communicative behaviour that serves the same function as the challenging behaviour. This process is central for fostering independent access to social environments and enhancing overall quality of life. FCT is unique in that the alternative behaviours consist of socially important forms of communication, such as vocalisations, manual signs, pictures, or speech-generating devices (Steinbrenner et al., 2020). Successful management of challenging behaviours often involves effective interprofessional collaboration (Sheridan & Kratochwill, 2007; Reuter-Yuill et al., 2024).

Engaging in an interprofessional collaborative approach between SLPs and BAs offers numerous benefits, such as personal and professional growth, enhanced health and educational outcomes for clients, enriched experiences for both clients and practitioners, greater treatment fidelity, and the assurance of effective, individualised, evidence-based and responsive interventions. The following is an online survey distributed to all dually certified SLP-BCBA's ($n = 7$) in Sweden, highlighting the perceived benefits experienced by both SLPs and BAs. The survey included the question, 'What benefits do you see in being both an SLP and a behaviour analyst?' (Strömberg, 2024). All respondents were initially trained as SLPs and later obtained BA certification. All participants had experience working with children with autism. The survey responses predominantly highlighted how studying behaviour analysis to master's-level enhanced their speech-language pathology practice. The following are some of the responses from the survey (translated from Swedish):

> An SLP has knowledge of speech, language, and communication and how it can be described/diagnosed. As a behaviour analyst, you get effective tools to measure, teach and analyse skills within these areas.

> Another addition as a behaviour analyst is the focus on motivation and positive reinforcement. Not always assuming that the "inner" motivation to communicate is there. To not just think that a skill needs to be developed/learned, but to stop and think from the person's perspective—why? When should they use the skill?
>
> Behaviour analysis has given me the importance of looking at the function of communication—i.e., why and not just how (function before form).
>
> I would especially like to highlight the concepts of behavioural excesses/deficits, and motivating operations, that marry very well with all the SLP deep knowledge of communication and language and the interdisciplinary fields that form the ground.
>
> Yes, today the work with speech, language and communication without ABA would be perceived as very poor and almost impossible. (Strömberg, 2024)

In other words, behaviour analysis may enhance speech-language pathology practice by adding new tools to the toolbox and making the existing tools 'sharper' and more effective. That is, not only acquiring new skills but also getting better at what you are already doing.

13.5 Conclusions

In terms of interprofessional collaboration, it is beneficial to embrace a humble approach with other members of the team as it emphasises the acknowledgement that 'we don't know it all, nor can one person do it all'. Every member of the team contributes valuable insights to the overall outcome and, at the same time, has limitations in their knowledge and skill repertoires. Therefore, active collaboration becomes crucial to gaining a deeper understanding of others' perspectives. Research evidence within the respective disciplines is essential when collaborating to identify what is most effective, responsive, and meaningful for the people served.

Recognition of overlaps and differences in relation to theoretical as well as practical knowledge and skills promotes open and collaborative discussions when identifying goals, intervention strategies, support services, data collection procedures, methods for providing performance feedback, and conducting data analysis for progress monitoring. Clear, respectful discussions with a focus on evidence-based intervention foster a shared understanding of the intervention's impact on an individual's learning and responses. Evaluating the effectiveness of a specific intervention ultimately enables decisions on whether to continue, modify, or discontinue it (Slim & Reuter-Yuill, 2021; Spencer et al., 2020).

Understanding each other's terms and establishing a shared, agreed-upon terminology and language for describing processes is important as it fosters effective collaboration. This collective and dynamic process enhances awareness of the theoretical underpinnings of terms and their application. Most important is reaching consensus on shared ethical principles, guidelines, and a conceptual framework (Cox, 2012; Slim & Reuter-Yuill, 2021). When SLPs and BAs collectively adhere to shared values and a unified language, guided by consistent motivation, and well-aligned foundational principles, these alignments strengthen interprofessional collaborative practices. Culturally responsive collaboration increases fidelity of intervention and has a positive and enduring impact on the lives of those receiving services. By adopting a culturally responsive, person-centred, interprofessional collaborative approach, SLPs and BAs can achieve great benefits for both practitioners and clients.

References

American Psychiatric Association. (2022). *Diagnostic and statistical manual of mental disorders* (5th ed., text rev.).

American Speech-Language-Hearing Association. (2005). *Evidence-based practice in communication disorders* [Position Statement]. Available from www.asha.org/policy

American Speech-Language-Hearing Association. (2016). *Scope of practice in speech-language pathology* [Scope of Practice]. Available from www.asha.org/policy/

American Speech-Language-Hearing Association. (2022). *Speech-language pathology assistant scope of practice* [Scope of Practice]. Available from www.asha.org/policy

American Speech-Language-Hearing Association. (n.d.-a). *Augmentative and alternative communication (AAC).* https://www.asha.org/public/speech/disorders/aac/

American Speech-Language-Hearing Association. (n.d.-b). *Augmentative and alternative communication (AAC).* https://www.asha.org/njc/aac/

American Speech-Language-Hearing Association. (n.d.-c). *Augmentative and alternative communication* (Practice Portal). https://www.asha.org/practice-portal/professional-issues/augmentative-and-alternative-communication/#collapse_4

Baer, D. M., Wolf, M. M., & Risley, T. R. (1968). Some current dimensions of applied behavior analysis. *Journal of Applied Behavior Analysis, 1*(1), 91–97.

Behavior Analyst Certification Board. (2024a, January 23). *About the BACB.* https://www.bacb.com/about/

Behavior Analyst Certification Board. (2020). *Ethics code for behavior analysts.* https://bacb.com/wp-content/ethics-code-for-behavior-analysts/

Behavior Analyst Certification Board. (2023). *Registered behavior technician handbook.* https://www.bacb.com/wp-content/uploads/2022/01/RBTHandbook_231228-a.pdf

Behavior Analyst Certification Board. (2024b, January 23). *U.S. licensure of behavior analysts.* https://www.bacb.com/u-s-licensure-of-behavior-analysts/

Beukelman, D. R., & Light, J. C. (2020). *Augmentative & alternative communication: Supporting children and adults with complex communication needs.* Brookes Publishing Company.

Beukelman, D., & Mirenda, P. (2013). *Augmentative and alternative communication: Supporting children & adults with complex communication needs* (4th ed.). Paul H. Brookes Publishing.

Brodhead, M. T., Quigley, S. P., & Wilczynski, S. M. (2018). A call for discussion about scope of competence in behavior analysis. *Behavior Analysis in Practice, 11*(4), 424–435.

Burkholder, E. O., & Peláez, M. (2000). A behavioral interpretation of Vygotsky's theory of thought, language, and culture. *Behavioral Development Bulletin, 9*(1), 7–9. https://doi.org/10.1037/h0100530

Contreras, B. P., Hoffman, A. N., & Slocum, T. A. (2021). Ethical behavior analysis: Evidence-based practice as a framework for ethical decision making. *Behavior Analysis in Practice, 15*(2), 619–634. https://doi.org/10.1007/s40617-021-00658-5

Cooper, J., Heron, T., & Heward, W. (2020). *Applied behavior analysis* (3rd ed.). Pearson Education Ltd..

Cox, D. J. (2012). From interdisciplinary to integrated care of the child with autism: The essential role for a code of ethics. *Journal of Developmental Disorders, 42*, 2729–2738. https://doi.org/10.1007/s10803-012-1530-z. PMID: 22527703.
Daly, K., & Celiberti, D. (2021). It takes a village to stand for science: Showcasing some allies. *Science in Autism Treatment, 18*(12).
Dillenburger, K., Röttgers, H.-R., Dounavi, K., Sparkman, C., Keenan, M., Thyer, B., & Nikopolous, C. (2014). Multidisciplinary teamwork in autism: Can one size fit all? *The Australian Educational and Developmental Psychologist, 31*(02), 97–112.
Drisko, J. W., & Friedman, A. (2019). Let's clearly distinguish evidence-based practice and empirically supported treatments. *Smith College Studies In Social Work, 89*(3–4), 264–281. https://doi.org/10.1080/00377317.2019.1706316
Gerenser, J. E., & Koenig, M. A. (2019). *ABA for SLPs: Interprofessional collaboration for autism support teams*. Paul H. Brookes Publishing Co.
Greenwell, T., & Walsh, B. (2021). Evidence-based practice in speech-language pathology: Where are we now? *Journal of Speech-Language pathology, 30*(1), 186–198.
Hall-Mills, S., Ireland, M., Flynn, P. F., & Hoffman, L. (2023). Evidence-based practice engagement in schools. *ASHA Journals*. Online resource. https://doi.org/10.23641/asha.23152817.v1
Hanley, G. P. (2012). Functional assessment of problem behavior: Dispelling myths, overcoming implementation obstacles, and developing new lore. *Behavior Analysis in Practice, 5*(1), 54–72. https://doi.org/10.1007/bf03391818
Heward, W. L., Critchfield, T. S., Reed, D. D., Detrich, R., & Kimball, J. W. (2022). ABA from A to Z: Behavior science applied to 350 domains of socially significant behavior. *Perspectives on Behavior Science: An Official Journal of the Association for Behavior Analysis International, 45*(2), 327–359. https://doi.org/10.1007/s40614-022-00336-z
Higginbotham, J., & Satchidanand, A. (2019). *From triangle to diamond: Recognizing and using data to inform our evidence-based practice*. ASHA Journals: Academy. https://academy.pubs.asha.org/2019/04/from-triangle-to-diamond-recognizing-and-using-data-to-inform-our-evidence-based-practice
Hume, K., Steinbrenner, J. R., Odom, S. L., Morin, K. L., Nowell, S. W., Tomaszewski, B., Szendrey, S., McIntyre, N. S., Yücesoy-Özkan, S., & Savage, M. N. (2021). Evidence-based practices for children, youth, and young adults with autism: Third generation review. *Journal of Autism and Developmental Disorders, 51*(11), 4013–4032. https://doi.org/10.1007/s10803-020-04844-2
Iwata, B. A., DeLeon, I. G., & Roscoe, E. M. (2013). Reliability and validity of the functional analysis screening tool. *Journal of Applied Behavior Analysis, 46*, 271–284. https://doi.org/10.1002/jaba.31
Johnston, J. M. (2014). *Radical behaviorism for ABA practitioners*. Sloan Publishing.
Kasper, T., Slim, L., & Reuter-Yuill, L. (2024, March 6). *Buckle Up! steering towards effective SLP Collaboration*. Association for Behavior Analysis International (ABAI), *Verbal Behavior Matters Blog*.
Keenan, M., Dillenburger, K., Konrad, M.-H., Debetencourt, N., Vuksan, R., Kourea, L., Pancocha, K., Kingsdorf, S., Brandtberg, H. J., Ozkan, N., Abdelnour, H., Da Costa-Meranda, M., Schuldt, S., Mellon, R., Herman, A., Tennyson, A., Ayvazo, S., Moderato, P., Attard, N., et al. (2022). Professional development of behavior analysts in Europe: A snapshot for 21 countries. *Behavior Analysis in Practice, 16*(3), 709–729. https://doi.org/10.1007/s40617-022-00754-0
LaFrance, D. L., Weiss, M. J., Kazemi, E., Gerenser, J., & Dobres, J. (2019). Multidisciplinary teaming: Enhancing collaboration through increased understanding. *Behavior Analysis in Practice, 12*(3), 709–726. https://doi.org/10.1007/s40617-019-00331-y
Lemoncello, R., & Ness, B. (2013). Evidence-based practice & practice-based evidence applied to adult, medical speech-language pathology. *Perspectives on Gerontology, 18*(1), 14–26. https://doi.org/10.1044/gero18.1.14
Light, J., Barwise, A., Gardner, A. M., & Flynn, M. (2021). Personalized early AAC intervention to build language and literacy skills: A case study of a 3-year-old with complex communication needs. *Topics in Language Disorders, 41*, 209–231.

Maenner, M. J., Williams, A. R., Amoakohene, E., Hughes, M. M., McArthur, D., Williams, S., Patrick, M., DiRienzo, M., Washington, A., Shaw, K. A., Warren, Z., Vehorn, A., Bakian, A. V., Bilder, D. A., Gutierrez, J., Durkin, M. S., Furnier, S. M., Salinas, A., Fitzgerald, R. T., et al. (2023). Prevalence and characteristics of autism spectrum disorder among children aged 8 years—Autism and developmental disabilities monitoring network, 11 sites, United States, 2020. *MMWR. Surveillance Summaries, 72*(2). https://doi.org/10.15585/mmwr.ss7202a

Matson, J. L., & Vollmer, T. R. (1995). *User's guide: Questions about behavioral function (QABF)*. Scientific Publishers.

McLaughlin, S. F. (2010). Verbal behavior by B.F. Skinner: Contributions to analyzing early language learning. *The Journal of Speech and Language Pathology–Applied Behavior Analysis, 5*(2), 114–131. https://doi.org/10.1037/h0100272

Melanson, I. J., & Fahmie, T. A. (2023). Functional analysis of problem behavior: A 40-year review. *Journal of Applied Behavior Analysis, 56*(2), 262–281. https://doi.org/10.1002/jaba.983

Muskens, J. B., Velders, F. P., & Staal, W. G. (2017). Medical comorbidities in children and adolescents with autism spectrum disorders and attention deficit hyperactivity disorders: A systematic review. *European Child & Adolescent Psychiatry, 26*(9), 1093–1103. https://doi.org/10.1007/s00787-017-1020-0

O'Neill, R. E., Horner, R. H., Albin, R. W., Sprague, J. R., Storey, K., & Newton, J. S. (1997). Functional assessment and program development for problem behavior: A practical handbook. Pacific Grove, CA: Brooks/Cole Publishing.

Olswang, L. B., & Bain, B. (1994). Data collection: Monitoring children's treatment progress. *American Journal of Speech-Language Pathology, 3*(3), 55–66.

Paul, R., Norbury, C., & Gosse, C. (2018). *Language disorders from infancy through adolescence: Listening, speaking, reading, writing, and communicating* (5th ed.). Elsevier.

Prelock, P. A., & McCauley, R. J. (2021). Treatment of Autism Spectrum Disorders: Evidence-Based Intervention Strategies for Communication and Social Interactions. Paul H. Brookes Publishing Co.

Reuter-Yuill, L., Kasper, T., Slim, L., & Shillingsburg, A. (2024). Augmentative and alternative communication (AAC). In J. C. Vladescu & A. N. Kisamore (Eds.), *Promoting language for learners with autism Spectrum disorder: A guide for applied behavior analysis practitioners*. Routledge/Taylor & Francis.

Saini, V., Fisher, W. W., Retzlaff, B. J., & Keevy, M. (2020). Efficiency in functional analysis of problem behavior: A quantitative and qualitative review. *Journal of Applied Behavior Analysis, 53*(1), 44–66. https://doi.org/10.1002/jaba.583

Sheridan, S. M., & Kratochwill, T. R. (2007). *Conjoint behavioral consultation: Promoting family-school connections and interventions*. Springer Science+Business Media, LLC.

Skinner, B. F. (1957). *Verbal behavior*. Prentice-Hall, Inc.

Slim, L., & Reuter-Yuill, L. M. (2021). A behavior-analytic perspective on interprofessional collaboration. *Behavior Analysis in Practice, 14*(4), 1238–1248. https://doi.org/10.1007/s40617-021-00602-7

Slim, L. (2021, November 14). *Authentic Interprofessional collaboration: Reflections from self to others* [webinar]. Manhattan Psychology Group (MPG).

Slocum, T. A., Detrich, R., Wilczynski, S. M., Spencer, T. D., Lewis, T., & Wolfe, K. (2014). The evidence-based practice of applied behavior analysis. *The Behavior Analyst, 37*(1), 41–56. https://doi.org/10.1007/s40614-014-0005-2

Speech Pathology Applied Behavior Analysis Special Interest Group of Association of Behavior Analysis International. (2023, December). *Volume 3 Newsletter.*

Spencer, T., Slim, L., Cardon, T., & Morgan, L. (2020). *ABAI Interprofessional collaborative practice between behavior analysts and speech-language pathology*. Workgroup of ABAI Practice Board.

Steinbrenner, J. R., Hume, K., Odom, S. L., Morin, K. L., Nowell, S. W., Tomaszewski, B., Szendrey, S., McIntyre, N. S., Yücesoy-Özkan, S., & Savage, M. N. (2020). *Evidence-based practices for children, youth, and young adults with autism*. The University of North Carolina at Chapel Hill, Frank Porter Graham Child Development Institute, National Clearinghouse on Autism Evidence and Practice Review Team.

Strömberg, D. (2019). Developing and maintaining competence at the workplace: Staff training and supervision at a habilitation center for children with autism in Stockholm, Sweden. In *Presentation at the 45th Association for Behavior Analysis International Annual Convention.*

Strömberg, D. (2024). *Unpublished raw data on benefits of dual certification for Swedish SLP-BCBA's.*

Sutton, A. (2008). Language acquisition theory and AAC intervention. *Perspectives on Augmentative and Alternative Communication, 17*(2), 56–61. https://pubs.asha.org

Tiger, J. H., Hanley, G. P., & Bruzek, J. (2008). Functional communication training: A review and practical guide. *Behavior Analysis in Practice, 1*(1), 16–23. https://doi.org/10.1007/BF03391716

Tonér, S. (2023). Ständigt lärande organisation på autismcenter små barn i Stockholm. *Logopeden, 3*, 14–17.

Zákon Č. 96/2004 Sb (amended 2017). https://www.zakonyprolidi.cz/cs/2004-96#cast1

Zeidan, J., Fombonne, E., Scorah, J., Ibrahim, A., Durkin, M. S., Saxena, S., Yusuf, A., Shih, A., & Elsabbagh, M. (2022). Global prevalence of autism: A systematic review update. *Autism Research, 15*(5), 778–790. https://doi.org/10.1002/aur.2696

Chapter 14
Faculty–Student Collaboration in the Dissemination of Applied Behavior Analysis-Based Interventions

Michelle P. Kelly, Sarah C. Mead Jasperse, and Adel A. Wahdain

Abstract Collaboration and dissemination are both encouraged professional activities for behavior analysts, and, often, dissemination becomes a collaborative activity. For a variety of reasons, behavior analytic faculty may choose their students to be their dissemination collaborators. This may happen because the faculty member is the lone person in their specialty, because the students are local to the region and have more expertise and knowledge of the dominant culture, or simply because they want to mentor their students to be effective disseminators. The purposes of this chapter are (a) to provide an overview of a "collaborate to disseminate" model within the field of behavior analysis; (b) present 16 actionable strategies for how faculty and students can bridge theory and practice both inside and outside the classroom, and work together to disseminate information about applied behavior analysis-based interventions across the academic domains of research, teaching, and service; and (c) illustrate these concepts through a series of student–faculty dissemination activities in the United Arab Emirates as a case example.

Keywords Academia · Autism spectrum disorder · Higher education · Mentoring · Partnership · Service

As behavior analysts residing and working in a country that has a relatively new behavior analytic community, we are often asked for advice and tips regarding effective and ethical dissemination practices. The first and second authors of this chapter have been faculty members in at least three behavior analysis programs each (in the Republic of Ireland, the Kingdom of Saudi Arabia, the United Arab Emirates

M. P. Kelly (✉) · S. C. Mead Jasperse
Emirates College for Advanced Education, Abu Dhabi, United Arab Emirates
e-mail: mkelly@ecae.ac.ae; Sarah.Mead@ecae.ac.ae

A. A. Wahdain
Hemam for Inclusive Education – Al Azza, Ministry of Education, Abu Dhabi, United Arab Emirates
e-mail: adel.wahdain@moe.gov.ae

S. Halder et al. (eds.), *Applied Behavior Analysis-Based Interventions for Autism Spectrum Disorder*, https://doi.org/10.1007/978-981-95-2889-9_14

[UAE], and the United States) and have found that the most successful dissemination efforts have involved collaboration with students and graduates (including the third author).

When the science of behavior analysis is not well established in an academic setting, the role of students as allies with more expertise and knowledge of the dominant culture becomes increasingly important. This is especially true for a lone behavior analyst on faculty. If faculty and students can come together to disseminate the science in a collaborative manner, the benefits for the wider community can be significant. By working together, they can build local capacity for providing applied behavior analysis (ABA) services and expand the reach of behavior analysis within and beyond the field of autism spectrum disorder (ASD) intervention. Such partnerships offer numerous opportunities for both faculty and students to engage in meaningful and impactful work.

The purposes of this chapter are (a) to provide an overview of a "collaborate to disseminate" model in the field of behavior analysis, (b) provide 16 actionable suggestions regarding how faculty and students can bridge theory and practice in (and beyond) the classroom and collaborate to disseminate about ABA-based interventions, and (c) describe a series of faculty–student dissemination activities in the UAE.

14.1 Dissemination as a Professional Activity for Applied Behavior Analysts

Dissemination as a process involves targeting the distribution of information and intervention materials to specified audiences (Schillinger, 2010). For the purposes of this chapter, dissemination is not limited to scientific dissemination via journal publications and conference presentations, but, instead, refers to the widespread sharing of information about the science of behavior analysis to and beyond the behavior analytic community. These dissemination efforts are necessary for the growth and expansion of the field in socially meaningful ways. "Effective dissemination is a matter of effective behavior: the effective behavior of the disseminator to motivate, teach, or signal the effective behavior of the consumer" (Flynn et al., 2023, p. 25).

Dissemination to both clinical professionals (e.g., behavior analysts, social workers, speech and language pathologists) and non-clinical professionals (e.g., clients, parents, policymakers) has been an encouraged professional activity since shortly after the founding of the field of behavior analysis (Garcia et al., 2023). Morris (1985) summarized many of the issues related to dissemination that were occurring around that time, including inaccuracies in the media, misconceptions held by the public, and related policy and funding concerns, and these issues continue to be of concern today (Kelly et al., 2019).

As the profession of behavior analysis developed, compliance documents delineated an expectation for active dissemination efforts. For example, the Behavior

Analyst Certification Board (BACB, 2014, 2020) has included mention of the importance of actively engaging in dissemination and the call for ethical behavior in all dissemination efforts, underscoring the attention given to dissemination efforts within the field. There have been published accounts of large-scale dissemination endeavors (e.g., Fixsen & Blase, 1993) as well as publications that provide guidance for professionals who wish to further their own dissemination efforts (e.g., Helton & Alber-Morgan, 2018). Kelly et al. (2019) outlined the history, successes, challenges, and ethics of effective dissemination and summarized the efforts of several professional associations in the field of behavior analysis, including the BACB (www.bacb.com), the Association for Behavior Analysis International (ABAI; www.abainternational.org), and the European Association for Behavior Analysis (EABA; www.europeanaba.org).

There are also other professional entities contributing to behavior analysis dissemination efforts, including the nonprofit Association of Professional Behavior Analysts (APBA; https://www.apbahome.net/) founded in 2007, whose mission is "to promote and advance the science-based practice of behavior analysis by advocating for public policies and informing, supporting, and protecting practitioners and consumers." Another important organization to highlight is the Association for Science in Autism Treatment (ASAT; https://asatonline.org/). Founded in 1998, ASAT's mission is to "promote safe, effective, science-based treatments for people with autism by disseminating accurate, timely, and scientifically sound information." They fulfill their mission via their website, monthly newsletter, externship program, as well as their media watch initiative that offers responses to accurate and inaccurate portrayals of autism intervention in the media.

14.1.1 Online Dissemination

The focus on media is more apparent in the BACB's (2020) most recent ethics code, which now includes definitions of "social media channel" and "website" in the glossary and dedicates subcodes 5.10 and 5.11 to ethical behavior when using these platforms. Kelly et al. (2019) provided an overview of online successes in dissemination with examples of popular websites and podcasts. When considering dissemination as a professional activity for both behavior analytic faculty and students, it would be unwise to overlook the significance of digital platforms, including social media sites like X, Facebook, Instagram, TikTok, and LinkedIn. These platforms offer a long list of advantages, including cost-effectiveness, the ability to reach other professionals instantaneously, and the capacity to engage different generations, particularly younger ones, who may not typically participate in discussions about developments in the field. Additionally, these digital platforms facilitate real-time professional peer review and dialogue (Flynn et al., 2023; O'Leary et al., 2017).

There is a growing number of ABA personalities who manage websites, social media accounts, and podcasts with the aim of sharing information and raising awareness about behavior analytic topics, including ABA-based interventions for autism spectrum disorder (ASD) (Parry-Cruwys et al., 2023). "It could be argued that the representation of our field in the social media realm shapes the cultural landscape of ABA as much as research publications. Those interested in consuming ABA services as parents or individuals, in learning about ABA as students, or in opposing ABA as critics are all more likely to encounter representations of ABA online rather than through published print media" (Parry-Cruwys et al., 2023, p. 244). It is, thus, prudent for behavior analysts to be aware and knowledgeable of the advantages, disadvantages, and ethical challenges of social media, as well as latest social media iterations and offerings.

14.2 Collaboration as a Professional Activity for Applied Behavior Analysts

Collaboration refers to the process in which two or more individuals, groups, or organizations work jointly to accomplish a task, pursue a common objective, or participate in shared decision-making to address complex challenges (Slim & Reuter-Yuill, 2021). A foundational principle outlined by the BACB (2020) that all behavior analysts should abide by is to benefit others, and one way this can be done is by "effectively and respectfully collaborating with others in the best interest of those with whom they work" (p. 4). ABA practitioners working with individuals with ASD are likely to work with many nonbehavior analytic colleagues, including teachers, nurses, social workers, psychologists, policymakers, and speech-language pathologists. Therefore, it is important to have a strong collaborative repertoire with the skill of effective cross-disciplinary collaboration with others who may have differing ideologies, ethics standards, and intervention approaches (Dillenburger et al., 2014).

Slim and Reuter-Yuill (2021) outlined core competency domains that promote effective collaboration and strengthen partnerships, including the need for shared values and ethics. Within the values and ethics domain, sub-competencies are met by engaging in culturally attuned practices, demonstrating cultural humility, and participating in reciprocal exchanges that establish and strengthen a collaborative culture. Referring specifically to international collaboration and dissemination in behavior analysis, Kelly et al. (2019) emphasized the importance of understanding the cultural contexts in which the dissemination will occur and communicating effectively with the intended audience.

14.3 A Collaborate to Disseminate Model: Overview and Rationale

We suggest that behavior analytic faculty use a "collaborate to disseminate" model with their students and graduates (see Fig. 14.1). This model can be conceptualized as a process in which two or more people work together to achieve the shared goal of disseminating the science of behavior analysis to target audiences through collaborative activities. If faculty and students can build an effective collaborative relationship, this may ultimately help benefit society in meaningful ways by disseminating the benefits of our science, including ABA-based interventions for ASD, in practice (Spencer et al., 2021).

Slim and Reuter-Yuill (2021) provide an overview of collaborative service delivery models in clinical settings, healthcare, and education and suggest that the rising interest in multidisciplinary, interdisciplinary, and transdisciplinary models in other fields provides a unique opportunity for the dissemination of ABA. The question is, do behavior analysts have collaborative repertoires that are strong enough to capitalize upon these potential dissemination opportunities?

One resource that may be helpful for behavior analysts seeking self-development in the area of collaboration is ABAI Practice Board's document about interprofessional collaborative practice (Spencer et al., 2021). This document recommended that professionals adopt the World Health Organization's (WHO, 2010) Framework for Action on Interprofessional Education and Collaborative Practice (IPEC) and uphold interprofessional practice and interprofessional education to build competency (Spencer et al., 2021). Given that behavior analysts have not always been successful at establishing and sustaining collaborative relationships (Taylor et al., 2019), it is important that we do not attenuate dissemination opportunities for the science of behavior analysis and, instead, continue to focus upon building our own competencies in collaboration (Slim & Reuter-Yuill, 2021).

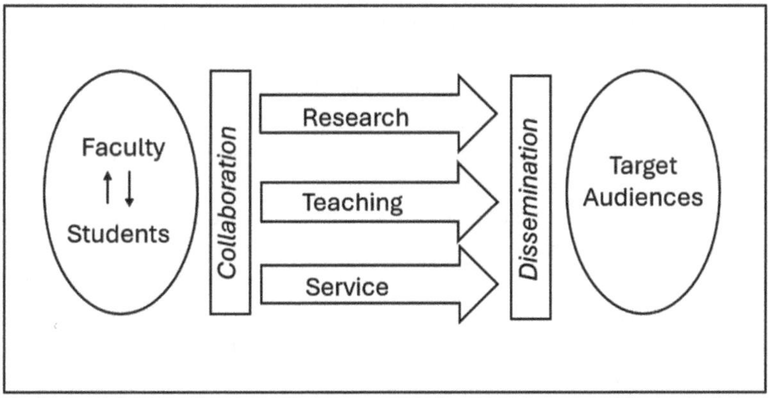

Fig. 14.1 Collaborate to disseminate model for faculty and students across academic domains

Spencer et al. (2021) outlined some of these competencies, including the need to work together with mutual respect and shared values, acknowledge our collaborators' roles and abilities, and communicate in a professional, positive, and constructive manner that supports a team approach. Although ABAI's resource document specifically addresses interprofessional collaborative practice between behavior analysts and speech-language pathologists, the competencies outlined may also be valuable for behavior analytic faculty in collaborating effectively with their students. Such collaboration can ultimately benefit society by enhancing the impact of dissemination efforts.

14.3.1 Student–Faculty Collaboration to Disseminate Behavior Analysis

Effective collaborative practices require the application of each team member's knowledge and skills to ensure effective, cohesive execution of an integrated plan (Slim & Reuter-Yuilli, 2021). When the plan is to disseminate the science of behavior analysis, a collaborate to disseminate model is useful. This idea is not new. Rather, faculty and students have been successfully collaborating across a number of domains for decades. Like any activity of a graduate student, dissemination activities typically begin within the mentor–mentee relationship of an advisor (faculty member) and advisee (student). Ideally, faculty should start students on this path early so they will continue to prioritize dissemination across their career.

Martens (2018) published recommendations regarding how faculty advisors can effectively collaborate with their students to shape their behavior so that students can take responsibility for their own learning and professional development. With respect to dissemination, this collaborative process becomes critical because the target audiences of the dissemination activities may have very limited exposure to behavior analytic content. Mentors must ensure that the content is accurate and the mentee is well-prepared to disseminate. This is especially challenging for faculty when students are new to the science and are disseminating in a language the faculty cannot understand. The mentee, in a collaborative dissemination activity as described above, must ensure that the method of dissemination is a good match for the local audience and that the content is culturally and linguistically appropriate.

Table 14.1 outlines the recommended action steps and target audience for effective collaboration in dissemination across research, teaching, and service. While not exhaustive, this table is intended as a starting point to encourage more effective collaboration between faculty and students in disseminating the science of behavior.

In an effort to provide specific suggestions for collaborative activities between behavior analytic faculty and students, the remainder of this chapter will examine each action listed in Table 14.1 and outline a case example of collaboration in the dissemination of behavior analysis in the Middle East across the domains of research, teaching, and service (see Kelly et al., 2016, 2024 for an overview of ABA

Table 14.1 Action steps and target audience for effective collaboration in dissemination across academic domains

Domain	Action item	Action description	Target audience
A. Dissemination in research domain	1. Research funding.	Support students to access grants to fund research and attendance and participation at conferences to disseminate their results	Community at large; conference attendees
	2. Conference presentations.	Mentor students through presenting their graduate research outcomes at ABA and non-ABA conferences	
	3. Journal clubs.	Provide opportunities for students to participate and present at journal clubs	Journal club attendees (students and professionals)
	4. Research publications.	Assist students in publishing research	Research consumers
	5. Research assistants.	Recruit student research assistants for faculty-led research	
	6. Research translation.	Prompt students to translate seminal research into their native language	Community at large
B. Dissemination in teaching domain	7. Program planning.	(i) Incorporate service requirement as a graduation criterion. (ii) Incorporate comprehensive instruction regarding all aspects of behavior analysis.	Students; community at large
	8. Curriculum development.	Develop curricula that promote an inclusive, equitable, and just environment	Students
	9. Student assessments.	Create assignments that include an opportunity for students to disseminate the science of behavior analysis	Community at large
	10. In-class translation.	Request in-class translation to ensure fluency of behavior analytics concepts and principles	Students
	11. Guest lectures.	Provide opportunities for students to guest lecture in other departments	Nonbehavior analytic faculty and students

(continued)

Table 14.1 (continued)

Domain	Action item	Action description	Target audience
C. Dissemination in service domain	*Service to the community*		
	12. Partner engagement.	Assist students in finding opportunities to engage with community partners at hosted events and programs	Community at large
	13. Community presentations.	Encourage and support students to present seminars and workshops (in-person or online) to behavior analysts and nonbehavior analysts in the community	Community-based behavior analysts; community at large
	Service to the profession		
	14. Professional membership.	Encourage students to seek student membership in behavior analytic entities	Community at large
	15. Using social media platforms.	Model for students how to actively and appropriately engage in reliable ABA-related pages and groups across social media platforms	Social media users
	16. Formal translation.	Provide opportunities for students to translate ABA-related documents and resources into their native language	Community at large

in the Gulf region). Although an in-depth, critical analysis of the social processes of collaboration and dissemination as they pertain to behavior analysis is likely warranted, this is not the focus of this chapter. Instead, our intention in this chapter is to offer general, actionable guidance to the reader with suggestions that may require tailoring to specific educational and cultural settings.

14.4 A Case from the United Arab Emirates: Emirates College for Advanced Education

In 2014, the first Verified Course Sequence (VCS) in ABA in the UAE was established as part of a Bachelor of Education program at Emirates College for Advanced Education (ECAE; www.ecae.ac.ae) in the capital city of Abu Dhabi. In 2019, a 1-year Postgraduate Diploma and a 2-year Master of Education were launched providing VCSs that met the academic requirements for the Board Certified Assistant Behavior Analyst (BCaBA) and BCBA credentials, respectively.[1] Herein, we describe some examples from the development of our program at ECAE, where

[1] Note: These VCSs are currently not active and remain on hold with ABAI.

UAE national students and expatriate faculty developed a respectful and productive alliance. The faculty continues to learn to work in a Middle Eastern culture, appreciating the impact of local traditions and customs on teaching, learning, research, and dissemination (see Olsen & Kelly, 2020; AlQahtani, 2023). Meanwhile, the students have learned to navigate the world of behavior analysis by analyzing and questioning how the methods and guidelines "fit" with the populations they serve now and into the future.

14.5 Faculty–Student Collaboration in Behavior Analytic Research, Teaching, and Service

Hayes (2018) discussed how being a successful academic requires accomplishments across the three domains of research, teaching, and service. The three-pronged approach to professional activities also provides structure to how faculty and students may engage in collaborative dissemination activities (see Fig. 14.1). Emphasis is typically placed on research for both faculty and graduate students, where promotion is contingent on a specified number of high-impact publications and graduation is contingent on the successful defense of a dissertation or thesis, but dissemination may occur across any of the domains.

14.5.1 Dissemination in the Research Domain (Table 14.1, A)

Dissemination should be established as the standard expectation for all research (Taylor, 2019). The 2013 Declaration of Helsinki states that researchers have a duty to make publicly available the results of their research on human participants, whether the results are positive, negative, or inconclusive (World Medical Association, 2025). The British Educational Research Association (BERA, 2024) outlines that this responsibility to disseminate research is for the benefit of educational professionals, policymakers, and the wider public. This leads us to the question—what can faculty do in order to collaborate with students to disseminate their research on ABA-based interventions for ASD? This becomes especially important when students have conducted research in their native languages or where the student has more expertise and knowledge of the dominant culture where the data were collected.

14.5.1.1 Research Funding (A1)

One barrier for students wishing to conduct research in ABA-based interventions for ASD is the cost involved in pursuing and continuing postgraduate training. Faculty may be able to help alleviate this financial burden by encouraging students to access external grants. One suggestion is for faculty to support and collaborate with students in applying for the Innovative Student Research Grant in Diversity, Equity, and Inclusion offered by the Society for the Advancement of Behavior Analysis (Society for the Advancement of Behavior Analysis [SABA], 2025a). For example, a doctoral student was the recipient of this award in 2022 for her research on evaluating culturally sensitive ABA services to Spanish-speaking caregivers of children with ASD who live in Puerto Rico (SABA, 2025b).

Once research data are collected and analyzed, faculty should advocate for their students by striving to dedicate college/university funding for student attendance at national and international conferences to disseminate their findings related to ABA-based interventions for ASD. As above, faculty may also be able to support by encouraging students to access external grants. One example of this is the SABA (2025c) student presenter grants that helpfully covers the registration cost for the annual ABAI convention. In 2025, SABA awarded grants to 133 students from Brazil, Canada, Great Britain, Ireland, Japan, Mexico, Puerto Rico, Spain, and the United States.

14.5.1.2 Conference Presentations (A2)

Another way to be successful within the domain of research dissemination is to present at conferences, which may include sharing one's own data-based dissemination efforts. Faculty can assist students by (a) actively seeking presentation opportunities where their own research and their students' research might fit; (b) sharing calls for proposals; (c) working collaboratively on the development and submission of abstracts; (d) seeking funding opportunities for conference attendance, as discussed above; (e) working collaboratively on the development and presentation of conference materials; and (f) publicizing the successful achievements of the student presenter. This process, of course, is commonplace in well-established behavior analytic programs in geographic regions where conferences are plentiful, but for students in the Middle East or other regions where behavior analytic conferences are rarely available locally or nationally, this is more challenging.

As behavior analysis develops globally, the surge of newly established conferences, such as the First Saudi Applied Behavior Analysis Symposium at Dar Al-Hekma (2023) University, will enable students to benefit from such public platforms to present their data. Furthermore, as conferences moved to a virtual platform during the COVID-19 pandemic, students were afforded the opportunity to present at international conferences without struggling to meet the financial and time demands of flying around the world. If students are first-time presenters, presenting their research in poster format might be a prudent way to introduce them to the potentially daunting task of presenting to expert behavior analysts (Flynn et al., 2023), especially if presentations are not in their native language.

It is recommended that we strive to disseminate our research outside the box in nonbehavior analytic journals and conferences to increase awareness of the science with nonbehavioral colleagues, as well as potentially creating opportunities to establish training, practice, and collaborative research efforts. This is particularly important for behavior analysts working in countries where ABA services may not be as widely known and understood. Faculty and students are also encouraged to collaborate on delivering workshops and data-driven presentations at conferences. These forums provide an opportunity to effectively demonstrate the practical application of behavior analysis across disciplines and foster dialogue with a diverse, nonbehavior analytic audience.

If prospective graduate students have the opportunity to select from a range of prospective mentors, it would be wise to seek training with advisors who are actively disseminating in nonbehavior analytic forums/contexts (Friman, 2014; Reed, 2014; Schlinger, 2014). One way faculty can collaborate with students to work towards this goal is to encourage students to join organizations and attend conferences outside behavior analysis (Morris, 2014). While it may be challenging for faculty and students to use appropriate verbal behavior with diverse audiences and remain mindful of the recipients' backgrounds and experiences with our science (Kelly et al., 2019), faculty must continue, or begin, to guide students in presenting at non-ABA conferences. Faculty need to be dialoguers, not just speakers, demonstrating to students how to maintain open lines of communication with nonbehavior analysts. This includes being open to discussing both the merits of our science (Kelly et al., 2019) and the current state of ABA (Hanley, 2021; Suckle et al., 2025).

14.5.1.3 Journal Clubs (A3)

According to Morris (2014), it is best to begin with simple, small-scale actions and build from the ground up. Perhaps presenting at national or international forums or conferences is too big or too intimidating for some graduate students or perhaps completely inaccessible if the required financial supports are not available. If this is the case, faculty could help identify other dissemination outlets, such as university research forums and journal clubs in which students can practice disseminating research content.

14.5.1.4 Research Publications (A4)

In deciding where to publish student data, Morris (2014) recommends that we "publish outside the box to the strengths you have acquired inside the box" (p. 91). To adequately prepare students to publish in ABA journals, faculty should design programs that incorporate a research component as well as assessments and training across courses that assist in shaping research skills. Ideally, faculty would strive to maintain postgraduation connections with their students and research advisees, whereby they can continue to advise and consult on research-related matters (e.g., sourcing a relevant journal for publication). It is important that faculty continue to work with students after collaborative papers have been published, given that "the most important work begins after your paper is accepted for publication. That is, spreading your findings across the globe" (Garcia et al., 2023, p. 227).

It is advisable that students be fluent when speaking about behavior analysis in technical language to an expert audience before demonstrating their ability to use nontechnical language with people outside the science (Friman, 2017). Teaching students to become good behavioral translators and ambassadors is certainly not easy (Foxx, 1996), but all behavior analytic instructors should ensure that they themselves, along with their students, are able to influence the world beyond behavior analysis (Morris, 2014). To achieve this, faculty should include diverse readings from nonbehavior analytic journals (e.g., *Autism, Journal of Autism and Developmental Disorders, Research in Autism Spectrum Disorders, Review Journal of Autism and Developmental Disorders*) across all program courses.

Faculty should also ensure that both their students and they publish across disciplines, where appropriate, to maximize the widespread dissemination of their research beyond behavior analysts. This may mean that faculty diversify their research methodologies to demonstrate the impact of ABA-based interventions (see Hozella et al., 2023) by using case studies (e.g., Healy et al., 2008), surveys (e.g., Mitteer et al., 2024), or qualitative research (see Burney et al., 2024). It might also be the case that students instead publish their data as gray literature given that "Grey literature has a role in increasing the breadth of voices represented in the behavioral sciences as well as addressing some of the inequities to accessing relevant and timely research" (Ulm & Shaffer, 2023, p. 261). Examples of these dissemination efforts might include the production of infographics, op-eds, policy briefs, preprints, working papers, and magazine or newspaper articles (Ulm & Shaffer, 2023).

14.5.1.5 Research Assistants (A5)

Recruiting behavior analytic students as research assistants for faculty-led research is likely something faculty already do or plan to do. This affords students the opportunity to gain experience with the publication process and how to publish within high-caliber behavior analytic and ASD journals. Given the power differential between faculty and students, it is important that faculty engage in ethical dissemination by, for example, considering authorship conventions when engaging in this scholarship partnership with their students (Giuliano, 2019; Torres et al., 2023).

How can we take this collaboration to the next level? Faculty should encourage behavior analytic students to also apply to be research assistants in projects led by faculty outside of our field working with participants with ASD. This will empower students with the skills of multidisciplinary collaboration as well as provide a potential opportunity for them to enhance the research with their behavioral perspective.

14.5.1.6 Research Translation (A6)

Non-English-speaking behavior analytic students face many challenges when trying to publish in English-language journals, including the need to write in technically correct English, adhering to editorial rules and standards, and engaging in written discussions with journal editors about reviewers' feedback (Zhang et al., 2023). That said, in Article 71 of their Ethical Guidelines for Educational Research (5th ed.), BERA (2024) states: "Where research is conducted in a setting in which English is not the prevalent (or only) language, researchers should make the fruits of their research available in languages that make it locally accessible." Therefore, from an ethics standpoint, faculty should guide students to translate their own research related to ABA-based interventions for ASD into their native language so that important outcomes can be fully understood and appreciated. As artificial intelligence tools continue to advance, this task is becoming increasingly feasible and efficient (Amano et al., 2025). One potential barrier is copyright agreements, and, therefore, approval should be sought from the initial publishing body before seeking to publish a translated version of the manuscript. An exciting recent development for faculty and students is that the *Journal of Applied Behavior Analysis* has started translating some of its seminal articles into other languages, including Spanish and Chinese (Wiley, 2025).

14.5.1.7 Dissemination in the Research Domain: Case Examples from the Emirates College for Advanced Education

Master of Education in ABA (MEd. in ABA) students at ECAE presented at the online, sixth annual conference of the Association for Behavior Analysis Australia (2024) providing them with the opportunity to disseminate the data collected during their research thesis assessment. The pressure of presenting live, especially as non-native English speakers, was eased by the option to pre-record their presentations. This allowed students to refine their delivery by recording multiple versions of different slides and enabled their research supervisors to provide extensive feedback, ensuring that the presentations met the high standards required for such an event. Ideally, conference organizers will continue to offer such virtual options to encourage international dissemination and afford behavior analytic students and faculty around the world greater opportunities to attend and present at such prestigious conferences.

An Emirati ECAE student co-founded an ABA Journal Club (www.instagram.com/abajournal_club/) in 2020 to review and discuss peer-reviewed articles in both English and Arabic. These online sessions are supported by ECAE faculty to provide an open, safe environment for students (and other interested individuals) to discuss articles and practice speaking about research using technical and non-technical language with fellow audience members interested in the science. If no journal club exists in a particular region, faculty could encourage students to establish one. While faculty can offer guidance and consultation, these clubs should ideally be student-led to foster greater audience engagement.

14.5.2 Dissemination in the Teaching Domain (Table 14.1, B)

As faculty with a formal role in teaching others, it is crucial that we strive to be the most effective educators possible. Recognizing the importance of a strong teaching repertoire, faculty should expose their students to every teaching opportunity that arises, both within and beyond their behavior analytic programs, to further improve how they build and disseminate our science (Rehfeldt, 2021).

14.5.2.1 Program Planning (B7)

When planning programs, it is suggested that faculty consider incorporating a service requirement for graduation (see Section C for more details) so that establishing operations are strengthened for students to initiate collaboration with faculty on ongoing dissemination efforts.

A critical component of training students to effectively disseminate behavior analysis is the inclusion of comprehensive instruction on the experimental analysis of behavior, along with the philosophical and theoretical foundations of the field, verbal behavior, and radical behaviorism within graduate programs (Schlinger, 2015). These programs should equip students with the ability to speak fluently about all three branches of the science: theoretical, experimental, and applied. St. Peter (2013) emphasized the importance of training the next generation of behavior analysts to be proficient collaborators. This includes teaching graduate students how to communicate effectively with stakeholders outside the field of behavior analysis and how to critically engage with research from other disciplines.

14.5.2.2 Curriculum Development (B8)

Despite its importance, and unlike supervision requirements, behavior analysts are not expected to undergo specific training to become effective disseminators (Zhang et al., 2023). During the planning phase for new courses, faculty should ensure that students are actively taught effective dissemination skills. This includes developing soft skills like public speaking and presentation techniques, as well as using various modalities to convey information, such as presentation slides, videos, podcasts, blogs, and academic social networks (Keenan, 2016; Zhang et al., 2023).

Development of the necessary cultural awareness skills is also an important consideration as faculty plan new and/or updated courses in their program (Fong et al., 2016). One effective approach to achieve this is by integrating courses that specifically focus on culture and cultural adaptations in behavior analytic procedures (Sivaraman & Fahmie, 2020a, 2020b; Tsami et al., 2019). These courses would directly align with the BACB's (2020) core principle of ensuring competence for both faculty and students as they would "increase their knowledge and skills related to cultural responsiveness and service delivery to diverse groups" (p. 4). The course could begin by prompting students to engage in both self-reflection and self-critique to empower them to be lifelong, reflective learners, practitioners, and researchers (Tervalon & Murray-Garcia, 1998). Of course, this self-assessment exercise should also be completed by faculty (and at the institutional level; Tervalon & Murray-Garcia, 1998) to assess their own cultures, values, and biases. This becomes especially important if university instructors are teaching students whose geographic, linguistic, and cultural backgrounds differ from their own and they are engaging in extracurricular dissemination activities as well.

14.5.2.3 Student Assessment (B9)

Behavior analysts should promote the science of behavior by making information about it available to the public (Kelly et al., 2019). Faculty can encourage students to proactively disseminate the science of behavior by tying this ethical responsibility into program curricula. As faculty create syllabi and course outlines, they can create assignments that include an opportunity for students to disseminate the science of behavior analysis, multilingually if possible. A good example of this can be found in the work of Nava et al. (2019) in which graduate students created culturally responsive multimedia content to be used in undergraduate behavior analysis classes. This content included videos and pictures corresponding to four topics (respondent conditioning, reinforcement, antecedent control, extinction and punishment) and showed examples of the behavioral principles in their everyday lives.

14.5.2.4 In-Class Translation (B10)

Friman (2017) advises behavior analytic faculty to teach students to be bilingual so that students can speak about the science using both technical and nontechnical language. One way to enhance this is by integrating available translations of behavior analysis terminology into our curriculum. ABAI chapters (e.g., Association for Behavior Analysis-United Arab Emirates) may have these translations available. Faculty can also request students to complete in-class translation to ensure fluency of behavior analytic concepts and principles. This can be done in a whole group format or in break-out rooms or small group discussions where students feel comfortable sharing experiences and freely discussing in their native language (Najdowski et al., 2021).

14.5.2.5 Guest Lectures (B11)

It is recommended that faculty model effective dissemination efforts by availing themselves to guest lecture in other programs/departments (e.g., education, special education, psychology, medicine, business). The ABAI directory of instructors (ABAI, 2025a) helps advance the science of behavior analysis by listing instructors who may be available for teaching-related services internationally. Faculty could also work with graduates to guest lecture to newer student cohorts within their own behavior analysis programs and/or encourage them to guest lecture across disciplines.

14.5.2.6 Dissemination in the Teaching Domain: Case Example from the Emirates College for Advanced Education

The first author collaborated with her undergraduate ABA students on an in-class project during their ethics course to submit an application for the DBA-SIG's Dissemination of Behavior Analysis 2020 Grant, which they successfully won. This student-led project involved the creation of a brand-new website (abauae.net) that aimed to (a) disseminate the science of human behavior to the public at large in the UAE as well as all Arabic-speaking individuals interested in behavior analysis globally; (b) provide easy-to-understand explanations of behavior analysis in the Emirati dialect of the Arabic language; (c) create and publish short videos that describe and demonstrate ABA-related material; (d) collate readily available Arabic resources and make them easily available; and (e) promote ABA-related events and activities occurring in the UAE.

As part of their MEd. in ABA, students completed a course titled "The Applications of Behavior Analysis." This course featured an assessment where students collaborated in small groups to design and create dissemination projects (Murray et al., 2021). These projects included developing Arabic podcasts, YouTube channels, TikTok videos, and workshops, with some of them available to the public on abauae.net.

14.5.3 Dissemination in the Service Domain (Table 14.1, C)

Although service requirements for graduation are encouraged and viewed positively, they may be virtually nonexistent for graduate students (Schulz et al., 2021). This is currently the case in many universities around the world (including ECAE) where students can successfully graduate with degrees without evidence of completing any service at all to the college, community, or profession, across their entire program. One example of integrating service learning into graduate requirements can be seen at Dar Al-Hekma University in Jeddah, Kingdom of Saudi Arabia, where the first author previously worked. This university requires undergraduate students to complete 100 h of community service and graduate students to complete 10 h as part of their graduation requirements (L. Baowaidan, personal communication, August 29, 2024). We would suggest that behavior analytic programs around the world consider making students more accountable by incorporating this additional graduation criterion to further motivate students to initiate collaboration with faculty on ongoing dissemination efforts.

Since many institutions do not have service requirements for graduate students, both students and faculty may need to actively seek additional opportunities. This can help ensure they are well-prepared for success in teaching, service delivery, and contributing to the college, community, and profession (Schulz et al., 2021), fostering their role as responsible and engaged citizens (Rehfeldt, 2021). "A record of service for the profession, for the university, for the community shows concern for the group" (Hayes, 2021) and indicates an interest in the successful dissemination of the science of behavior analysis. However, Hayes (2021) recommends that sustained involvement in a single area is a better indicator of service responsibility than attempting to engage in numerous activities superficially. She also advises students to avoid the appearance of merely checking boxes for their curriculum vitae.

14.5.3.1 Partner Engagement (C12)

When designing courses and programs, it is recommended that behavior analytic faculty consider incorporating service learning (Rehfeldt, 2021), also known as "community engagement pedagogies" (Bandy, 2011). Service learning is a pedagogy integrating academically relevant service activities that address human and community needs into a course and may strengthen the student–faculty relationship (Bandy, 2011). Faculty could connect with groups that work on outreach initiatives such as a University Service-Learning Committee (if such a group exists) to identify potential projects with organizations in the local community (see American School of Dubai, 2025; Suffolk University, 2025). If such a committee does not exist at an institution, faculty could take the initiative to establish it by utilizing reliable online resources as a guide. For instance, they might refer to the freely available Service Learning Manual published by the Community Partnerships Department at the Chicago School of Professional Psychology (2021).

One way faculty could potentially assess students within this service learning model is to assign participatory action research (PAR) that is based on reflection, data collection, and action (Baum et al., 2006). PAR is a methodology that enables faculty and student researchers to partner with communities and "seeks to understand and improve the world by changing it" (Baum et al., 2006, p. 854). This is an important, socially valid outcome resulting from effective faculty–student collaborative efforts to promote our science.

14.5.3.2 Community Presentations (C13)

Behavior analytic faculty and students can collaborate to disseminate behavior analysis by presenting seminars and workshops (in-person or online) to the community at large. It is important for faculty to provide plentiful opportunities for students to engage in meaningful, in-depth learning and training activities beyond the classroom. The target audience may be behavior analysts or nonbehavior analysts depending on the topic and objectives of the event. Service to the profession often forms part of the requirements for promotion and tenure for behavior analytic faculty and has beneficial effects for the individual, the institution, and the profession of behavior analysis as a whole.

14.5.3.3 Professional Membership (C14)

Service-related professional activities may include participating or holding office in professional associations and societies (Miller, 1987). This service may of course be extended to students by encouraging them to seek student membership in behavior analytic entities such as ABAI (2025b), APBA (2025) and local, national, and/or regional chapters (ABAI, 2025c).

14.5.3.4 Social Media Platforms (C15)

Due to the phenomenal growth and development of social media in recent years, students should also be directed to actively engage in reliable ABA-related pages and groups across all platforms (e.g., ABA Middle East, www.facebook.com/groups/ABAMiddleEast) while adhering to the important recommendations by O'Leary et al. (2017).

14.5.3.5 Formal Translation (C16)

Faculty and students can also benefit the profession of behavior analysis by working together to coordinate and execute the translation of ABA-related documents and resources from English into other languages (see Virues-Ortega et al., 2015 for considerations). Translation requires the translator to have both subject matter expertise and an understanding of the cultural context of the languages involved. Non-English-speaking ABA students may possess these essential skills, which are crucial for accurate and meaningful translation (Zhang et al., 2023).

Completing formal translation can be very challenging as it takes time, effort, and can be costly. Some suggestions for how to address these barriers include (a) incorporate translation costs within research/grant funding applications; (b) reach out to local ABA chapters to see if they have resources to help with these translation efforts; (c) apply for an International Development Grant from the SABA (2025d).

14.5.3.6 Dissemination in the Service Domain: Case Examples from the Emirates College for Advanced Education

One example can be seen when Kelly et al. (2020) presented an online panel entitled "ABA Ethics in the UAE: The Next Generation's Perspective" to more than 100 attendees from across the Gulf region. After studying and thoroughly considering ethics in their ethics and professionalism course, especially within the context of the UAE, a panel of six graduate ABA students discussed core ethical approaches, principles, and rights during this free online continuing education event. The students made suggestions for how to promote an ethical culture at work and how to disseminate the science of behavior analysis during the COVID-19 pandemic. Specific attention was paid to the local context, including discussion of the cultural appropriateness of the BACB ethics code, and analysis of ethical dilemmas involving fad treatments for ASD.

Another example is the International Development Grant awarded to the second author in 2023, to create a series of ABA training videos that are appropriate for and freely accessible to an Arab Muslim audience (SABA, 2025e). Here, the faculty member recruited a graduate of ECAE to provide the Arabic voice-over for these videos. The goal of this project is to create training resources that will have a lasting impact by providing materials suitable for instructors or faculty who need resources tailored for Arab Muslim communities.

14.6 Conclusion

This chapter reviewed the collaborate to disseminate model in the field of behavior analysis. Practical suggestions (or reminders) were offered regarding how faculty and students can collaborate with the intention of reinvigorating a focus on dissemination in behavior analytic programs across the three prongs of professional activities: research, teaching, and service. A case study of a college in the UAE offered successful examples of proactive dissemination of ABA in the Gulf region in the Middle East.

Going forward, further conceptual investigation of both collaboration and dissemination within the science of behavior analysis is warranted with potential to develop a framework that would help operationalize dissemination and the ideas and practices related to collaboration. As faculty and students plan future efforts for the dissemination of ABA-based interventions for ASD, it might be useful to state clearly the purpose of the efforts (including the potential to impact policy), the processes to be used, and the challenges that might be faced. Similarly, it may be a worthwhile endeavor to analyze different understanding, possibilities, and modes of collaboration as influenced by different dissemination purposes, processes, and challenges. It would also be beneficial to expand the analysis of collaboration beyond the faculty–student relationship to include various contexts, such as interactions between students, collaborations between students and community groups, and interdisciplinary efforts.

References

AlQahtani, O. (2023). The UAE and gulf countries' cultural characteristics and their influence on autism. *Review Journal of Autism and Developmental Disorders, 12*, 163–167. https://doi.org/10.1007/s40489-023-00373-7

Amano, T., Bowker, L., & Burton-Jones, A. (2025). AI-mediated translation presents two possible futures for academic publishing in a multilingual world. *PLoS Biol 23*(6), e3003215. https://doi.org/10.1371/journal.pbio.30

American School of Dubai. (2025). *Service learning*. https://www.asdubai.org/learning/service-learning

Association for Behavior Analysis Australia. (2024). https://auaba.com.au/

Association for Behavior Analysis International [ABAI]. (2025a). *Search instructor.* https://www.abainternational.org/education/instructor-directory.aspx

Association for Behavior Analysis International [ABAI]. (2025b). *Student/Transitional student members.* https://www.abainternational.org/membership/studenttransitional-student-members.aspx

Association for Behavior Analysis International [ABAI]. (2025c). *Chapters.* https://www.abainternational.org/constituents/chapters/chapters-home.aspx

Association of Professional Behavior Analysts [APBA]. (2025). *Membership information.* https://www.apbahome.net/membership-information

Bandy, J. (2011). What is service learning or community engagement? *Vanderbilt University Center for Teaching.* https://www.utrgv.edu/ceo/_files/documents/service-learning-and-community-engagement.pdf

Baum, F., MacDougall, C., & Smith, D. (2006). Participatory action research. *Journal of Epidemiology and Community Health, 60*(10), 854–857. https://doi.org/10.1136/jech.2004.028662

Behavior Analyst Certification Board [BACB]. (2014). *Professional and ethical compliance code for behavior analysts.* Author.

Behavior Analyst Certification Board [BACB]. (2020). *Ethics code for behavior analysts.* Author.

Burney, V., Arnold-Saritepe, A., & McCann, C. M. (2024). How can qualitative methods be applied to behavior analytic research: A discussion and suggestions for implementation. *Behavior Analysis in Practice, 17*, 431–441. https://doi.org/10.1007/s40617-024-00917-1

British Educational Research Association [BERA]. (2024). *Ethical guidelines for educational research(5thed.).* www.bera.ac.uk/publication/ethicalguidelines-for-educational-research-2024

Dar Al-Hekma. (2023). *Dar Al-Hekma university is proud to announce its first Saudi virtual applied behavior analysis symposium.* https://www.dah.edu.sa/en/research/conferences/Pages/About-the-MABA-symposium.aspx

Dillenburger, K., Röttgers, H.-R., Dounavi, K., Sparkman, C., Keenan, M., Thyer, B., & Nikopoulos, C. (2014). Multidisciplinary teamwork in autism: Can one size fit all? *The Australian Educational and Developmental Psychologist, 31*(2), 97–112. https://doi.org/10.1017/edp.2014.13

Fixsen, D. L., & Blase, K. A. (1993). Creating new realities: Program development and dissemination. *Journal of Applied Behavior Analysis, 26*(4), 597–615. https://doi.org/10.1901/jaba.1993.26-597

Flynn, S., Evans, L., & Sessanga, H. (2023). Types of dissemination. In A. K. Griffith & T. C. Ré (Eds.), *Disseminating behavioral research* (pp. 25–37). Springer. https://doi.org/10.1007/978-3-031-47343-2_2

Fong, E. H., Catagnus, R. M., Brodhead, M. T., Quigley, S., & Field, S. (2016). Developing the cultural awareness skills of behavior analysts. *Behavior Analysis in Practice, 9*(1), 84–94. https://doi.org/10.1007/s40617-016-0111-6

Foxx, R. M. (1996). Translating the covenant: The behavior analyst as ambassador and translator. *The Behavior Analyst, 19*(2), 147–161. https://doi.org/10.1007/BF03393162

Friman, P. C. (2014). Publishing outside the box: Attaining mainstream prominence requires demonstration of mainstream relevance. *The Behavior Analyst, 37*(2), 73–76. https://doi.org/10.1007/s40614-014-0014-1

Friman, P. C. (2017). In B. Zey (Chair), *Dissemination: A collaborative effort* [Panel discussion]. 43rd Annual Convention of the Association for Behavior Analysis International, https://www.abainternational.org/events/program-details/event-detail.aspx?sid=51677&by=ByArea#s325_0

Garcia, Y., Muñoz-Martínez, A., Andrews, M., & Junca, E. (2023). Now your manuscript is accepted…what's next? In A. K. Griffith & T. C. Ré (Eds.), *Disseminating behavioral research* (pp. 221–231). Springer. https://doi.org/10.1007/978-3-031-47343-2_13

Giuliano, T. A. (2019). Guiding undergraduates through the process of first authorship. *Frontiers in Psychology*. https://doi.org/10.3389/fpsyg.2019.00857

Hanley, G. (2021). *A perspective on today's ABA from Dr. Hanley*. https://practicalfunctionalassessment.com/2021/05/05/a-perspective-on-todays-aba-by-dr-greg-hanley/

Hayes, L. J. (2018). Research, etc. *Behavior Analysis in Practice, 11*(3), 187–188. https://doi.org/10.1007/s40617-018-0231-2

Hayes, L. J. P. (2021). In J. A. Schulz (Chair), *Success in academia: Developing teaching and service repertoires* [Panel discussion] 47th annual convention of the Association for Behavior Analysis International. https://www.abainternational.org/events/program-details/event-detail.aspx?sid=72271&by=ByArea#s126_0

Healy, O., O'Connor, J., Leader, G., & Kenny, N. (2008). Three years of intensive applied behavior analysis: A case study. *Journal of Early and Intensive Behavior Intervention, 5*(1), 4–22. https://doi.org/10.1037/h0100407

Helton, M. R., & Alber-Morgan, S. R. (2018). Helping parents understand applied behavior analysis: Creating a parent guide in 10 steps. *Behavior Analysis in Practice, 11*(4), 496–503. https://doi.org/10.1007/s40617-018-00284-8

Hozella, W., Schneider, R., Tammik, J., & Beaver, B. (2023). Introduction to dissemination in behavioral sciences. In A. K. Griffith & T. C. Ré (Eds.), *Disseminating behavioral research* (pp. 3–23). Springer. https://doi.org/10.1007/978-3-031-47343-2_17

Keenan, M. (2016). The scientific image in behavior analysis. *The Behavior Analyst, 39*, 7–8. https://doi.org/10.1007/s40614-016-0059-4

Kelly, M. P., Alhammadi, A. A. E. A., Aljasmi, A. A. I., Almahri, F. A. M., Alsaadi, M. K. S. K., Maliki, A. I., Al Marzouqi, M. M. S. (2020). *ABA ethics in the UAE: The next generation's perspective* [Webinar]. Emirates College for Advanced Education. https://www.youtube.com/watch?reload=9&v=rzQWtJUyN2E

Kelly, M. P., Alireza, I., Busch, H. E., Northrop, S., Al-Attrash, M., Ainsleigh, S., & Bhuptani, N. (2016). An overview of autism and applied behavior analysis in the Gulf cooperation Council in the Middle East. *Review Journal of Autism and Developmental Disorders, 3*(2), 154–164. https://doi.org/10.1007/s40489-016-0073-1

Kelly, M. P., Alireza, I., Azzaam, S., Baowaidan, L. M., Gabr, A. A., Taqi, R., & Yateem, S. N. (2024). Applied behavior analysis and autism spectrum disorder in the Gulf region in the Middle East. *Journal of Developmental and Physical Disabilities, 36*, 591–614. https://doi.org/10.1007/s10882-023-09931-7

Kelly, M. P., Martin, N., Dillenburger, K., Kelly, A. N., & Miller, M. M. (2019). Spreading the news: History, successes, challenges, and the ethics of effective dissemination. *Behavior Analysis in Practice, 12*(2), 440–451. https://doi.org/10.1007/s40617-018-0238-8

Martens, B. K. (2018). The student should help the teacher: A view from 30 years as an ABA trainer. *Behavior Analysis in Practice, 11*(3), 184–186. https://doi.org/10.1007/s40617-018-0220-5

Miller, R. I. (1987). *Evaluating faculty for promotion and tenure.* Jossey-Bass Publishers.

Mitteer, D. R., Boyle, M. A., & Craig, A. R. (2024). Reinforcement-schedule thinning practices during functional communication training: A survey of behavior analysts. *Behavioral Interventions.* https://doi.org/10.1002/bin.2002

Morris, E. K. (1985). Public information, dissemination, and behavior analysis. *The Behavior Analyst, 8*(1), 95–110. https://doi.org/10.1007/BF03391916

Morris, E. K. (2014). Stop preaching to the choir, publish outside the box: A discussion. *The Behavior Analyst, 37*(2), 87–94. https://doi.org/10.1007/s40614-014-0011-4

Murray, C. M., Kelly, M. P., & Mead Jasperse, S. C. (2021). Student-faculty collaboration in dissemination of behavior analysis in The United Arab Emirates. In D. Mudgal (chair), *bringing ABA to the world: Changes across cultures, borders, and disciplines* [symposium] 47th Annual Convention of the Association for Behavior Analysis International. https://www.abainternational.org/events/program-details/event-detail.aspx?sid=71986&by=ByArea#s249_0

Najdowski, A. C., Gharapetian, L., & Jewett, V. (2021). Toward the development of antiracist and multicultural graduate training programs in behavior analysis. *Behavior Analysis in Practice, 14*(2), 462–477. https://doi.org/10.1007/s40617-020-00504-0

Nava, C. E., Fahmie, T. A., Jin, S., & Kumar, P. (2019). Evaluating the efficacy, preference, and cultural responsiveness of student-generated content in an undergraduate behavioral course. *Behavior Analysis in Practice, 12*(4), 747–757. https://doi.org/10.1007/s40617-019-00344-7

O'Leary, P. N., Miller, M. M., Olive, M. L., & Kelly, A. N. (2017). Blurred lines: Ethical implications of social media for behavior analysts. *Behavior Analysis in Practice, 10*(1), 45–51. https://doi.org/10.1007/s40617-014-0033-0

Olsen, P. M., & Kelly, M. P. (2020). Applied behavior analysis with Arab-Muslim populations: The importance of cultural awareness. In B. M. Connors & S. T. Capell (Eds.), *Multiculturalism and diversity in applied behavior analysis: Bridging theory and application* (pp. 83–97). Taylor & Francis/Routledge. https://doi.org/10.4324/9780429263873

Parry-Cruwys, D., MacDonald, J., Parry-Cruwys, R., & Cicoria, M. (2023). Nontraditional options for dissemination. In A. K. Griffith & T. C. Ré (Eds.), *Disseminating behavioral research* (pp. 243–257). Springer. https://doi.org/10.1007/978-3-031-47343-2_15

Reed, D. D. (2014). Determining how, when, and whether you should publish outside the box: Sober advice for early career behavior analysts. *The Behavior Analyst, 37*(2), 83–86. https://doi.org/10.1007/s40614-014-0012-3

Rehfeldt, R. A. (2021). In J. A. Schulz (Chair), *Success in academia: Developing teaching and service repertoires* [Panel discussion] 47th Annual Convention of the Association for Behavior Analysis International. https://www.abainternational.org/events/program-details/event-detail.aspx?sid=72271&by=ByArea#s126_0

Schillinger, D. (2010). In P. Fleisher & E. Goldstein (Eds.), *An introduction to effectiveness, dissemination, and implementation research: A resource manual for community engaged research.* University of California, Clinical and Translational Science Institute.

Schlinger, H. D., Jr. (2014). Publishing outside the box: Unforeseen dividends of talking to strangers. *The Behavior Analyst, 37*(2), 77–81. https://doi.org/10.1007/s40614-014-0010-5

Schlinger, H. D., Jr. (2015). Training graduate students to effectively disseminate behavior analysis and to counter misrepresentations. *Behavior Analysis in Practice, 8*(1), 110–112. https://doi.org/10.1007/s40617-014-0028-x

Schulz, J. A., Hayes, L. J. P., Rehfeldt, R. A., & Twyman, J. S. (2021). *Success in academia: Developing teaching and service repertoires* [Panel discussion] 47th Annual Convention of the Association for Behavior Analysis International. https://www.abainternational.org/events/program-details/event-detail.aspx?sid=72271&by=ByArea#s126_0

Sivaraman, M., & Fahmie, T. A. (2020a). A systematic review of cultural adaptations in the global application of ABA-based telehealth services. *Journal of Applied Behavior Analysis, 53*(4), 1838–1855. https://doi.org/10.1002/jaba.763

Sivaraman, M., & Fahmie, T. A. (2020b). Evaluating the efficacy and social validity of a culturally adapted training program for parents and service providers in India. *Behavior Analysis in Practice, 13*(4), 849–861. https://doi.org/10.1007/s40617-020-00489-w

Slim, L., & Reuter-Yuill, L. M. (2021). A behavior-analytic perspective on interprofessional collaboration. *Behavior Analysis in Practice, 14*, 1238–1248. https://doi.org/10.1007/s40617-021-00602-7

Society for the Advancement of Behavior Analysis [SABA]. (2025a). *Innovative student research grant in diversity, equity, and inclusion.* https://saba.abainternational.org/grants/innovative-student-research-grant-dei/

Society for the Advancement of Behavior Analysis [SABA]. (2025b). *2022: Anniette Maldonado.* https://saba.abainternational.org/grants/innovative-student-research-grant-dei/anniette-maldonado/

Society for the Advancement of Behavior Analysis [SABA]. (2025c). *Senior student presenter grant.* http://saba.abainternational.org/grants/senior-student-presenter-grant.aspx

Society for the Advancement of Behavior Analysis [SABA]. (2025d). *International development grant.* https://saba.abainternational.org/grants/International-Development-Grant

Society for the Advancement of Behavior Analysis [SABA]. (2025e). *2023: Sarah Mead Jasperse.* https://saba.abainternational.org/grants/international-development-grant/sarah-mead-jasperse/

Spencer, T. D., Slim, L., Cardon, T., & Morgan, L. (2021). *Interprofessional collaborative practice between behavior analysts and speech-language pathologists.* Association for Behavior Analysis. https://www.abainternational.org/media/180194/abai_interprofessional_collaboration_resource_document.pdf

St. Peter, C. C. (2013). Changing course through collaboration. *The Behavior Analyst, 36*(1), 155–160. https://doi.org/10.1007/BF03392299

Suckle, E., Chown, N., Tarbox, J., & Mathur, S. K. (2025). Speaking across the autism worldview divide: A dialogue between critical autism studies and behaviour analytic scholars. *Disability & Society, 40*(12), 3263–3285. https://doi.org/10.1080/09687599.2025.2478049

Suffolk University. (2025). *Service-learning designation.* https://www.suffolk.edu/student-life/student-involvement/community-public-service/service-learning/service-learning-designation

Taylor, J. (2019). Reporting research findings to participants is an ethical imperative. *BMJ, 367*, l6324. https://doi.org/10.1136/bmj.l6324. PMID: 31685487.

Taylor, B. A., LeBlanc, L. A., & Nosik, M. R. (2019). Compassionate care in behavior analytic treatment: Can outcomes be enhanced by attending to relationships with caregivers? *Behavior Analysis in Practice, 12*(3), 654–666. https://doi.org/10.1007/s40617-018-00289-3

Tervalon, M., & Murray-Garcia, J. (1998). Cultural humility versus cultural competence: A critical distinction in defining physician training outcomes in multicultural education. *Journal of Health Care for the Poor and Underserved, 9*(2), 117–125. https://doi.org/10.1353/hpu.2010.0233

The Chicago School of Professional Psychology. (2021). *Service learning manual.* https://community.thechicagoschool.edu/handson/Pages/Service-Learning.aspx

Torres, K. M., Arrastía-Chisholm, M. C., & Tackett, S. (2023). Ethical dissemination. In A. K. Griffith & T. C. Ré (Eds.), *Disseminating behavioral research* (pp. 39–49). Springer. https://doi.org/10.1007/978-3-031-47343-2_3

Tsami, L., Lerman, D., & Toper-Korkmaz, O. (2019). Effectiveness and acceptability of parent training via telehealth among families around the world. *Journal of Applied Behavior Analysis, 52*(4), 1113–1129. https://doi.org/10.1002/jaba.645

Ulm, A. D., & Shaffer, E. (2023). Grey literature. In A. K. Griffith & T. C. Ré (Eds.), *Disseminating behavioral research* (pp. 259–268). Springer. https://doi.org/10.1007/978-3-031-47343-2_16

Virues-Ortega, J., Martin, N., Schnerch, G., Garcia, J., & Mellichamp, F. (2015). A general methodology for the translation of behavioral terms into vernacular languages. *The Behavior Analyst, 38*, 125–135.

Wiley. (2025). *Journal of Applied Behavior Analysis translated.* https://onlinelibrary.wiley.com/page/journal/19383703/homepage/jaba-translated

World Health Organization [WHO]. (2010). *Framework for action on interprofessional education and collaborative practice.* https://www.who.int/publications/i/item/framework-for-action-on-interprofessional-education-collaborative-practice
World Medical Association. (2025). *WMA declaration of Helsinki-Ethical principles for medical research involving human subjects.* https://www.wma.net/policies-post/wma-declaration-of-helsinki-ethical-principles-for-medical-research-involving-human-subjects/
Zhang, D., Lin, F. Y., & Martin, N. (2023). International dissemination of behavior analysis. In A. K. Griffith & T. C. Ré (Eds.), *Disseminating behavioral research* (pp. 269–282). Springer. https://doi.org/10.1007/978-3-031-47343-2_17

Chapter 15
Empowering Families: The Role of ABA and Evidence-Based Parent-Implemented Interventions in Autism Support

Yu-Shan Ding and Hui-Ting Wang

Abstract Parent-implemented interventions (PIIs) have recognition as a practical and evidence-based practice, allowing parents to extend therapeutic gains from clinical to natural settings. This literature review examines the evolution, benefits, and effectiveness of PIIs, particularly considering the increasing relevance of telehealth methods. The shift from professional-led to parent-implemented intervention emphasizes empowering parents as co-educators, enabling continuous and consistent practice of intervention strategies in a child's daily environment.

The review highlights that PII not only improves children's social skills, communication abilities, and adaptive behaviors but also enhances parental well-being by reducing stress and increasing confidence. The collaborative relationship between therapists and parents, combined with structured coaching and feedback, supports positive changes in parent–child interactions and family dynamics. However, challenges such as ensuring intervention fidelity, adapting to different cultural contexts, and maintaining long-term benefits post-intervention remain. Addressing these challenges involves tailored training for parents, ongoing support, and developing flexible intervention models that accommodate varying family needs and preferences. This review underscores the importance of integrating PII into broader autism intervention strategies to promote development for children with autism and their families.

Keywords ASD · Coaching · Feedback · Parent-implemented interventions

According to the Centers for Disease Control and Prevention (CDC), approximately 1 in 36 children is diagnosed with autism spectrum disorder (ASD), as reported by estimates from the CDC's Autism and Developmental Disabilities Monitoring (ADDM) Network (Maenner, 2023). ASD is a developmental disability characterized by persistent challenges in social interaction and restricted, repetitive patterns

Y.-S. Ding · H.-T. Wang (✉)
Department of Special Education, National Taiwan Normal University, Taipei, Taiwan
e-mail: tinaw@ntnu.edu.tw

S. Halder et al. (eds.), *Applied Behavior Analysis-Based Interventions for Autism Spectrum Disorder*, https://doi.org/10.1007/978-981-95-2889-9_15

of behavior and interests (Keen et al., 2016). The high prevalence of ASD has heightened global awareness and underscored the need for effective interventions. Children with autism face lifelong challenges that impact both themselves and their families (Hume et al., 2021). Thus, it is essential to direct resources toward effective therapies, given that each intervention requires substantial time and financial investment. Applied behavior analysis (ABA) is a scientific paradigm that has accumulated massive evidence on teaching children with autism (Cooper et al., 2020; Lovaas, 1987; Makrygianni & Reed, 2010). Evidence-based autism interventions, mostly ABA-based interventions, are crucial for the well-being of both individuals with autism and their families.

As current research trend not only focuses toward supporting children with autism, but also begins to recognize the importance of involving key individuals in the child's environment, particularly parents. Upon learning that their child has ASD, families often need to adjust and develop strategies such as "accepting the diagnosis" and "seeking resources." Accepting the diagnosis involves understanding the child's symptoms, their characteristics, and methods of care and education. Seeking resources includes accessing psychological support for parents, improving parent–child interactions, reassessing overall family time management and financial planning, and exploring available therapeutic institutions and programs. In these circumstances, it is natural for professionals to view parents as co-educators, collaborating to maximize the child's developmental progress.

Parent-implemented intervention (PII) has gained increasing recognition as an evidence-based teaching approach within the ASD field (Hume et al., 2021). Following systematic training, coaching, and guidance provided by qualified professionals, parents can either start embedding educational objectives within routine-based activities, or extending therapeutic effects achieved from professional therapists in primary clinic setting to family setting such as home and community environment, thereby fostering gradual and sustained improvements in their child's behavior (Ding et al., n.d; Ding et al., 2025). The family setting is the child's natural environment, should be able to characterize by predictable, structured, and repetitive daily routines. Such an environment is conducive to establishing reliable systems for the child and allows for the continuous practice of newly acquired skills until they become ingrained and generalized (Ding, 2020; Ingersoll & Gergans, 2007). Parents can use everyday activities as intervention materials, which not only reinforces the child's learning but also enhances parents' sense of self-efficacy in their parenting roles. Numerous studies have shown that this approach can effectively reduce caregiving burdens and improve the ecological validity of interventions (Kasperzack et al., 2020; Liu & Schertz, 2022; Pellecchia et al., 2020).

This literature review focuses on parent-implemented interventions for children with autism, especially how ABA took place. It begins by exploring the historical development of parent involvement in ASD interventions, followed by an analysis of the benefits of such approaches. Subsequently, it reviews various parent intervention programs described in the literature, highlighting how natural evolution and the impact of the COVID-19 pandemic. In resource-rich areas, PII can serve as a supplementary and alternative therapeutic option, while in resource-limited and remote regions, as well as in low- and middle-income countries, parent themselves may become the only available therapeutic source, especially after COVID-19. It has made remote parent-implemented interventions a viable modern alternative. When discussing intervention programs, it is natural to consider their effectiveness. This review, therefore, examines outcomes for children, parents, and families, with particular attention to the generalization of effects in naturalistic settings. Ultimately, this literature review aims to deepen the understanding of ABA in parent-implemented interventions in ASD and promote their broader application.

15.1 Parent-Implemented Intervention

There are various terminologies used in parent services for children with autism, each emphasizing different aspects of parental involvement and support. *Parent-implemented intervention* involves parents progressing from being educated and supported to becoming the primary intervention implementer of their children with autism. *Parent education* typically includes courses that cover understanding and recognizing autism traits, developmental tasks, and stages of child development. These sessions are usually conducted without the target child being present. *Parent support* refers to psychological adjustment courses for parents, which may take the form of support groups led by counselors or therapists. The primary aim of these sessions is to help parents cope with the diagnosis and reduce stress, again, without the child being present.

In contrast, parent-implemented intervention involves parents undergoing a systematically planned series of courses that target specific goals for their child (Berkowitz & Graziano, 1972). These goals may include managing challenging behaviors or enhancing social and communication skills. After one-on-one or group training sessions, parents practice the techniques learned by interacting directly with their children. Therapists often observe these sessions in person or review recordings to provide positive or constructive feedback. In this context, parents act as the direct educators of their children, which is how this literature review defines parent-implemented intervention.

Different cultural backgrounds and parental gender roles may influence the content of parent-implemented intervention (PII) programs, requiring adaptations to align with regional practices and beliefs (Casillas et al., 2017; Wang & Casillas, 2012). For instance, in some cultures, including Taiwan, parents often prefer and emphasize parent-led, cognitively focused parent–child interactions. These approaches, while culturally ingrained, may not always be scientifically supported in achieving academic or other developmental outcomes.

One PII study conducted in Taiwan implemented the Project ImPACT (Ingersoll & Dvortcsak, 2010), a parent-implemented intervention program originally developed in the United States. This program required additional explanations, culturally relevant examples, and clarification of the underlying principles to better suit Taiwanese families (Ding, 2020; Ding et al., 2025). Although there were minimal cultural adaptations to transition from the scientifically supported child-led approach to the culturally preferred parent-led model, the findings revealed significant challenges. Specifically, "following the child's lead" was identified as the most difficult skill to master. It was also the first and most fundamental skill taught, requiring the longest latency to achieve criterion among the four targeted skills (following the child's lead, imitation, animation, and modeling/expanding language).

15.2 History

PII initially emerged from researchers' efforts to enhance children's developmental progress by facilitating the generalization and maintenance of learned behaviors in natural settings. These approaches were also motivated by resource limitations, as autism therapy was often concentrated in university research centers, making access quite difficult. Additionally, the trend toward deinstitutionalization and the empowerment of parents as equal partners in the therapeutic process supported this shift. Furthermore, early detection, intervention, and the establishment of empirically validated treatments provided a strong foundation for involving parents directly in the therapeutic process.

In 1966, the first documented instance of a parent acting as a co-educator involved a mother of a 6-year-old autistic boy who felt helpless in managing her son's behavior. The therapist suggested learning tantrum management strategies, leading the mother to observe therapist–child interactions through a two-way mirror. The practitioner explained every strategy and trained the mother to conduct those skills at home. Over 3 months of close working with the practitioner, with twice-weekly sessions, the mother was trained to record the frequency, duration, and triggers of tantrums. This process marked the first instance of extending therapeutic practices beyond the clinic. Results showed notable improvements in the child's behavior, demonstrating the effectiveness of parent involvement (Wetzel et al., 1966).

In another study, parents were engaged as co-educators. During a period when autism was widely regarded as unteachable, Risley (1968) designed interventions in both a laboratory and home setting for a 6-year-old girl with brain damage and autism. The interventions aimed to eliminate inappropriate climbing and aggressive behaviors toward her younger sibling. Once these challenging behaviors were reduced, milk was introduced as the sole reinforcer. Throughout the intervention, the mother meticulously recorded the child's behavioral issues at home and documented the implementation of punishment methods. After the child's dangerous behaviors were nearly eliminated, the mother, following a single session of guidance from the experimenter, began imitation training at home. Over 115 training sessions (totaling 41 h), the mother successfully established five new imitative behaviors (pounding on walls, stomping feet, standing up, raising arms, and putting on a hat), in addition to two previously established imitative behaviors, achieving consistent demonstration of all seven behaviors during randomized modeling trials. The experimenter conducted home visits, and all observational data between the mother and the experimenter were fully consistent. Although the punishment methods used in this study are now widely considered unethical and are legally prohibited in contemporary practice, the study holds historical significance. It highlights the potential for parents to serve as co-educators, taking responsibility for implementing and maintaining interventions while providing valuable feedback. For example, the mother noted that spanking was the least acceptable form of punishment during the intervention process.

Previous studies inviting parents to serve as observer-learners and implement intervention techniques as co-educators at home focused on single-family interventions. Given the significant heterogeneity within the autism spectrum, this study emphasized empowering parents as direct interventionists, positioning them as "parent-therapists" with the research team serving as consultants. In 1973, Lovaas further explored parent-implemented interventions by studying 20 children with autism, dividing them into four groups: inpatient with parental observation, inpatient with parental involvement, and two outpatient groups with parental involvement. Interventions included behavior shaping and language training, targeting behaviors such as self-stimulation, echolalia, appropriate speech, nonverbal social behaviors, and appropriate play, with follow-up assessments conducted 1–4 years later. Findings revealed that children who returned to the hospital regressed in behavior, while those who stayed with their parents retained and even advanced their progress. This study highlighted the critical role of parents in maintaining therapeutic gains, especially when parents received adequate training (Lovaas et al., 1973). These studies were also the first ABA-based PII in the history (Lovaas et al., 1973; Risley, 1968; Wetzel et al., 1966).

Research findings indicate that one of the most effective conditions is parents to demonstrate a highly engaged, nurturing, and expectation-driven parenting approach. Parents are required to invest significant time and effort in intentionally teaching their children. This aligns with Ferster's (1961) observation that when parents are preoccupied merely with household tasks, they may miss valuable opportunities to provide positive reinforcement for their children (Feinstein, 2011).

15.3 Theoretical Approach of Parent-Implemented Intervention (PII)

Contemporary methods for treating ASD have shaped the approaches used in parent-implemented interventions (PIIs), beginning with operant learning strategies in the 1960s. This shift moved from mere "parent involvement" to structured "parent training." Lovaas was a pioneer in using applied behavior analysis (ABA) as an intervention method to teach children with autism. However, subsequent research in laboratory settings revealed that some controlled conditions could not be replicated in a child's natural environment, leading to the development of more naturalistic treatment approaches (Nordquist & Wahler, 1973). The realization that many interventions focusing on single skills (Sarokoff & Sturmey, 2004), such as discrete trial training (DTT; Lovaas, 1987), failed to generalize effectively in natural settings prompted a wave of advocacy for early childhood intervention. This shift in perspective emphasized the importance of early developmental milestones, particularly in language and social communication, transforming the child from a passive recipient to an active participant. It also requires that the instructor (whether a therapist or parent) be more responsive, depending on their ability to observe and respond to the child's focus of attention (Rogers et al., 2005).

Therefore, researchers later recognized that ABA-based interventions targeting individual skills or behavior reduction could be effectively combined with developmental approaches that align with typical child development trajectories. This synergy led to the emergence of Naturalistic Developmental Behavioral Interventions (NDBIs), a model conceptualized and formalized by Schreibman et al. (2015). NDBIs strategically align with a child's developmental sequence and utilize everyday life contexts to promote generalization and maintenance of newly acquired skills. Pivotal response training (PRT; Koegel & Koegel, 2006) has been a prominent example of this approach, emphasizing motivation and child choice, while other models such as the Early Start Denver Model (ESDM; Rogers & Dawson, 2010), Joint Attention Symbolic Play Engagement and Regulation (JASPER; Kasari et al., 2006), Enhanced Milieu Teaching (EMT; Kaiser & Roberts, 2013), and Reciprocal Imitation Training (RIT; Ingersoll, 2010) further expanded this framework. Collectively, these approaches have advanced intervention practices by blending the structured, evidence-based strategies of ABA with developmentally appropriate, child-centered methodologies in PIIs.

There were additional NDBI studies. For example, Brian et al. (2016) conducted a randomized controlled trial (RCT) focusing on young children suspected of having ASD and their mothers. The 12-week intervention included one-on-one parent training using the parent-mediated NDBI program, Social ABCs. Post-intervention results for children aged 18–30 months showed significant improvements in responsiveness and overall functional vocalization. There was a notable increase in shared smiling between parent and child. However, at a 3-month follow-up, both shared smiling and social orientation had decreased, suggesting that maintaining interaction quality and quantity at a certain level may be necessary for sustained benefits. The study also found that children's learning outcomes were associated with the fidelity of the parents' implementation. The one-on-one coaching model included demonstrations and practice during the baseline period, followed by 8 weeks of real-time guidance in the home environment. In the final 4 weeks, researchers transitioned to a consulting role (Brian et al., 2016). These characteristics are common in PII, including one-on-one coaching, instructional components such as explanation, demonstration, practice, and feedback, with parent–child interaction videos used for assessment. While on-site one-on-one demonstration and guidance provide immediate feedback and are convenient for families near research centers, online platforms offer an alternative access point for those in resource-scarce areas. Typically, instructional components consist of at least three to four different strategies.

15.3.1 Telehealth Intervention

Considering the prevalence of ASD and the established benefits of early intervention for infants suspected of having ASD (Guthrie et al., 2023; Lovaas, 1987), families living in remote areas or those with limited resources face significant challenges. These include overcoming travel costs and coordinating family schedules, or low standard of healthcare system, poverty, and lack of professional training in low- and middle-income countries (LAMICs), which can greatly hinder parents' access to intervention resources. Since 2017, researchers have focused on these issues, drawing inspiration from the long-established concept of telehealth in public health systems. Telehealth has the potential to reduce the likelihood of delayed diagnoses and interventions due to these logistical barriers. It can provide synchronous or asynchronous access to training, assessments, and screening information, allowing parents to choose convenient times that fit their schedules. Additionally, telehealth overcomes geographical and temporal limitations, enabling a wider range of experts and family members to participate in the intervention process (Pan et al., 2023) or a remedial solution for task-sharing method as recommended for LAMICs (Le et al., 2022). The outbreak of COVID-19 necessitated a rapid shift across various fields to online activities. With in-person contact restricted, online platforms became the alternative. Research has shown that the effectiveness of remote interventions can be comparable to that of face-to-face interventions (Hao et al., 2021).

Telehealth-based PII for ASD typically includes real-time online meetings for group training and education between professionals and parents, demonstration videos of intervention strategies for asynchronous viewing and repeated practice by parents, and websites for information retrieval. Cloud storage is often used for submitting parent–child interaction assignments. Mobile applications may also be utilized for monitoring and reminders, and written materials are typically provided for parental reference (Pacia et al., 2022). To alleviate the burden on researchers and therapists, telehealth allows for self-paced learning, offering parents an alternative to guided instruction (Hong et al., 2018). During the peak of the pandemic, Kunze et al. (2021) recruited six parent–child pairs for an online parent intervention program. These participants were on waiting lists for early intervention following diagnosis and resided in remote areas or had low-resource backgrounds. The intervention aimed to improve higher-order restrictive and repetitive behaviors and interests (RRBIs). Participants used tablets, smartphones, or laptops equipped with cameras and headsets; researchers provided a tripod and Yamay M98 Bluetooth™ headset. The instructional process included demonstration videos, parent–child practice, feedback, and discussions. Four evidence-based as well as ABA-based practices were employed: modeling, prompting, differential reinforcement of alternative behaviors, and Response Interruption and Redirection (RIRD). The results indicated increased behavioral flexibility and reduced rigidity in children. Parents used intervention strategies most consistently by the fifth session, resulting in marked improvements in their children's behaviors. However, prompting was the strategy parents most frequently forgot to use (Kunze et al., 2021).

Additionally, an Italian study highlighted reasons for refusing online courses, including a preference for face-to-face learning, a perceived lack of warmth, unstable Internet connections, and reluctance to change established habits (Salomone & Maurizio Arduino, 2017). These findings suggest that online programs need to prioritize building harmonious collaborative relationships from the outset and emphasize the advantages of online learning, such as the convenience of not needing to hire a babysitter while parents participate in training at home.

15.4 The Training Components of Parent-Implemented Intervention (PII)

Parent-implemented interventions (PIIs) originated from ABA approaches pioneered by Risley (1968). These early interventions trained parents for 10 h per month, transitioning to weekly sessions after 2 months, to implement strategies such as social reinforcement and 1-min free play. Consistent with existing literature, these methods increased compliance, enhanced imitative behaviors, and reduced behavioral issues and emotional outbursts among children with autism (Risley, 1968; Wetzel et al., 1966). A key advantage of PIIs is their application in natural settings, where reinforcements and activities occur naturally within the home environment. Over time, PII programs evolved to address parents' specific needs, shifting from focusing solely on reducing problem behaviors to fostering adaptive skill development. Modern PIIs incorporate instructional components such as modeling, problem-solving, role-play, feedback, parent education model (Alexander et al., 2015; Ding et al., in preparation).

Feedback is a cornerstone of PIIs, serving as a critical predictor of how consistently parents use intervention strategies mid-program (Sone et al., 2023). Delivered during real-time practice or through reviews of recorded parent–child interactions, feedback helps parents refine their techniques and maintain fidelity (Ding et al., in preparation). Small group discussions, often conducted without children present, complement these efforts by addressing course-related questions, facilitating the development of home-based strategies, and providing social support, thereby enhancing intervention effectiveness. Even the most streamlined PII programs include multiple instructional components, ensuring a multifaceted approach to parent training.

Prompting also plays a dual role in PIIs, serving as both a coaching tool for parents and a strategy parents use with their children. Therapists prompt parents during training sessions to guide their implementation of intervention strategies, particularly in telehealth contexts where real-time feedback is provided (Hamberger et al., 2022). Parents are also taught systematic prompting procedures—such as least-to-most (LTM), most-to-least (MTL), or progressive-prompt delay (PPD)—to support their children's learning (Ousley et al., 2023). Among these, parents often prefer LTM prompting (Halbur et al., 2020), though it is frequently forgotten without reinforcement (Kunze et al., 2021). Repeated reminders from therapists are often necessary to ensure consistent use (Erturk et al., 2021).

An equally important but often overlooked component is teaching parents how to fade prompts to foster their child's independent skill development. Despite its significance, research on prompt fading strategies in parent training remains limited, highlighting a gap in current practices. By combining structured feedback, collaborative coaching methods such as small group discussions, and comprehensive instruction on prompting and prompt fading, PIIs can maximize their impact, empowering parents while promoting positive outcomes for children.

15.5 Outcomes

PIIs are evidence-based strategies in autism education that emphasize the critical role of parental involvement in promoting children's developmental progress (Tarver et al., 2019). Historically, the focus of these interventions was primarily on measuring child-specific outcomes, such as improvements in language, social engagement, adaptive skills, and reductions in problem behaviors. Parents were initially seen as facilitators who implemented professional-designed strategies to achieve developmental gains for their children, with minimal attention paid to the parents' own experiences or needs (Lovaas, 1987). Research during this early period demonstrated that children benefited significantly when their families were involved, particularly in settings that encouraged the natural generalization of skills across home and community contexts (Carr et al., 2016).

As the field matured, researchers began to recognize the indirect benefits for parents of participating in interventions. Studies highlighted improvements in parental well-being, including reduced stress, enhanced psychological resilience, and greater acceptance of autism diagnoses (Karst & Van Hecke, 2012; Weiss et al., 2012). These findings underscored the reciprocal relationship between parent and child outcomes, as greater parental competence and confidence in managing their child's behaviors often led to better developmental results for the child, further alleviating parental stress and enhancing family functioning (Jurek et al., 2023; Robertson et al., 2017).

In recent decades, the focus of research has expanded to include the direct measurement of parental behavior and skill acquisition, reflecting a shift toward treating parents as active agents of change rather than passive facilitators. Studies began to evaluate parents' ability to implement intervention strategies with fidelity, such as imitating their child's behaviors, following their child's lead, and using evidence-based teaching techniques (McDuffie & Yoder, 2010; Roberts & Kaiser, 2011). This new emphasis acknowledged that equipping parents with these skills not only benefits the child but also strengthens the parents' self-efficacy and capacity to maintain intervention strategies over time (Russell & Ingersoll, 2021).

Parallel to these developments, researchers have also turned their attention to family-level outcomes, recognizing the family as a child's natural ecological environment. While early interventions did not explicitly target family dynamics, subsequent studies highlighted how PIIs could reduce family chaos, improve parent–child relationships, and foster positive parenting practices (Wallace-Watkin et al., 2023). Additionally, interventions have been shown to empower families by enhancing their knowledge of autism, increasing their ability to advocate for resources, and improving social interactions among siblings (Jurek et al., 2023). These outcomes contribute to a more harmonious family environment, ultimately enhancing family quality of life (Wainer et al., 2021).

By addressing the interconnected domains of children, parents, and families, PIIs provide a comprehensive approach to autism intervention. They promote developmental gains for children, empower parents through skill-building and stress reduction, and create more cohesive and supportive family systems. The collaborative efforts of parents and professionals ensure that these interventions facilitate meaningful, sustainable change, improving the quality of life for all members of the family.

The following sections describe children's outcomes, parent outcomes, and family outcomes, respectively.

15.5.1 Children's Outcomes

Parent-implemented interventions (PIIs), predominantly grounded in behavioral analysis theory, initially focused on addressing specific child behaviors, such as reducing dangerous climbing or aggressive actions and teaching isolated skills like motor imitation. Early research demonstrated that applying natural reinforcement in real-life settings enhanced the generalization of intervention outcomes, allowing children to transition from resource-limited hospital settings to supportive home environments (Lovaas et al., 1973). Over time, the scope of interventions expanded from addressing problem behaviors to fostering a wide range of skills essential for daily life, including social engagement (Brookman-Frazee, 2004; Stone-Heaberlin et al., 2023), communication (Charlop-Christy & Carpenter, 2000), language (Hardan et al., 2015), imitation (Cardon, 2012), and adaptive behaviors (Rogers et al., 2022).

A systematic review by Gerow et al. (2024) identified the most commonly used intervention strategies in PIIs, including antecedent-based interventions, differential reinforcement, functional communication training, prompting, and reinforcement. These evidence-based approaches address disruptive behaviors and support skill development. Additionally, structured programs like Discrete Trial Training (DTT) (Stone-Heaberlin et al., 2023), the Early Start Denver Model (ESDM), and Improving Parents as Communication Teachers (ImPACT) have been widely applied to improve social engagement and communication in children with autism. Regarding adaptive skills, programs such as the Incredible Years (IY-ASD) target self-regulation and behavior management, teaching techniques like setting clear boundaries and proactive discipline strategies to reduce misbehaviors and foster independence (Orantes et al., 2023).

Promoting social engagement often focuses on training specific target behaviors such as eye contact, object imitation, and joint attention. Parent-responsive interventions, including Joint Attention, Symbolic Play, Engagement, and Regulation (JASPER) (Kasari et al., 2015), emphasize synchronized parental responsiveness, such as mirrored pacing and environmental arrangement, to increase child-initiated interactions (Shire et al., 2015). These strategies have proven effective in enhancing social participation and engagement.

In the domain of language and communication, parental verbal responsiveness—such as follow-in directives and expansions—has been shown to significantly improve expressive vocabulary and language use (McDuffie & Yoder, 2010). A meta-analysis by Roberts and Kaiser (2011) further confirmed that parent-implemented interventions can achieve language improvements comparable to therapist-led approaches. These strategies, applied during natural parent–child interactions, facilitate the generalization of language skills across diverse contexts.

Parent-implemented interventions have also demonstrated success in addressing behavioral challenges. For instance, programs like the 24-week parent training model by Bearss et al. (2015) showed sustained reductions in disruptive behaviors, such as tantrums and self-injury, at follow-ups (Bearss et al., 2015). These interventions are further enhanced when supported by telecommunication methods, offering parents accessible problem-solving channels during the process (Gerow et al., 2024).

Overall, PII programs provide comprehensive support for children with autism by promoting adaptive, social, communication, and behavioral skills. Future research should continue exploring subgroup-specific adaptations to maximize the effectiveness of these interventions across diverse populations.

15.5.2 Parent Outcomes

Parent-implemented interventions (PIIs) have increasingly recognized the pivotal role of parents in achieving meaningful outcomes for children with autism spectrum disorder (ASD). Early research primarily focused on the indirect effects of parental involvement, such as its impact on child-specific outcomes, including skill generalization and behavioral improvements. Over time, studies began to explore the direct impact of interventions on parents themselves, addressing their mental health, self-efficacy, and capacity to sustain therapeutic strategies.

Parental well-being is now widely acknowledged as a critical factor influencing both the success of interventions and overall family dynamics. Parents of children with autism often experience heightened stress compared to parents of typically developing children or those with other developmental disabilities (Weiss et al., 2012). This stress can undermine parent–child interactions, affecting the child's developmental progress. Conversely, higher parental self-efficacy has been shown to enhance parents' ability and motivation to consistently implement intervention techniques, fostering better outcomes for both parents and children (Sofronoff & Farbotko, 2002).

Direct measures of parental behavior, such as their ability to imitate their child, follow the child's lead, and apply evidence-based strategies, have become a significant area of focus. Studies have shown that interventions targeting these skills can lead to reductions in disruptive child behaviors, improved parent–child interactions, and increased parental satisfaction with the intervention process (Bearss et al., 2015). Programs like ImPACT Online have demonstrated that fostering parental self-efficacy correlates with a successful application of strategies in natural settings, further reinforcing parents' role as active agents of change (Russell & Ingersoll, 2021).

Parental stress reduction is another key outcome of PIIs, often supported through mindfulness-based programs and problem-focused coping strategies. For instance, combining the Early Start Denver Model (ESDM) with Mindfulness-Based Stress Reduction (MBSR) has been shown to alleviate parental distress, improve parent–child interactions, and reduce symptoms of depression and anxiety, although sustained benefits may require longer-term support (Dykens et al., 2014). Problem-solving education and social support networks have also been identified as essential tools for helping parents manage stress and avoid burnout, further enhancing their engagement in interventions (Canfield et al., 2023).

Beyond enhancing personal well-being, PIIs frequently empower parents to adopt advocacy roles within the ASD community. These interventions provide parents with essential knowledge and practical skills, enabling them to navigate complex service systems and support networks effectively. This empowerment extends beyond individual families, contributing to a broader societal understanding of autism and promoting inclusive practices.

Parental empowerment is a critical outcome of these interventions. Many parents report increased confidence in their ability to support their child after engaging in PIIs. They develop a deeper understanding of the importance of interaction and language development and learn how following their child's interests can enhance engagement. This improved sense of competence equips parents with strategies to better facilitate their child's developmental progress.

Furthermore, this empowerment often transcends the personal sphere, motivating parents to become advocates for autism awareness. By sharing their experiences and acquired knowledge, they support other families facing similar challenges, thereby strengthening the ASD community (Jurek et al., 2023).

By addressing both the practical and psychological needs of parents, PIIs ensure that parental outcomes are not only an integral component of intervention success but also a foundation for sustainable and meaningful improvements across the child's ecological system.

15.5.3 Family Outcomes

The family plays a central role in the ecological system of children with autism spectrum disorder, making it a critical context for the success of PIIs. Currently, PIIs are designed to establish a collaborative relationship with families by thoroughly understanding their priorities. These family priorities are systematically integrated into intervention goals, ensuring that the entire intervention process is guided by the family's core values and specific needs. This family-centered approach not only enhances the relevance and effectiveness of the intervention but also promotes greater family engagement, ownership, and the long-term sustainability of the strategies employed.

By aligning intervention goals with family priorities, PIIs create a supportive and responsive framework that acknowledges and respects the unique dynamics, strengths, and challenges of each family. This alignment fosters a sense of partnership between families and professionals, ultimately leading to better developmental outcomes for children with autism and greater confidence and competence for their caregivers.

While many early PIIs primarily targeted child-specific or parent-specific outcomes, contemporary research has increasingly recognized the broader impact of these interventions on overall family functioning. By fostering positive family dynamics and alleviating stressors, PIIs contribute significantly to enhancing the quality of family life, promoting resilience, and supporting the well-being of all family members.

One of the key benefits of PIIs is the reduction of family chaos, which can stem from the challenges of raising a child with autism. Structured interventions help families establish routines, enhance communication, and create a more orderly environment (Karst et al., 2015). In addition, interventions often equip families with knowledge about autism and advocacy skills, enabling them to access resources, navigate support systems, and advocate effectively for their child's needs (Minjarez et al., 2013). These outcomes not only benefit the immediate family but also strengthen the family's role as a cohesive support system.

PIIs also promote positive parent–child interactions by increasing parental responsiveness and reducing negative or passive parenting behaviors (Edmunds et al., 2019). As parents acquire intervention skills, these improvements often extend to other family members, including siblings. For example, siblings of children with autism may experience enhanced social interactions and improved relationships as a result of their parents' participation in PIIs (Yoder et al., 2021).

Family functioning is typically measured through tools that assess parent–child relationships, family dynamics, and marital satisfaction. For example, the Family Environment Scale and the Family Quality of Life Survey are commonly used to evaluate these dimensions (Park et al., 2003). Studies have shown that PIIs lead to improvements in family cohesion, reduced stress, and enhanced marital satisfaction, particularly in families where both parents actively participate (Hartley et al., 2012).

Programs such as The Incredible Years (IY-ASD) have demonstrated measurable success in improving family outcomes by reducing negative parenting practices and fostering positive interactions. These interventions help parents adopt proactive discipline strategies and manage challenging behaviors, creating a more harmonious family environment over time (Wahdan et al., 2023).

By addressing family dynamics alongside individual child and parent outcomes, PIIs provide a comprehensive approach to supporting families of children with autism. This holistic focus ensures that families not only become active participants in their child's intervention but also experience improvements in their own quality of life, promoting long-term well-being for all members.

15.6 Discussion

This chapter has explored the transformative potential of evidence-based, parent-implemented interventions (PIIs) rooted in ABA to empower families of children with autism. From Risley's (1968) early work, inviting parents into the intervention process, to contemporary approaches that leverage technology and collaborative coaching, PIIs have evolved to become a cornerstone of autism support. These interventions not only promote skill development in children but also empower parents and strengthen family dynamics, highlighting their integral role in fostering meaningful and sustainable outcomes.

15.6.1 Empowering Families Through Evolutionary Progress

Initially, PIIs focused primarily on child-specific outcomes, targeting behavioral improvements and isolated skills. Over the years, the field expanded its focus, acknowledging the critical importance of parental well-being, skill development, and family dynamics. Modern PIIs leverage Internet-based platforms, coaching frameworks, and collaborative strategies to equip parents with the tools they need to support their child's development effectively (Carruthers et al., 2023). These advancements have enabled families to transition from passive participants to active agents of change in the therapeutic process.

Despite these achievements, PIIs face ongoing challenges. Tailoring interventions to diverse family contexts requires careful consideration of cultural, economic, and logistical factors. Questions regarding who should deliver parent training, how programs should be structured, and when and where they should be implemented remain central to optimizing intervention outcomes. These questions underscore the need for flexible, individualized approaches that respect families' unique circumstances and priorities.

Acknowledging these diverse needs, recent research has proposed tiered intervention models to address varying levels of family readiness and resource availability. For instance, a three-tiered parent education model (Ding et al., 2025) offers a progressive framework that ranges from self-directed learning to group sessions and individualized coaching. This model highlights the potential of tiered systems in accommodating different family needs while maintaining cost-effectiveness and intervention fidelity. While the findings are promising, further research and replication are required to validate their broader applicability.

15.6.2 Key Insights: Parents as Partners in Intervention

A recurring theme in PIIs is the reciprocal relationship between parent and child outcomes. Parents who exhibit high responsiveness and implement interventions with fidelity often see immediate improvements in their child's behavior and skill acquisition. However, sustaining these changes requires addressing barriers such as stress, limited support, and misaligned expectations (Carruthers et al., 2023).

Effective PIIs also emphasize collaborative goal-setting, enabling parents to co-create intervention plans that align with their values and daily routines (Ingersoll & Dvortcsak, 2019; Siller & Morgan, 2018). For example, programs like ImPACT Online and Mindfulness-Based Stress Reduction (MBSR) have shown promise in reducing parental stress while enhancing self-efficacy and engagement (Dykens et al., 2014; Russell & Ingersoll, 2021). Follow-up strategies, such as periodic check-ins and booster sessions, can further ensure the sustainability of intervention gains, particularly as parents navigate caregiving demands.

15.6.3 Strengthening Family Dynamics

PIIs extend their impact beyond individual parent and child outcomes to include broader family dynamics. By reducing family chaos, improving communication, and fostering cohesive routines, these interventions create a more stable and supportive home environment (Karst et al., 2015). Positive spillover effects, such as improved social interactions among siblings and enhanced marital satisfaction, underscore the systemic benefits of PIIs.

Tailored interventions, particularly tiered models, hold promise for addressing family-specific challenges, such as time constraints or financial stress. The three-tiered framework (Ding et al., 2025) incorporates culturally relevant modifications, such as localized materials and respite care options, to reduce barriers and enhance engagement. This approach underscores the importance of adaptability in PII frameworks to ensure their effectiveness across diverse populations.

15.7 Future Directions: Advancing the Field of PIIs

To further empower families and enhance the impact of PIIs, several key areas warrant attention:

15.7.1 Customization and Individualization

Interventions should be tailored to accommodate parents' unique learning styles, family routines, and cultural contexts. Collaborative goal-setting and adaptive frameworks can ensure interventions remain relevant and impactful. Incorporating instructional components, such as modeling, feedback, and homework, should also be customized to align with family-specific dynamics and capacities.

15.7.2 Enhanced Professional Training

Incorporating adult learning principles into pre-service training for professionals delivering PIIs is essential. Coaching models emphasizing collaborative planning, reflection, and decision-making should be systematically analyzed to optimize outcomes. Additionally, specific training in delivering and balancing real-time practice, role-play, and feedback during sessions is critical to ensure parents gain confidence in implementing learned strategies. Instruction on teaching prompt fading techniques should be expanded to address current gaps in training.

15.7.3 Sustainability Through Follow-Up

Post-intervention strategies, such as regular follow-ups and booster sessions, can help parents retain and refine their skills, ensuring long-term sustainability of intervention benefits. These follow-ups should reinforce key instructional components, such as feedback and prompt fading, to prevent skill attrition and maintain fidelity in implementation.

15.7.4 Leveraging Technology

Online platforms, teleconsultations, and digital tools should be further explored to increase accessibility and provide real-time support for families, particularly those in underserved regions. Integrating technology to deliver structured instructional components, such as video modeling, remote feedback on homework, and collaborative small group discussions, can enhance accessibility and support.

15.7.5 Broader Inclusion of Family Dynamics

Future research should explore the systemic impact of PIIs, examining how interventions influence family relationships, including sibling interactions and marital satisfaction, to provide a holistic understanding of their benefits. Special attention should be given to how family members can collaboratively engage in PII practices, such as sharing responsibility for modeling and reinforcement.

15.7.6 Empowering Parental Advocacy

Interventions should equip parents with the knowledge and confidence to advocate for their child's needs, fostering a sense of empowerment that extends beyond the home to schools, communities, and policymaking arenas. Incorporating strategies like reflection and collaborative small group discussions within PIIs can build parents' advocacy skills by enhancing their understanding of intervention principles and fostering peer learning.

15.8 Conclusion

Parent-implemented interventions represent a vibrant and evolving field that empowers families to take an active role in supporting their child's development. Grounded in the principles of ABA and evidence-based practices, these interventions offer a dynamic framework for addressing the diverse needs of children, parents, and families. By incorporating tiered systems, leveraging technology, and addressing cultural and contextual factors, future efforts can refine and expand the role of PIIs. A stronger emphasis on the integration of instructional components, such as feedback and prompt fading, will enhance both the scalability and inclusivity of these interventions. Acknowledging emerging frameworks, such as the three-tiered model (Ding et al., 2025), provides a promising direction for enhancing the scalability and inclusivity of PIIs, ensuring families are not only supported but also empowered to thrive.

Acknowledgments We utilized ChatGPT, an AI language model developed by OpenAI, for language editing and correction purposes in the preparation of this manuscript. The AI-assisted edits focused solely on improving grammar, vocabulary, and overall readability. All academic content, ideas, and interpretations remain our own.

References

Alexander, J. L., Ayres, K. M., & Smith, K. A. (2015). Training teachers in evidence-based practice for individuals with autism spectrum disorder: A review of the literature. *Teacher Education and Special Education, 38*(1), 13–27. https://doi.org/10.1177/0888406414544551

Bearss, K., Burrell, T. L., Stewart, L., & Scahill, L. (2015). Parent training in autism spectrum disorder: What's in a name? *Clinical Child And Family Psychology Review, 18*, 170–182. https://doi.org/10.1016/0005-7967(72)90054-X

Berkowitz, B. P., & Graziano, A. M. (1972). Training parents as behavior therapists: A review. *Behaviour Research and Therapy, 10*(4), 297–317. https://doi.org/10.1016/0005-7967(72)90054-X

Brian, J. A., Smith, I. M., Zwaigenbaum, L., Roberts, W., & Bryson, S. E. (2016). The social ABCs caregiver-mediated intervention for toddlers with autism spectrum disorder: Feasibility, acceptability, and evidence of promise from a multisite study. *Autism Research, 9*(8), 899–912. https://doi.org/10.1002/aur.1582

Brookman-Frazee, L. (2004). Using parent/clinician partnerships in parent education programs for children with autism [article]. *Journal of Positive Behavior Interventions, 6*(4), 195–213. https://doi.org/10.1177/10983007040060040201

Canfield, C. F., Miller, E., Zhang, Y., Shaw, D., Morris, P., Galan, C., & Mendelsohn, A. L. (2023). Tiered universal and targeted early childhood interventions: Enhancing attendance across families with varying needs. *Early Childhood Research Quarterly, 63*, 362–369. https://doi.org/10.1016/j.ecresq.2023.01.004

Cardon, T. A. (2012). Teaching caregivers to implement video modeling imitation training via iPad for their children with autism. *Research in Autism Spectrum Disorders, 6*(4), 1389–1400. https://doi.org/10.1016/j.rasd.2012.06.002

Carr, T., Shih, W., Lawton, K., Lord, C., King, B., & Kasari, C. (2016). The relationship between treatment attendance, adherence, and outcome in a caregiver-mediated intervention for low-resourced families of young children with autism spectrum disorder. *Autism, 20*(6), 643–652. https://doi.org/10.1177/1362361315598634

Carruthers, S., Mleczko, N., Page, S., Ahuja, S., Ellis, C., Howlin, P., Leadbitter, K., Taylor, L., Slonims, V., & Charman, T. (2023). Using implementation science frameworks to explore barriers and facilitators for parents' use of therapeutic strategies following a parent-mediated autism intervention. *Autism, 27*(4), 1011–1025. https://doi.org/10.1177/13623613221125630

Casillas, N., Vigil, D. C., & Wang, H.-T. (2017). Latino and non-Latino white parents' experiences raising their child with ASD: An exploratory study. *The Qualitative Report, 22*(8), 2173–2195. https://doi.org/10.46743/2160-3715/2017.3261

Charlop-Christy, M. H., & Carpenter, M. H. (2000). Modified incidental teaching sessions: A procedure for parents to increase spontaneous speech in their children with autism. *Journal of Positive Behavior Interventions, 2*(2), 98–112. https://doi.org/10.1177/109830070000200203

Cooper, J. O., Heron, T. E., & Heward, W. L. (2020). *Applied behavior analysis*. Pearson. https://doi.org/10.1901/jaba.1989.22-454

Ding, Y.-S. (2020). *Applying three tier model of parent education with ImPact curriculum to improve social communication of Taiwanese parents with Young children with autism Spectrum disorder*. [Unpublished master's thesis]. University of National Taiwan Normal University. https://doi.org/10.6345/NTNU202001723

Ding, Y.-S., Wang, H.-T., & Lin, F. Y. (n.d.). *Parent-implemented interventions for children with autism: A systematic review*. In Preparation.

Ding, Y.-S., Wang, H.-T., & Lin, F. Y. (2025). Incorporating a Three-Tier yParent Education Model into ImPACT Curriculum in Taiwan. *Journal of Child and Family Studies, 4*, 1163–1177.

Dykens, E. M., Fisher, M. H., Taylor, J. L., Lambert, W., & Miodrag, N. (2014). Reducing distress in mothers of children with autism and other disabilities: A randomized trial. *Pediatrics, 134*(2), e454–e463. https://doi.org/10.1542/peds.2013-3164

Edmunds, S. R., Kover, S. T., & Stone, W. L. (2019). The relation between parent verbal responsiveness and child communication in young children with or at risk for autism spectrum disorder: A systematic review and meta-analysis. *Autism Research, 12*(5), 715–731. https://doi.org/10.1002/aur.2100

Erturk, B., Hansen, S. G., Machalicek, W., & Kunze, M. (2021). Parent-implemented early social communication intervention for young children with autism spectrum disorder. *Journal of Behavioral Education, 30*(4), 641–663.

Feinstein, A. (2011). *A history of autism: Conversations with the pioneers*. John Wiley & Sons. https://doi.org/10.1111/j.1467-8578.2011.00503.x

Gerow, S., Exline, E., Swafford, L., Cosottile, D., Conroy, M., Machalicek, W., Davis, T. N., Wei, Q., & James, A. (2024). Addressing challenging behavior and social–emotional skills in home-based services: A systematic review. *Journal of Positive Behavior Interventions, 26*(4), 241–256. https://doi.org/10.1177/10983007231224048

Guthrie, W., Wetherby, A. M., Woods, J., Schatschneider, C., Holland, R. D., Morgan, L., & Lord, C. E. (2023). The earlier the better: An RCT of treatment timing effects for toddlers on the autism spectrum. *Autism: The International Journal of Research & Practice, 1*. https://doi.org/10.1177/13623613231159153

Halbur, M. E., Kodak, T., Wood, R., & Corrigan, E. (2020). An evaluation of parent preference for prompting procedures. *Journal of Applied Behavior Analysis, 53*(2), 707–726. https://doi.org/10.1002/jaba.616

Hamberger, R. J., Evmenova, A. S., Coogle, C. G., & Regan, K. S. (2022). Parent coaching in natural communication opportunities through bug-in-ear technology. *Topics in Early Childhood Special Education, 42*(3), 234–245.

Hao, Y., Franco, J. H., Sundarrajan, M., & Chen, Y. (2021). A pilot study comparing tele-therapy and in-person therapy: Perspectives from parent-mediated intervention for children with autism Spectrum disorders [report]. *Journal of Autism and Developmental Disorders, 51*(1), 129. https://doi.org/10.1007/s10803-020-04439-x

Hardan, A. Y., Gengoux, G. W., Berquist, K. L., Libove, R. A., Ardel, C. M., Phillips, J., Frazier, T. W., & Minjarez, M. B. (2015). A randomized controlled trial of pivotal response treatment group for parents of children with autism. *Journal of Child Psychology and Psychiatry, 56*(8), 884–892. https://doi.org/10.1111/jcpp.12354

Hartley, S. L., Barker, E. T., Baker, J. K., Seltzer, M. M., & Greenberg, J. S. (2012). Marital satisfaction and life circumstances of grown children with autism across 7 years. *Journal of Family Psychology, 26*(5), 688–697. https://doi.org/10.1037/a0029354

Hong, E. R., Neely, L., Gerow, S., & Gann, C. (2018). The effect of caregiver-delivered social-communication interventions on skill generalization and maintenance in ASD. *Research in Developmental Disabilities, 74*, 57–71. https://doi.org/10.1016/j.ridd.2018.01.006

Hume, K., Steinbrenner, J. R., Odom, S. L., Morin, K. L., Nowell, S. W., Tomaszewski, B., Szendrey, S., McIntyre, N. S., Yücesoy-Özkan, S., & Savage, M. N. (2021). Evidence-based practices for children, youth, and young adults with autism: Third generation review. *Journal of Autism and Developmental Disorders*, 1–20. https://doi.org/10.1007/s10803-022-05438-w

Ingersoll, B. (2010). Brief report: Pilot randomized controlled trial of reciprocal imitation training for teaching elicited and spontaneous imitation to children with autism. *Journal of Autism and Developmental Disorders, 40*(9), 1154–1160.

Ingersoll, B., & Dvortcsak, A. (2010). Teaching social communication to children with autism: A manual for parents (Vol. 2). Guilford Press.

Ingersoll, B., & Dvortcsak, A. (2019). *Teaching social communication to children with autism and other developmental delays (2-book set): The project ImPACT guide to coaching parents and the project ImPACT manual for parents*. Guilford Publications.

Ingersoll, B., & Gergans, S. (2007). The effect of a parent-implemented imitation intervention on spontaneous imitation skills in young children with autism [article]. *Research in Developmental Disabilities, 28*(2), 163–175. https://doi.org/10.1016/j.ridd.2006.02.004

Jurek, L., Leadbitter, K., Falissard, B., Colin, C., Touzet, S., & Geoffray, M.-M. (2023). Parental experience of parent-mediated intervention for children with ASD: A systematic review and qualitative evidence synthesis [Article]. *Autism: The International Journal of Research & Practice, 27*(3), 647–666. https://doi.org/10.1177/13623613221112204

Kaiser, A. P., & Roberts, M. Y. (2013). Advances in early communication and language intervention. *Journal of Early Intervention, 35*(2), 106–124. https://doi.org/10.1177/1053815113504826

Karst, J. S., & Van Hecke, A. V. (2012). Parent and family impact of autism spectrum disorders: A review and proposed model for intervention evaluation. *Clinical Child and Family Psychology Review, 15*, 247–277. https://doi.org/10.1007/s10567-012-0119-6

Karst, J. S., Van Hecke, A. V., & Carson, A. M. (2015). Parent and family outcomes of PEERS: A social skills intervention for adolescents with autism Spectrum disorder [Journal Articles; Reports–Research]. *Journal of Autism and Developmental Disorders, 45*(3), 752–765. https://doi.org/10.1007/s10803-014-2231-6

Kasari, C., Freeman, S., & Paparella, T. (2006). Joint attention and symbolic play in young children with autism: A randomized controlled intervention study. *Journal of Child Psychology and Psychiatry, 47*(6), 611–620. https://doi.org/10.1111/j.1469-7610.2005.01567.x

Kasari, C., Gulsrud, A., Paparella, T., Hellemann, G., & Berry, K. (2015). Randomized comparative efficacy study of parent-mediated interventions for toddlers with autism. *Journal of Consulting and Clinical Psychology, 83*(3), 554. https://doi.org/10.1037/a0039080

Kasperzack, D., Schrott, B., Mingebach, T., Becker, K., Burghardt, R., & Kamp-Becker, I. (2020). Effectiveness of the stepping stones triple P group parenting program in reducing comorbid behavioral problems in children with autism. *Autism, 24*(2), 423–436. https://doi.org/10.1177/1362361319866063

Keen, D., Webster, A., & Ridley, G. (2016). How well are children with autism spectrum disorder doing academically at school? An overview of the literature. *Autism, 20*(3), 276–294. https://doi.org/10.1177/1362361315580962

Koegel, R. L., & Koegel, L. K. (2006). *Pivotal response treatments for autism: Communication, social, & academic development*. Paul H. Brookes Publishing.

Kunze, M. G., Machalicek, W., Wei, Q., & St. Joseph, S. (2021). Coaching via telehealth: Caregiver-mediated interventions for young children on the waitlist for an autism diagnosis using single-case design. *Journal of Clinical Medicine, 10*(8), 1654. https://doi.org/10.3390/jcm10081654

Le, P. D., Eschliman, E. L., Grivel, M. M., Tang, J., Cho, Y. G., Yang, X., Tay, C., Li, T., Bass, J., & Yang, L. H. (2022). Barriers and facilitators to implementation of evidence-based task-sharing mental health interventions in low- and middle-income countries: A systematic review using implementation science frameworks. *Implementation Science, 17*, 4.

Liu, X., & Schertz, H. H. (2022). Parents outcomes of parent-mediated intervention for toddlers with autism [journal articles; reports–research]. *Grantee Submission, 42*(3), 259–268. https://doi.org/10.1177/02711214211019117

Lovaas, O. I. (1987). Behavioral treatment and normal educational and intellectual functioning in young autistic children. *Journal of Consulting and Clinical Psychology, 55*(1), 3–9. https://doi.org/10.1037/0022-006X.55.1.3

Lovaas, O. I., Koegel, R., Simmons, J. Q., & Long, J. S. (1973). Some generalization and follow-up measures on autistic children in behavior therapy 1. *Journal of Applied Behavior Analysis, 6*(1), 131–165. https://doi.org/10.1901/jaba.1973.6-131

Maenner, M. J. (2023). Prevalence and characteristics of autism spectrum disorder among children aged 8 years—Autism and Developmental Disabilities Monitoring Network, 11 sites, United States, 2020. *MMWR. Surveillance Summaries, 72*. https://doi.org/10.15585/mmwr.ss7202a1

Makrygianni, M. K., & Reed, P. (2010). A meta-analytic review of the effectiveness of behavioural early intervention programs for children with autistic spectrum disorders. *Research in Autism Spectrum Disorders, 4*(4), 577–593. https://doi.org/10.1016/j.rasd.2010.01.014

McDuffie, A., & Yoder, P. (2010 Aug). Types of parent verbal responsiveness that predict language in young children with autism spectrum disorder. *Journal of Speech, Language, and Hearing Research, 53*(4), 1026–1039. https://doi.org/10.1044/1092-4388(2009/09-0023)

Minjarez, M. B., Mercier, E. M., Williams, S. E., & Hardan, A. Y. (2013). Impact of pivotal response training group therapy on stress and empowerment in parents of children with autism. *Journal of Positive Behavior Interventions, 15*(2), 71–78. https://doi.org/10.1177/1098300712449055

Nordquist, V. M., & Wahler, R. G. (1973). Naturalistic treatment of an autistic child. *Journal of Applied Behavior Analysis, 6*(1), 79–87. https://doi.org/10.1901/jaba.1973.6-79

Orantes, D., Rohacek, A., & Antshel, K. M. (2023). ADHD, distractibility, and ABA. In *Handbook of applied behavior analysis for children with autism: Clinical guide to assessment and treatment* (pp. 391–414). Springer.

Ousley, C. L., Raulston, T. J., & Gilhuber, C. S. (2023). Telecoaching for parents of Young autistic children using strength-based video feedback. *Journal of Autism and Developmental Disorders*, 1–16. https://doi.org/10.1007/s10803-023-06199-w

Pacia, C., Holloway, J., Gunning, C., & Lee, H. (2022). A systematic review of family-mediated social communication interventions for Young children with autism. *Review Journal of Autism and Developmental Disorders, 9*(2), 208–234. https://doi.org/10.1007/s40489-021-00249-8

Pan, C.-Y., Kuo, T.-Y., & Kuo, F.-L. (2023). Meta-analysis of effectiveness of parent-mediated telehealth interventions in children with autism spectrum disorder. *Research in Autism Spectrum Disorders, 107*. https://doi.org/10.1016/j.rasd.2023.102209

Park, J., Hoffman, L., Marquis, J., Turnbull, A. P., Poston, D., Mannan, H., Wang, M., & Nelson, L. (2003). Toward assessing family outcomes of service delivery: Validation of a family quality of life survey. *Journal of Intellectual Disability Research, 47*(4–5), 367–384. https://doi.org/10.1046/j.1365-2788.2003.00497.x

Pellecchia, M., Beidas, R. S., Mandell, D. S., Cannuscio, C. C., Dunst, C. J., & Stahmer, A. C. (2020). Parent empowerment and coaching in early intervention: Study protocol for a feasibility study. *Pilot and Feasibility Studies, 6*, 22. https://doi.org/10.1186/s40814-020-00568-3

Risley, T. R. (1968). The effects and side effects of punishing the autistic behaviors of a deviant child 1. *Journal of Applied Behavior Analysis, 1*(1), 21–34. https://doi.org/10.1901/jaba.1968.1-21

Roberts, M. Y., & Kaiser, A. P. (2011). The effectiveness of parent-implemented language interventions: A meta-analysis. *American Journal of Speech-Language Pathology, 20*(3), 180–199. https://doi.org/10.1044/1058-0360(2011/10-0055)

Robertson, R. E., Sobeck, E. E., Wynkoop, K., & Schwartz, R. (2017). Participant diversity in special education research: Parent-implemented behavior interventions for children with autism [journal articles; reports–research; information analyses]. *Remedial and Special Education, 38*(5), 259–271. https://doi.org/10.1177/0741932516685407

Rogers, S. J., Cook, I., & Meryl, A. (2005). Imitation and play in autism. *Handbook of autism and pervasive developmental disorders, 1*, 382–405.

Rogers, S. J., & Dawson, G. (2010). *Early start Denver model for young children with autism: Promoting language, learning, and engagement*. Guilford Press.

Rogers, S. J., Stahmer, A., Talbott, M., Young, G., Fuller, E., Pellecchia, M., Barber, A., & Griffith, E. (2022). Feasibility of delivering parent-implemented NDBI interventions in low-resource regions: A pilot randomized controlled study. *Journal of Neurodevelopmental Disorders, 14*, 1–14. https://doi.org/10.1186/s11689-021-09410-0

Russell, K. M., & Ingersoll, B. (2021). Factors related to parental therapeutic self-efficacy in a parent-mediated intervention for children with autism spectrum disorder: A mixed methods study. *Autism, 25*(4), 971–981. https://doi.org/10.1177/1362361320974233

Salomone, E., & Maurizio Arduino, G. (2017). Parental attitudes to a telehealth parent coaching intervention for autism spectrum disorder [journal article]. *Journal of Telemedicine & Telecare, 23*(3), 416–420. https://doi.org/10.1177/1357633X16642067

Sarokoff, R. A., & Sturmey, P. (2004). The effects of behavioral skills training on staff implementation of discrete-trial teaching. *Journal of Applied Behavior Analysis, 37*(4), 535–538. https://doi.org/10.1901/jaba.2004.37-535

Schreibman, L., Dawson, G., Stahmer, A. C., Landa, R., Rogers, S. J., McGee, G. G., Kasari, C., Ingersoll, B., Kaiser, A. P., & Bruinsma, Y. (2015). Naturalistic developmental behavioral interventions: Empirically validated treatments for autism spectrum disorder. *Journal of Autism and Developmental Disorders, 45*(8), 2411–2428. https://doi.org/10.1007/s10803-015-2407-8

Shire, S. Y., Goods, K., Shih, W., Distefano, C., Kaiser, A., Wright, C., Mathy, P., Landa, R., & Kasari, C. (2015). Parents' adoption of social communication intervention strategies: Families including children with autism Spectrum disorder who are minimally verbal [report]. *Journal of Autism and Developmental Disorders, 45*(6), 1712. https://doi.org/10.1007/s10803-014-2329-x

Siller, M., & Morgan, L. (2018). Systematic review of research evaluating parent-mediated interventions for young children with autism: Years 2013 to 2015. In *Handbook of parent-implemented interventions for very young children with autism* (pp. 1–21).

Sofronoff, K., & Farbotko, M. (2002). The effectiveness of parent management training to increase self-efficacy in parents of children with Asperger syndrome. *Autism, 6*(3), 271–286. https://doi.org/10.1177/1362361302006003005

Sone, B. J., Lee, J., Grauzer, J., Kaat, A., & Roberts, M. Y. (2023). Identifying effective strategies to instruct parents during parent-implemented intervention: The role of parent practice with feedback [Article]. *Early Childhood Research Quarterly, 62*, 394–404. https://doi.org/10.1016/j.ecresq.2022.09.010

Stone-Heaberlin, M., Hartley, N., Lynch, J. D., Fisher, A. P., & Justice, N. (2023). Implementation of a parent-mediated discrete trial teaching intervention for children with autism spectrum disorder. *Behavior Analysis in Practice, 16*(1), 302–306. https://doi.org/10.1007/s40617-022-00735-3

Tarver, J., Palmer, M., Webb, S., Scott, S., Slonims, V., Simonoff, E., & Charman, T. (2019). Child and parent outcomes following parent interventions for child emotional and behavioral problems in autism spectrum disorders: A systematic review and meta-analysis. *Autism, 23*(7), 1630–1644. https://doi.org/10.1177/1362361319830042

Wahdan, M. M., Malak, M. Z., Al-Amer, R., Ayed, A., Russo, S., & Berte, D. Z. (2023). Effect of incredible years autism spectrum and language delays (IY-ASD) program on stress and behavioral management skills among parents of children with autism spectrum disorder in Palestine. *Journal of Pediatric Nursing, 72*, 45–52. https://doi.org/10.1016/j.pedn.2023.03.018

Wainer, A. L., Arnold, Z. E., Leonczyk, C., & Valluripalli Soorya, L. (2021). Examining a stepped-care telehealth program for parents of young children with autism: A proof-of-concept trial. *Molecular Autism, 12*(1), 32. https://doi.org/10.1186/s13229-021-00443-9

Wallace-Watkin, C., Sigafoos, J., & Waddington, H. (2023). Barriers and facilitators for obtaining support services among underserved families with an autistic child: A systematic qualitative review. *Autism, 27*(3), 588–601. https://doi.org/10.1177/13623613221123712

Wang, H.-T., & Casillas, N. (2012). Asian American parents' experiences of raising children with autism: Multicultural family perspective. *Journal of Asian and African Studies, 48*(5), 594–606. https://doi.org/10.1177/0021909612467421

Weiss, J. A., Cappadocia, M. C., MacMullin, J. A., Viecili, M., & Lunsky, Y. (2012). The impact of child problem behaviors of children with ASD on parent mental health: The mediating role of acceptance and empowerment. *Autism, 16*(3), 261–274. https://doi.org/10.1177/1362361311422708

Wetzel, R. J., Baker, J., Roney, M., & Martin, M. (1966). Outpatient treatment of autistic behavior. *Behaviour Research and Therapy, 4*(3), 169–177. https://doi.org/10.1016/0005-7967(66)90063-5

Yoder, P. J., Stone, W. L., & Edmunds, S. R. (2021). For which younger siblings of children with autism spectrum disorder does parent-mediated intervention work? *Autism: The International Journal of Research & Practice, 25*(1), 58–69. https://doi.org/10.1177/1362361320943373

Chapter 16
Breaking Barriers: Implementing Applied Behavior Analysis Practices in Low- and Middle-Income Countries

Rompiendo barreras: Implementación de prácticas del análisis conductual aplicado en países de ingresos bajos y medios

Ronaldo L. Rodas Jara, Laura Regina Gómez, Hui-Ting Wang, Liza R. Rodas Jara, and Adriana Kaori Terol

Abstract Applied Behavior Analysis (ABA) is one of the most studied and proven methods for helping people with autism spectrum disorders (ASD) and similar developmental issues make important and positive changes in their behavior. Despite decades of evidence, low- and middle-income countries (LMICs) severely limit access to ABA-informed interventions. Families in these settings often face delayed identification and diagnosis, scarce access to specialized practitioners, and minimal public-sector funding. These structural barriers are compounded by cultural and linguistic discontinuities that can reduce acceptability and feasibility—and, when poorly addressed, may lead to unintended consequences that conflict with families' priorities.

This chapter examines theoretical foundations and empirical evidence relevant to implementing ABA in resource-constrained LMICs. We emphasize how workforce

R. L. Rodas Jara (✉)
Universidad Iberoamericana, Asunción, Paraguay
e-mail: ronaldo.rodas@unibe.edu.py

L. R. Gómez
University of Florida, Gainesville, FL, USA

H.-T. Wang
Department of Special Education, National Taiwan Normal University, Taipei, Taiwan

L. R. Rodas Jara
Investigadora Independiente (Independent Researcher), Caaguazú, Paraguay

A. K. Terol
University of California, Davis, CA, USA

S. Halder et al. (eds.), *Applied Behavior Analysis-Based Interventions for Autism Spectrum Disorder*, https://doi.org/10.1007/978-981-95-2889-9_16

shortages, culturally grounded adaptation, and system-level resource constraints interact in practice. We also review delivery models that integrate caregiver-led interventions, community-embedded partnerships, and technology-facilitated training and supervision. Finally, we propose practical, policy-relevant recommendations aimed at culturally responsive, ethically sound, and economically sustainable services that build local capacity and improve long-term outcomes for individuals with autism, other developmental disabilities, and their families.

Keywords Applied Behavior Analysis · Autism spectrum disorder · Developmental disabilities · Low- and middle-income countries · Implementation barriers · Cultural adaptation · Caregiver-mediated interventions · Technology-assisted training

Resumen El Análisis Conductual Aplicado (ABA) es uno de los enfoques con mayor respaldo empírico para promover cambios conductuales socialmente significativos en personas con trastorno del espectro autista (TEA) y otras condiciones del neurodesarrollo. A pesar de décadas de evidencia, el acceso a intervenciones informadas por ABA sigue siendo muy limitado en países de ingresos bajos y medios (PIBM). En estos contextos, las familias suelen enfrentar demoras en la identificación y el diagnóstico, escasez de profesionales especializados y financiamiento público insuficiente. Además, hay diferencias culturales y lingüísticas que pueden hacer que las intervenciones sean menos aceptables y efectivas. Si no se manejan bien, esto puede llevar a resultados inesperados que pueden chocar con las prioridades de las familias.

Este capítulo revisa las bases teóricas y la evidencia práctica para implementar ABA en PIBM con recursos limitados. Se enfoca en cómo se relacionan la falta de personal, la adaptación cultural y las limitaciones de recursos en el sistema. Asimismo, se revisan modelos de prestación que integran intervenciones lideradas por cuidadores, alianzas comunitarias y mecanismos de capacitación y supervisión apoyados por tecnología. Finalmente, se sugieren recomendaciones prácticas y de política que se centran en servicios que sean culturalmente adecuados, responsables éticamente y sostenibles económicamente. Estas recomendaciones buscan fortalecer la capacidad local y mejorar los resultados a largo plazo para personas con TEA, otras discapacidades del desarrollo y sus familias.

Palabras clave Análisis conductual aplicado · Trastorno del espectro autista · Trastornos del neurodesarrollo · Países de bajos y medios ingresos · Barreras de implementación · Adaptación cultural · Intervenciones mediadas por cuidadores · Capacitación asistida por tecnología

Applied behavior analysis (ABA) fundamentally operates as a science grounded in the systematic examination and intentional modification of human behavior. It employs rigorous data-informed methodologies to investigate and illuminate the functional interconnections binding behavioral patterns to the environmental contexts in which they emerge (Cooper et al., 2019; Foxx, 2008). Over several decades of implementation and refinement, ABA-based interventions have consistently demonstrated efficacy as validated, evidence-based approaches for enhancing developmental trajectories and behavioral functioning in children and adolescents living with autism and an array of other developmental disabilities (Gitimoghaddam et al., 2022; Wong et al., 2015).

Despite the growing evidence base, a major implementation gap persists. This gap is critical because many children who could really benefit from early help and behavior support programs still live in poor areas, where these services are either scattered among different systems or completely missing.

The World Bank uses gross national income (GNI) per capita to group low- and middle-income countries (LMICs). Many of these countries still have deeply rooted structural problems that make it challenging to find developmental disabilities and give the right support. The World Bank uses gross national income (GNI) per capita to group low- and middle-income countries (LMICs). Many of these countries still have deeply rooted structural problems that make it hard to find developmental disabilities and give the right support. Research studies looking at service delivery in these situations have consistently highlighted how vital it is to make sure that children from low-income backgrounds with developmental disabilities have fair access to education and receive early help when needed.

This chapter pursues four interrelated objectives: (a) synthesizing current knowledge regarding the prevalence of developmental disabilities in LMICs and delineating the measurement and diagnostic challenges that persist; (b) summarizing the empirical evidence concerning culturally responsive adaptation strategies and diverse service delivery models suited to ABA-based interventions in resource-limited contexts; (c) identifying and analyzing key barriers to successful ABA implementation and tracing their ripple effects throughout communities and family systems; and (d) formulating evidence-based policy recommendations and practical strategies designed to foster sustainable, locally owned ABA program development.

16.1 Developmental Disability in Low- and Middle-Income Countries: Prevalence, Identification, and Diagnostic Challenges

Developmental disabilities (DDs) encompass a spectrum of conditions, including autism spectrum disorder (ASD), attention-deficit/hyperactivity disorder (ADHD), intellectual disability (ID), and specific learning disorder (SLDs). These conditions share a common characteristic: they significantly impair an individual's ability to function effectively across personal, social, academic, and occupational domains (American Psychiatric Association, 2013). According to estimates from the World

Health Organization (WHO), tens of millions of children worldwide experience moderate-to-severe developmental disabilities, with a disproportionately large proportion residing in low- and middle-income countries (LMICs) (World Health Organization, 2011).

16.1.1 Prevalence Estimation Challenges

Estimating the true prevalence of developmental disabilities in low- and middle-income (LMIC) populations presents methodological and practical difficulties that extend far beyond those found in wealthy areas. The scarcity of specialized diagnostic services in many regions means that many children with developmental concerns never encounter professionals trained to recognize and classify such conditions (Durkin, 2002; Kieling et al., 2011). Additionally, standardized assessment tools, which can be costly, need special training to use and understand, may not be suitable for different cultures and languages, and can differ greatly from one place to another. Cultural variations in how parents, educators, and community members conceptualize, interpret, and communicate concerns about child development substantially complicate prevalence estimation efforts (Durkin, 2002).

Preventable factors that disproportionately increase the burden of developmental disabilities affect low-resource communities. Complications during the perinatal period, early childhood infections (including those that are vaccine-preventable), and malnutrition significantly contribute to the prevalence of disabilities in economically disadvantaged populations (Baxter et al., 2014; Durkin, 2002). These modifiable risk factors suggest that improved public health interventions and nutritional support programs may partially reduce the disability burden observed in many LMICs.

16.1.2 Prevalence of Autism Spectrum Disorder and Intellectual Disability

Global prevalence estimates for ASD frequently cite a figure that approximates 1% of the child population. However, this figure obscures a troubling reality: region-specific estimates within LMICs remain sparse, inconsistently defined, and methodologically heterogeneous, making it exceedingly difficult to make meaningful cross-regional comparisons (Elsabbagh et al., 2012). The estimated worldwide prevalence of intellectual disability is approximately 5%, although considerable geographical variation exists (Polanczyk et al., 2007). Emerging evidence reveals a consistent pattern: IDRs tend to be significantly higher in low-income countries than in high-income countries. For instance, research comparing prevalence across contexts has revealed substantially elevated ID rates within LMICs relative to high-income countries (Maulik et al., 2011). This difference is probably due to real differences in health conditions and the fact that high-income countries often miss identifying cases, where better systems for early detection and intervention can lead to finding severe disabilities sooner.

16.2 ABA Adaptation for LMICs: Contextual Fit and Delivery Models

Although empirical literature examining ABA implementation within LMIC contexts remains in relatively early stages of development, emerging evidence strongly suggests that ABA-based strategies can produce meaningful improvements and demonstrate practical feasibility when deliberately and thoughtfully adapted to align with local contexts, values, and constraints (Abubakar & Kipkemoi, 2022). Service delivery frameworks that utilize existing community resources, especially those that prioritize peer-mediated learning and community-embedded, culturally relevant methodologies, show potential for broadening the impact of interventions and improving long-term sustainability in environments where trained behavior analysts and specialized professionals are significantly limited (Lee & Meadan, 2021; Wong et al., 2015).

16.2.1 Parent- and Caregiver-Mediated Interventions

Parent-mediated intervention (PMI) is a growing method where caregivers get organized training to use proven teaching techniques, help with communication skills, and support learning everyday life skills. PMIs are particularly well suited to LMIC contexts for multiple intersecting reasons: professional therapeutic services are chronically scarce; geographic distance and limited transportation infrastructure create nearly insurmountable barriers for family engagement with clinic-based services; and the costs associated with frequent, intensive professional contact are prohibitively high for most families (Lee & Meadan, 2021; Wong et al., 2015). By positioning caregivers as primary intervention agents, PMI models can dramatically expand service reach while simultaneously reducing per capita costs.

16.2.2 Cultural Responsiveness as a Core Design Principle

In ABA implementation, cultural responsiveness is fundamentally more than a superficial modification or esthetic adjustment to the existing intervention protocols. Rather, it constitutes a non-negotiable core principle that safeguards feasibility, ensures genuine acceptability by the communities it serves, and preserves the ethical integrity inherent in the intervention design and implementation processes. Culturally congruent adaptation typically necessitates substantive adjustments, including language translation, recalibration of intervention goals to reflect locally held values, modification of teaching materials and examples, and redesign of service delivery methods to accommodate existing family patterns and structural constraints (Divan et al., 2021). In certain cultural contexts, interventions emphasizing individual goal attainment and highly formalized and rigidly structured teaching protocols may require substantial reconceptualization to align with cultural values that emphasize interdependence and relational harmony.

Authentic cultural adaptation emerges through meaningful partnerships between external agents (researchers and program developers) and local stakeholders, including families, educators, clinicians, and community leaders, who collectively guide culturally grounded decisions regarding intervention targets, teaching methodologies, and successful measurement approaches (Divan et al., 2021; Pilkington et al., 2017). Successful cultural adaptations consistently incorporate the translation of all materials into local languages and dialects while rendering technical terminology comprehensible to lay audiences, deliberate alignment of trainers and supervisors with participants' linguistic and cultural backgrounds, and intentional substitution of culturally unfamiliar examples and visuals with locally meaningful alternatives that resonate with family and client experiences (Sivaraman & Fahmie, 2020).

Three key themes consistently appear in studies about successful adaptation efforts: building trust and real shared ownership with communities is essential; it's important to invest in training and supervision that can grow and last; and focusing on long-term success and fitting into existing systems is more important than just short-term achievements.

16.3 Barriers to the Implementation of ABA in LMICs and Downstream Impacts

Implementation barriers in the LMIC context rarely operate in isolation. Rather, they often group together into three connected areas that support each other: not having enough trained workers, differences in culture and language, and lack of resources and systems (Allen & Warzak, 2000; Durkin, 2002). Because these areas influence each other, trying to fix one problem without also addressing the others

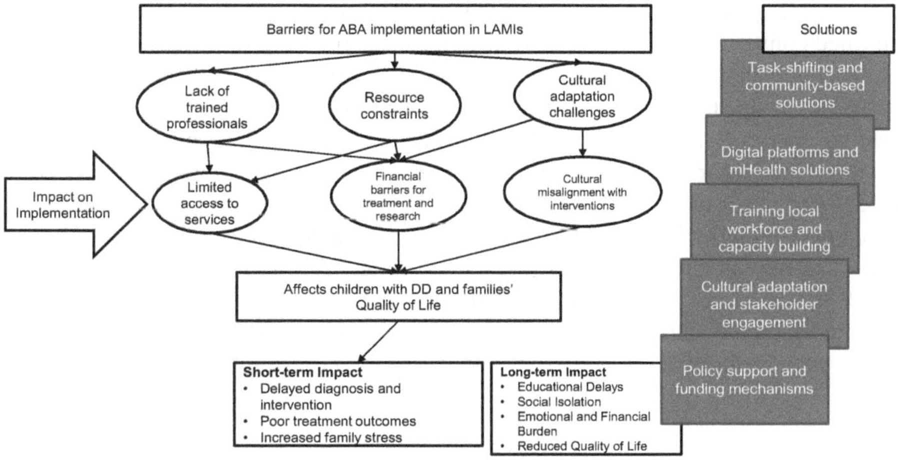

Fig. 16.1 Cultural adaptation funnel: From core ABA mechanisms to evidence-based practice in low- and middle-income countries (LMICs). *Note.* Delivery and materials undergo systematic modification through adaptation processes, whereas the core mechanisms of behavioral change remain intact

usually leads to only short-term changes, not lasting improvements in the quality of life and development for families, which is the main goal of these efforts.

Figure 16.1 illustrates the systemic relationships between these domains and their downstream cascading effects on families and individuals with autism and developmental disabilities.

16.3.1 Workforce Capacity and Supervision: A Critical Shortage

The most fundamental barrier to the implementation of ABA across LMICs is the acute and persistent scarcity of professionally trained individuals with expertise in behavioral analysis. Limited formal training and educator familiarity with ABA further constrain implementation capacity (Fennell & Dillenburger, 2018). The way professionals are spread out shows big differences; major cities usually have more specialized services for wealthier people, while many rural and remote areas hardly get any help at all (Divan et al., 2021). This uneven distribution is made worse by serious money problems; families looking for evaluations, expert advice, and ongoing support often have to pay a lot of money out of their own pockets for assessment fees, intervention materials, and regular consultations with professionals. These mounting costs exacerbate workforce shortages, further limiting families' ability to engage with services and creating perverse incentives that discourage individuals from entering the profession.

Scalable models have demonstrated an increasing potential within this constrained context. Such models rely on smartly shifting tasks and organized supervision systems that intentionally move the responsibility for providing key intervention strategies from highly trained specialists to carefully chosen and well-supervised non-specialists (Naithani et al., 2022; Lerman et al., 2020). Training teachers, community health workers, and parents who have personal experience in using structured behavioral techniques can greatly increase the availability of services while keeping the quality high, especially when combined with coaching that focuses on skills and regular checks to ensure standards are met. Even though there are still real challenges such as poor internet and limited access to devices in many low- and middle-income countries, using technology for remote supervision is showing that it can help overcome distance issues and lessen the need for travel.

16.3.2 Cultural Adaptation and Stigma: Deeper than Translation

Conversely, evidence-informed cultural adaptation demands genuine co-design partnerships with local stakeholders. This process involves iterative refinement and continuous information gathering through feedback loops involving families, educators, and community leaders.

Interventions that were first created and improved in wealthy countries often need to be completely rethought, going far beyond just translating the words, to be truly practical and accepted in low- and middle-income (LMIC) areas. While superficial language translation is necessary, it is insufficient when the underlying conceptual frameworks, metaphorical systems, and help-seeking practices substantially diverge across cultures. Teaching methods that focus on direct eye contact or strict, formal teaching rules may clash with values around respect, building relationships, and community-based care that are important in different cultures. Conversely, evidence-informed cultural adaptation demands genuine co-design partnerships with local stakeholders. This process involves iterative refinement and continuous information gathering from honest feedback loops that include families, educators, and community leaders.

The EVF provides a thorough, multidimensional framework for systematically directing adaptation initiatives across eight interconnected dimensions: language, individuals, metaphors, content, concepts, objectives, methodologies, and contexts (Bernal et al., 1995, 2009). Operationalizing this framework within LMIC contexts involves translating materials into local languages and dialects while ensuring that technical terminology remains accessible to individuals without formal training. The framework requires caregivers and community health workers to be co-trainers and co-designers, a practice that simultaneously increases community trust and enhances program sustainability. Culturally unfamiliar examples must be systematically replaced with locally meaningful alternatives, such as substituting soccer or traditional games with baseball references. Teaching materials should authentically reflect family routines and priorities and incorporate daily activities and valued practices (e.g., feeding animals in agrarian communities) to render interventions that are genuinely practical rather than abstractly theoretical.

Intervention goals need to be adjusted to truly reflect the community's cultural values, focusing on teamwork and family unity instead of individual independence, and prioritizing practical skills, like communication for expressing basic needs, that families see as most important. Delivery methods require adaptation to match local realities. For example, group-based sessions or home visits may be more feasible and culturally acceptable than clinic-based intensive programs when geographic distance and limited transportation present insurmountable obstacles. Finally, contextual factors, such as limited Internet connectivity, require practical consideration, with asynchronous video modules or printed instructional manuals serving as culturally acceptable alternatives to live telehealth coaching.

Addressing stigma is both critical and demanding. Widespread misunderstandings and folk theories about autism and neurodevelopmental disorders often lead to delays in diagnosis and a significant drop in service use. To effectively address this issue, we need to include community education campaigns that promote understanding of different developmental abilities, explain proven practices based on research, and respond to local worries about intervention goals. Evidence-based health initiatives, such as brief radio segments broadcast in local languages explaining the evidence supporting caregiver-mediated interventions, have demonstrated effectiveness in rural areas. Situational analyses from low-income settings (e.g., Ethiopia) highlight that workforce shortages, stigma, and limited service infrastructure often interact to delay identification and constrain service uptake (Tekola et al., 2016). Together, these various strategies make sure that interventions are easy to understand, fit well with the local culture, are ethically responsible, and can realistically work in areas with limited resources.

16.3.3 Resource and System Constraints: Sustainability Challenges

Traditional comprehensive ABA programs require substantial resources and investments. High ratios of direct service providers to clients, specialized materials and environmental modifications, and frequent intensive supervision contribute to substantial program expenses. Many low- and middle-income countries deal with overlapping problems: not enough government funding for disability services, reliance on temporary grants that can change with politics and donor interests, and poor inclusion of disability issues in national policies, which together make it hard to provide consistent and lasting services.

Resource scarcity directly contributes to multiple documented harms: delayed access to early intervention during critical developmental windows, substantial gaps in follow-up services after the initial diagnosis, and reduced effectiveness of interventions when programmatic approaches do not align with families' daily routines and stated priorities. These patterns can reliably generate elevated caregiver stress and deepen existing inequalities in educational and health outcomes, often widening disparities instead of reducing them.

16.4 Sustainable ABA Programs for Low- and Middle-Income Countries

True sustainability means making careful and planned efforts to build local skills to include ABA-informed services in current educational and health systems, instead of relying on outside funding and management that stop when the money runs out. Sustainable models always have three main parts: a comprehensive workforce development program, culturally appropriate and locally responsive supervision structures, and financing mechanisms that help families pay less (Abubakar & Kipkemoi, 2022; Divan et al., 2021).

16.4.1 Leveraging Digital Tools for Scaling and Reaching

Digital tools help programs grow by making it easier to train people from a distance, collect and analyze data more quickly, and provide effective remote supervision and coaching. Evidence from broader digital health and mobile health (mHealth) initiatives in low- and middle-income countries (LMICs) shows that better technology and easier-to-use platforms can greatly increase the number of people who use services and the effectiveness of interventions (Lee et al., 2016). However, when putting these tools into practice, it's important to pay attention to ongoing challenges, like poor or unstable Internet access, limited availability of devices, and different levels of digital skills in various communities.

16.4.2 Policy and Regulatory Frameworks

Policy development and implementation are the essential foundational elements for sustainable system changes. Governments can strengthen the field by formally recognizing ABA as evidence-based practice, establishing transparent training and supervision standards, and systematically integrating disability-related services into public health and education systems. Certification and licensure pathways that follow international standards can protect families from practitioners who are not effective or ethical while also encouraging consistency in ethical practice based on evidence. Evidence from implementation research in LMICs underscores that sustaining evidence-based interventions requires integration into routine systems, leadership support, and attention to local context (Hailemariam et al., 2012).

16.5 Collaborating with Community Stakeholders

Community collaboration increases program acceptability and ensures that intervention priorities accurately reflect the community's needs and values. The strategic engagement of diverse stakeholders, including families, local service providers, educators at all levels, and policymakers, demonstrates both program adoption and the likelihood of long-term sustainability (Divan et al., 2021; Pilkington et al., 2017).

Thorough research on how communities get involved in low- and middle-income countries shows that methods like forming groups of women, creating networks of community health workers, and having regular home visits have consistently led to better health for mothers and children, while also improving links between families and official health services. Similar community-based groups are expected to help with ABA implementation by incorporating caregiver training and regular support services into well-known local networks that the community trusts and engages with.

16.6 Effectiveness Evaluation: ABA Interventions in Low- and Middle-Income Countries

As ABA-informed service delivery models grow around the world, careful evaluation is becoming more important to show real results, find problems in how services are delivered, and help improve quality and programs over time. A complete evaluation should look at both clinical results (such as improvements in communication, adaptive behaviors, and involvement in community activities) and implementation outcomes (such as feasibility, acceptability, and fidelity). Establishing routine data systems and robust quality assurance processes will facilitate continuous, transparent monitoring of these multifaceted outcomes. Practical ways to put this into action include regularly monitoring progress using standardized methods, assessing adherence to core intervention components, and keeping detailed records of coaching sessions, training completion, and any adaptations made during implementation.

This emphasis on context-sensitive evaluation is crucial because contextual factors fundamentally influence the intervention effects. So, research in low- and middle-income countries should focus on practical trials and mixed methods that ensure strong scientific accuracy while also being useful and scalable in real-life situations.

16.7 Ethical Considerations in the Implementation of ABA in LMICs

Ethical implementation requires genuine cultural responsiveness, equitable allocation of inherently limited resources, and robust safeguards against exploitation and harm. Interventions must authentically align with local values and emphasize functional outcomes that meaningfully improve participation in valued activities and enhance the quality of life.

Group-based or caregiver-mediated intervention formats may enable more children to access services in contexts where specialist resources are profoundly limited, even if the intensity falls below that typical in high-resource settings. Ethical planning processes must explicitly and transparently consider the opportunity costs and distributed justice principles (McCabe et al., 2023).

Cultural humility, characterized by ongoing self-reflection, genuine shared decision-making, and respectful, authentic partnerships with communities, substantially mitigates inherent power imbalances in service delivery relationships (Wright, 2019). Continuous professional development and structured supervision constitute critical mechanisms for maintaining ethical standards and thoughtfully adapting interventions while preserving client dignity and respect.

16.8 ABA Knowledge Dissemination and Best Practices in Low- and Middle-Income Countries

Knowledge dissemination strategies should strategically prioritize accessible training materials, regional communities of practice, and collaborative partnerships to facilitate meaningful knowledge exchanges across diverse settings. Culturally relevant curricula and thoughtfully designed supervision models simultaneously support intervention fidelity and enable authentic local adaptation, thereby reflecting community needs and values.

Training carefully selected non-specialists to deliver autism interventions has demonstrated promise in resource-limited settings, particularly when coupled with structured implementation manuals and ongoing coaching support from qualified supervisors (Naithani et al., 2022). Although feasibility depends on the existing local infrastructure, technology-enabled learning approaches—encompassing asynchronous instructional modules, virtual coaching and supervision, and peer support networks—can substantially expand the reach of interventions (Rey & Omigbodun, 2015).

Open-access digital resources (e.g., freely accessible e-textbooks and training materials) can further support capacity building in low-resource settings by reducing cost barriers to continuing education and supervision (Rey & Omigbodun, 2015).

Establishing centers of excellence or regional resource hubs positioned to deliver specialized expertise, quality oversight, and technical support for emerging programs merits serious consideration. Collectively, culturally informed curricula and innovative delivery approaches can meaningfully enhance both the accessibility and sustainability of evidence-based global autism interventions.

16.9 Implications and Future Directions

Future research must prioritize culturally grounded adaptations that simultaneously preserve the core behavioral mechanisms that render ABA effective. This imperative requires genuine co-design with families and communities coupled with transparent documentation of modifications employing established adaptation frameworks (Wiltsey Stirman et al., 2019).

Task-shifting merits continued rigorous evaluation, encompassing studies examining training dosage requirements, optimal supervision structures, intervention fidelity maintenance, and client outcomes across diverse service sectors, including schools and primary care settings. Technology-enabled service delivery, encompassing telehealth coaching and mobile data systems, may substantially reduce geographic and economic barriers to service access, cost-effectiveness, and genuine sustainability merit examination under real-world LMIC constraints, such as unstable connectivity and limited device availability (Lee et al., 2016; Sivaraman & Fahmie, 2020).

In conclusion, research on policy should carefully explore how national laws, funding methods, and professional certification processes affect the availability of services and their quality. It should also find out which combinations of these policies best promote real inclusion in regular service systems.

Implicancias para las Políticas Públicas en Latinoamérica

Esta sección responde directamente a la importancia fundamental enfatizada en este capítulo respecto a la necesidad urgente de ofrecer recursos accesibles en idiomas locales. Considerando esta perspectiva crítica como una prioridad central del capítulo, hemos incluso intencionalmente traducido este apartado al español.

Para garantizar genuinamente la equidad en el acceso a servicios basados en ABA en América Latina, resulta necesario adoptar políticas públicas que cuidadosamente prioricen la formación profesional rigurosa de especialistas locales. Además, es importante la integración estratégica de intervenciones mediadas por cuidadores dentro de programas comunitarios existentes y el aprovechamiento deliberado de tecnologías digitales para capacitación sistemática y monitoreo oportuno. Se recomienda enérgicamente la creación de marcos regulatorios comprensivos que reconozcan y valoren activamente la diversidad cultural y lingüística característica de estos países, así como la implementación de incentivos concretos para fortalecer la colaboración genuina entre gobiernos nacionales, instituciones universitarias y organizaciones no gubernamentales dedicadas al refuerzo de prácticas basadas en evidencias culturalmente adaptadas a cada realidad regional específica.

Mediante la implementación deliberada de estas acciones integradas, resulta posible reducir significativamente las brechas actuales en identificación temprana, diagnóstico oportuno y tratamiento accesible, mientras se promueve simultáneamente la sostenibilidad a largo plazo y se mejoran los resultados demostrados para personas con TEA, otros trastornos del neurodesarrollo, y sus familias operando dentro de contextos de bajos recursos económicos.

16.10 Conclusion

Applied Behavior Analysis can improve the developmental trajectories and life outcomes of individuals living with autism and other developmental disorders in low- and middle-income countries. However, meaningfully expanding evidence-based services requires far more than simple replication or direct importation of service models developed within high-income settings. To make long-term use of these services successful, we need to build local skills through training, adapt methods to fit cultural and practical realities, and create real trust and ownership in the community by working together fairly.

When workforce development, adapting to cultural needs, making financing accessible, and supporting policies are all tackled together as a unified approach, ABA-informed techniques can be used ethically and effectively, even in very limited-resource environments. Continued collaborative efforts among academic researchers, practicing clinicians, policy advocates, and families are essential for meaningfully reducing persistent disparities and substantially increasing equitable access to high-quality evidence-based care.

16.11 Moving Beyond: A Call for Action

> *"Science cannot advance without cultural sensitivity and ethical responsibility." Our goal is to ensure that evidence-based practices respect diversity and promote human dignity in every context. This book concludes with the following mission: "Building and enhancing systems that respond to the real and individual needs of families around the world."*

> *"La ciencia no puede avanzar sin sensibilidad cultural y responsabilidad ética. Nuestro objetivo es garantizar que las prácticas basadas en evidencia respeten la diversidad y promuevan la dignidad humana en cada contexto. Este libro concluye; sin embargo, la misión continúa: construir y fortalecer sistemas que respondan a las necesidades reales e individuales de las familias en todo el mundo."*

Acknowledgments Grammarly was used to improve language editing, including readability, grammar, and syntax. The software had no involvement in the conceptualization, analysis, interpretation, or conclusions of this manuscript; all intellectual content is entirely the authors' own.

Appendix

ABA Implementation Framework for LMICs

Strategic Solutions for Sustainable Implementation

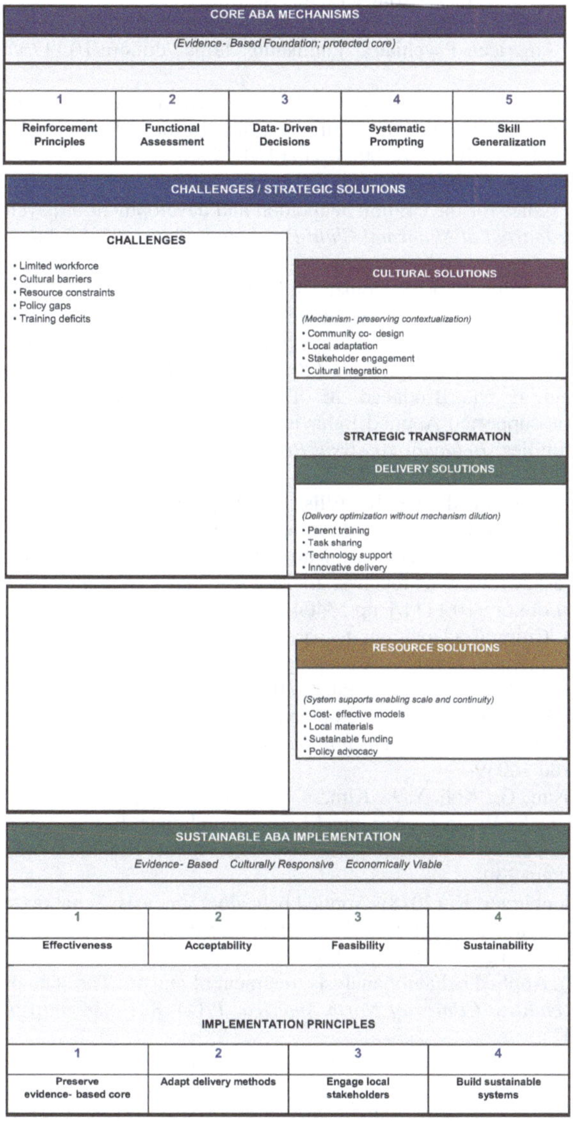

Fig. A1 ABA Implementation Framework for LMICs. The main proven methods are kept intact while tailored solutions tackle local issues to help ensure the implementation is effective, acceptable, practical, and long-lasting

References

Abubakar, A., & Kipkemoi, P. (2022). Commentary on early intervention for very young children with or at high likelihood of autism. *Developmental Medicine & Child Neurology, 64*(9), 1051–1052. https://doi.org/10.1111/dmcn.15258

Allen, K. D., & Warzak, W. J. (2000). The problem of parental nonadherence in clinical behavior analysis: Effective treatment is not enough. *Journal of Applied Behavior Analysis, 33*(3), 373–391. https://doi.org/10.1901/jaba.2000.33-373

American Psychiatric Association. (2013). *Diagnostic and statistical manual of mental disorders* (5th ed.). American Psychiatric Publishing. https://doi.org/10.1176/appi.books.9780890425590

Baxter, A. J., Brugha, T. S., Erskine, H. E., Scheurer, R. W., Vos, T., & Scott, J. G. (2014). Epidemiology and global burden of autism spectrum disorders. *Psychological Medicine, 45*(3), 601–613. https://doi.org/10.1017/S003329171400172X

Bernal, G., Bonilla, J., & Bellido, C. (1995). Ecological validity and cultural sensitivity for outcome research: Issues for the cultural adaptation and development of psychosocial treatments with Hispanics. *Journal of Abnormal Child Psychology, 23*(1), 67–82. https://doi.org/10.1007/BF01447045

Bernal, G., Jiménez-Chafey, M. I., & Domenech Rodríguez, M. M. (2009). Cultural adaptation of treatments: A resource for considering culture in evidence-based practice. *Clinical Psychology: Science and Practice, 16*(3), 284–304. https://doi.org/10.1111/j.1468-2850.2009.01170.x

Cooper, J. O., Heron, T. E., & Heward, W. L. (2019). *Applied behavior analysis* (3rd ed.). Pearson.

Dennison, A., Lund, E. M., Brodhead, M. T., Mejia, L., Armenta, A., & Leal, J. (2019). Delivering home-supported Applied Behavior Analysis therapies to culturally and linguistically diverse families. *Behavior Analysis Practice, 12*(4), 887–898. https://doi.org/10.1007/s40617-019-00374-1. PMID: 31976301.

Divan, G., Bhavnani, S., Leadbitter, K., Ellis, C., Dasgupta, J., Abubakar, A., Elsabbagh, M., Hamdani, S. U., Servili, C., Patel, V., & Green, J. (2021). Annual research review: Achieving universal health coverage for children with autism spectrum disorder in low- and middle-income countries: A review of reviews. *Journal of Child Psychology and Psychiatry, 62*(5), 514–535. https://doi.org/10.1111/jcpp.13404

DuBay, M. (2022). Cultural adaptations to parent-mediated autism spectrum disorder interventions for Latin American families: A scoping review. *American Journal of Speech-Language Pathology, 31*(3), 1517–1534. https://doi.org/10.1044/2022_AJSLP-21-00239

Durkin, M. (2002). Epidemiology of developmental disabilities in low-income countries. *Mental Retardation and Developmental Disabilities Research Reviews, 8*(3), 206–211. https://doi.org/10.1002/mrdd.10039

Elsabbagh, M., Divan, G., Koh, Y.-J., Kim, Y. S., Kauchali, S., Marcín, C., Montiel-Nava, C., Patel, V., Paula, C. S., Wang, C., Yasamy, M. T., & Fombonne, E. (2012). Global prevalence of autism and other pervasive developmental disorders. *Autism Research, 5*(3), 160–179. https://doi.org/10.1002/aur.239

Fennell, B., & Dillenburger, K. (2018). Applied behaviour analysis: What do teachers of students with autism spectrum disorder know? *International Journal of Educational Research, 87*, 110–120. https://doi.org/10.1016/j.ijer.2016.06.012

Foxx, R. M. (2008). Applied behavior analysis treatment of autism: The state of the art. *Child and Adolescent Psychiatric Clinics of North America, 17*(4), 821–834. https://doi.org/10.1016/j.chc.2008.06.007

Gitimoghaddam, M., Chichkine, N., McArthur, L. H., Sangha, S. S., & Symington, V. (2022). Applied behavior analysis in children and youth with autism spectrum disorders: A scoping review. *Perspectives on Behavior Science, 45*(3), 521–557. https://doi.org/10.1007/s40614-022-00338-x

Hailemariam, D., Berhane, Y., & Worku, A. (2012). Sustained implementation of evidence-based health interventions in low- and middle-income countries: A systematic review. *Implementation Science, 7*, Article 9. https://doi.org/10.1186/1748-5908-7-9.

Hastings, R. P., Robertson, J., & Yasamy, M. T. (2012). Interventions for children with pervasive developmental disorders in low- and middle-income countries. *Journal of Applied Research in Intellectual Disabilities, 25*(2), 119–134. https://doi.org/10.1111/j.1468-3148.2011.00680.x

Kieling, C., Baker-Henningham, H., Belfer, M., Conti, G., Ertem, I., Omigbodun, O., Rohde, L. A., Srinath, S., Ulkuer, N., & Rahman, A. (2011). Child and adolescent mental health worldwide: Evidence for action. *The Lancet, 378*(9801), 1515–1525. https://doi.org/10.1016/S0140-6736(11)60827-1

Lee, S. H., & Meadan, H. (2021). Parent-mediated intervention for young children with autism in low- and middle-income countries: A systematic review. *Early Childhood Education Journal, 49*(5), 895–907. https://doi.org/10.1007/s10643-020-01121-6

Lee, S. H., Nurmatov, U. B., Nwaru, B. I., Mukherjee, M., Grant, L., & Pagliari, C. (2016). Effectiveness of mHealth interventions for maternal, newborn and child health in low- and middle-income countries: Systematic review and meta-analysis. *Journal of Global Health, 6*(1), 010401. https://doi.org/10.7189/jogh.06.010401

Lerman, D. C., O'Brien, M. J., Neely, L., Call, N. A., Tsami, L., Schieltz, K. M., Berg, W. K., Graber, J., Huang, P., Kopelman, T., & Cooper-Brown, L. J. (2020). Remote coaching of caregivers via telehealth: Challenges and potential solutions. *Journal of Behavioral Education, 29*(2), 195–221. https://doi.org/10.1007/s10864-020-09378-2

Lopez, K., Magaña, S., Morales, M., & Iland, E. (2019). Parents taking action: Reducing disparities through a culturally informed intervention for Latinx parents of children with autism. In *Rethinking social work practice with multicultural communities* (pp. 31–49). Routledge.

Lygnegård, F., Moberg, J., & Dillenburger, K. (2013). Interventions for children with developmental disabilities living in poverty in low- and middle-income countries: A systematic review. *Journal of Applied Research in Intellectual Disabilities, 26*(6), 461–475. https://doi.org/10.1111/jar.12053

Maulik, P. K., Mascarenhas, M. N., Mathers, C. D., Dua, T., & Saxena, S. (2011). Prevalence of intellectual disability: A meta-analysis of population-based studies. *Research in Developmental Disabilities, 32*, 419–436. https://doi.org/10.1016/j.ridd.2010.12.018

McCabe, H. B., Ding, K., & Deng, Q. (2023). Ethics of resource allocation and intensity of applied behavior analytic services for children with autism in low- and middle-income countries: Commentary on a case study in China. *Perspectives on Behavior Science, 46*(2), 241–257. https://doi.org/10.1007/s40614-023-00366-z

Naithani, R., Patel, V., & Divan, G. (2022). Training non-specialists to deliver autism interventions in low-resource settings: A scoping review. *Autism Research, 15*(1), 38–54. https://doi.org/10.1002/aur.2647

Pilkington, G., Khatib, M. N., Panday, S., Simkhada, P., Hill, R., & Jones, L. (2017). *The effectiveness of community engagement and participation approaches in low and middle-income countries: Contextualisation of review findings to South Asia and Nepal*. EPPI-Centre, Social Science Research Unit, UCL Institute of Education, University College London. https://assets.publishing.service.gov.uk/media/5b10309040f0b634cfb50550/DFID_Community_Engagement_Contextualisation_LJMU_POST_COPY_EDIT.pdf

Polanczyk, G., de Lima, M. S., Horta, B. L., Biederman, J., & Rohde, L. A. (2007). The worldwide prevalence of ADHD: A systematic review and metaregression analysis. *American Journal of Psychiatry, 164*(6), 942–948. https://doi.org/10.1176/ajp.2007.164.6.942

Rey, J. M., & Omigbodun, O. O. (2015). International dissemination of evidence-based practice, open access and the IACAPAP textbook of child and adolescent mental health. *Child and Adolescent Psychiatry and Mental Health, 9*, Article 47. https://doi.org/10.1186/s13034-015-0084-1.

Sivaraman, M., & Fahmie, T. A. (2020). A systematic review of cultural adaptations in the global application of ABA-based telehealth services. *Journal of Applied Behavior Analysis, 53*(4), 1838–1855. https://doi.org/10.1002/jaba.763

Tekola, B., Baheretibeb, Y., Roth, I., Tilahun, D., Fekadu, A., Hanlon, C., & Hoekstra, R. A. (2016). Challenges and opportunities to improve autism services in low-income countries: Lessons from a situational analysis in Ethiopia. *Global Mental Health, 3*, e21. https://doi.org/10.1017/gmh.2016.17

Tsami, L., Lerman, D., & Toper-Korkmaz, O. (2019). Effectiveness and acceptability of parent training via telehealth among families around the world. *Journal of Applied Behavior Analysis, 52*(4), 1113–1129. https://doi.org/10.1002/jaba.645

Wiltsey Stirman, S., Baumann, A. A., & Miller, C. J. (2019). The FRAME: An expanded framework for reporting adaptations and modifications to evidence-based interventions. *Implementation Science, 14*, Article 58. https://doi.org/10.1186/s13012-019-0898-y.

Wong, C., Odom, S. L., Hume, K. A., Cox, A. W., Fettig, A., Kucharczyk, S., Brock, M. E., Plavnick, J. B., Fleury, V. P., & Schultz, T. R. (2015). Evidence-based practices for children, youth, and young adults with autism spectrum disorder: A comprehensive review. *Journal of Autism and Developmental Disorders, 45*(7), 1951–1966. https://doi.org/10.1007/s10803-014-2351-z

World Bank. (2018). *World Bank open data*. Retrieved from https://data.worldbank.org

World Health Organization. (2011). *World report on disability*. WHO.

Wright, P. I. (2019). Cultural humility in the practice of applied behavior analysis. *Behavior Analysis in Practice, 12*(4), 805–809. https://doi.org/10.1007/s40617-019-00343-8